WHEAT
BELLY
TOTAL
HEALTH

WHEAT BELLY TOTAL HEALTH

The Ultimate Grain-Free Health
and Weight-Loss Life Plan

WILLIAM DAVIS, MD

RODALE.

Exclusive direct mail edition is being published simultaneously by Rodale Inc. as *The Grain-Free Cure.*

© 2014 by William Davis, MD

Rodale books may be purchased for business or promotional use or for special sales. For information, please write to:
Special Markets Department, Rodale Inc., 733 Third Avenue, New York, NY 10017

Printed in the United States of America

Rodale Inc. makes every effort to use acid-free ∞, recycled paper ∞.

Book design by Amy King

Photos: page 89 (before) by Frank Garcia, (after) by Tami Calhoun; page 114 (before and after) by Nathan Pokocky; page 132 (before) by Tom Engstrom, (after) by Kersten Safford; page 160 (before and after) by Eric Drury; page 216 (before) by Nathan Frohnapple, (after) by Alexis Frohnapple

Library of Congress Cataloging-in-Publication Data is on file with the publisher.

ISBN 978-1-62336-408-3

Distributed to the trade by Macmillan

2   4   6   8   10   9   7   5   3   1   hardcover

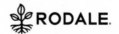

We inspire and enable people to improve their lives and the world around them.

rodalebooks.com

To all the readers who have the boldness,
courage, and conviction to rebel against conventional dietary advice
and discover what real *nutrition can do for human health*

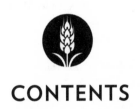

CONTENTS

ACKNOWLEDGMENTS

WHEN SOMETHING SPARKS a phenomenon as large and revolutionary as the Wheat Belly movement, it becomes bigger than any one person. While it began as my personal effort to understand why, when patients in my office removed all things wheat from their diet, astounding transformations in health developed, it has ballooned into a collection of projects that are, I believe, changing the way we all look at food and nutrition.

As Team Wheat Belly has grown, a number of people have proven crucial players who have helped advance this cause, in particular this new book, *Wheat Belly Total Health*, the largest and most comprehensive book project in the *Wheat Belly* line to date, as well as all the projects that complement this book.

Among those whose input was crucial to this and related projects:

My agent, Rick Broadhead, who fights for this cause as if his own. A more mild-mannered but fierce defender I could have never found.

My editors at Rodale, Jennifer Levesque and Anne Egan, helped craft this message to suit the needs of an audience eager to hear and understand more about why this counterintuitive approach works. Despite the changing landscape of book publishing, they have helped deliver the Wheat Belly message to a public barraged with competing, and often contrary, dietary messages. Vice President/Publisher of Rodale Books Mary Ann Naples and Vice President/Deputy Publisher Kristin Kiser have worked in the background to advance the Wheat Belly cause, proving instrumental to projects such as the Wheat Belly special to air on public television. My publicist at Rodale, Emily Eagan Weber, dealt masterfully with the vagaries of media and managed to keep this message in the public eye, while Chris DeMarchis dealt tirelessly with many of the book's logistical details.

This *Total Health* project did not occur in isolation but developed as part of a broad front of projects that all cross-fertilize each other, everyone involved making a contribution, direct or indirect, to the final project. Among the members of Team Wheat Belly are my longtime friend Chris Kliesmet, who has helped hone these ideas from day one; Gary and Patti Miller, who champion the food and education projects; Paul and Anne MacInnis, who manage my speaking engagements, tours, and media projects; and Cindy Ratzlaff, social media consultant, who has helped make the Wheat Belly online experience a more engaging, stimulating, and entertaining interaction.

Of course, my wife and companion, Dawn, who had to endure my endless hours of distraction of the sort that goes with writing a book, deserves many, many thank-yous for her patience and support. Now that the preoccupation of the writing process is over, there will be no more befuddled looks: You are now back in my focus.

INTRODUCTION

YOU'VE BEEN GRAINED.

Beaten, demoralized, discouraged, your life and health have been bankrupted by "healthy whole grains." The worst of the bunch is modern wheat: the Judas of dietary "wisdom," despot of the breakfast bowl, tyrant of the bakery cabinet, the semidwarf darling of agribusiness. Your eyes were sprouting cataracts, your arteries were stiffening, your skin was wrinkling and plagued with rashes, your joints were sore and arthritic, your organs were inflamed, your belly fat was expanding, your blood sugar was climbing, and man breasts may even have been sprouting. Your mind was clouded by fog, your medication list was growing, and your schedule was fouled by mad scrambles for the nearest bathroom—all while you were being driven to consume more and more of the food that *all* official providers of nutritional advice advised you to consume . . . until you put an end to the whole mess as a result of the revelations made in *Wheat Belly*.

You boldly removed foods that enjoy the blessings of agencies in the business of dispensing dietary advice. You defied the USDA and its MyPlate and MyPyramid. You scoffed at the urgings of the Surgeon General's office. You thumbed your nose at the advice of the American Heart Association, American Diabetes Association, and the Academy of Nutrition and Dietetics. You sniggered at the antics of the wheat lobby and wheat trade groups as they desperately launched wave after wave of damage control. You removed grains like a festering abscess that refused to heal until lanced, and you discovered that health and vigor began to reappear.

I've experienced this personally. When I removed all "healthy whole grains" from my life, it reversed my diabetes until I became confidently nondiabetic, I was freed from mind fog that persisted no matter how many cups of coffee I drank, and I found relief from the annoying symptoms of irritable bowel syndrome. My triglyceride level dropped from 350 to 42 mg/dl, my HDL increased from 27 to 97 mg/dl, and the dark thoughts and moods that I had struggled with for many years were simply erased. I did the *opposite* of widely accepted health advice and experienced a transformation in health.

Coming to the realization that conventional nutritional advice has as much value as old bubble gum stuck on the sidewalk can't help but make you skeptical about whether most sources of health advice are objective, unbiased, and based on science in the first place. At best, dietary advice was driven by incomplete or misinterpreted data, an army of dietitians and "experts" unwittingly doing the dirty work of distributing the information. At worst, it was advice that served the ambitions of agribusiness and other powerful interests, all working to commoditize the human diet—yes, *commoditize*, or derive maximal financial gain by persuading us that the human diet should be dependent on foods that are inexpensive, indifferent to quality, blind to source, traded and arbitraged on a massive scale, and hungrily desired by the masses. Yes, you were grained.

When we peel back the veneer of marketing, trumped-up science, the appeal of convenience, and the yank of addiction, we find that, as a civilization, we made an enormous dietary blunder about 10,000 years ago: We mistook the seeds of grasses—first consumed in desperation—as food. We then allowed this mistake to balloon, not only perceiving this mistake as the discovery of a dietary staple, but as a food *ideal* for human consumption. Recognizing the ills of modern wheat in *Wheat Belly* was the first step, but now we can take another major step and eliminate *all* grains. Once that is accomplished, we proceed even further along the path toward total health by identifying and undoing all the harmful effects we've accumulated during our grain-consuming years and that can persist even in the aftermath of grain removal. That's why I call this approach "Total Health."

In *Wheat Belly Total Health*, we are going to explore in greater detail why this dietary detour has caused more human disease and suffering than all the wars of the world combined. We'll discuss why and how experts joined in on this mass hysteria, even co-opting government agencies and policies into the delusion and creating an example of collective madness larger than the Salem witch trials or the fearmongering of the Red Scare, making absurd practices such as bleeding with leeches or frontal lobotomies seem quaint. We will then take this journey of discovery further, discussing how, after you undo this grain-induced mess, you can pick up the pieces and reconstruct diet and correct weight, hormonal status, and other facets of health you may have thought were out of reach.

There are aspects of life that are beyond your influence—genetics, family, and shoe size, for instance—but most of the factors that color your day-to-day existence are indeed under your control. Removing grains is the courageous first step, but there are plenty more steps to climb to fully undo the years of health abuse you've endured. In this book, there are wonderfully empowering strategies for you to consider to heal the wounds received during your grain-consuming days and unravel the tangle of health problems that developed. Once you're grain-free, you may be left with disruptions of bowel flora and digestive function, nutritional deficiencies, and chronic conditions like osteoporosis. These will all need to be addressed. You may find that medications previously prescribed to treat a long list of grain-related health conditions are no longer necessary. Some people take their diets on other unhealthy detours, such as by introducing gluten-free grains or unhealthy sweeteners, and discover that, while they may not be as bad off as when they consumed grains, they're striking compromises in health that *needn't* be struck. All these issues must be addressed to find your path back to total health, ungrained.

Brace yourself for revelations about diet and health that you've probably never heard, even if you were an avid reader of the original *Wheat Belly*. In *Wheat Belly Total Health*, I follow a no-holds-barred, sacred-cows-be-damned, reach-for-the-skies attitude. My goal is not to titillate, nor to astound, but to inform without the influence of agribusiness interests or the bias of flawed epidemiology. I'm going to ask tough questions while discarding preconceived notions to get to the root of dietary wisdom. There we discover that, minus grains, not only does a long list of chronic health conditions dissolve, but you are also capable of achieving new heights of health and life performance that you had only previously imagined were possible.

We relieve this emperor of his new clothes while watching his huge wheat belly and man breasts shrink, his swollen joints flex, and his seborrheic skin clear. We observe his further health gains by dodging all other grains, then reclothe him in fabrics truly fit for a king. That king will be you, in all your noble, grain-free glory.

THE GRAIN-FREE EXPERIENCE: A CROWD PLEASER

I could not have written *Wheat Belly Total Health* 3 years ago when the original *Wheat Belly* book came out. So many people have engaged in this lifestyle change, so many physicians and health-care professionals have come to embrace these concepts, so many new lessons have been learned as the worldwide rejection of the "healthy whole grain" message has grown that have crowd-sourced a steady stream of new and unexpected lessons. *Wheat Belly Total Health* distills the wisdom gained from the millions of people who have embraced grain-free living and rediscovered what it means to be fully healthy and alive. We are collectively undoing what humans have managed to botch for 300 generations, and we are doing it while dietitians, the USDA, and other defenders of the status quo harrumph, protest, and cast insults as they watch their last 40 years of work crumble beneath their feet.

The Information Age explodes with the empowered wisdom of crowds, shared at lightning speed and dispelling conventional "wisdom" as fast as sexting can take down a congressional career. We've learned, for instance, that wheat intolerance really means intolerance to *all* grains since, after all, they are all genetically related grasses. (Yes, *grasses*, just like the stuff in your backyard or what's munched on by goats and horses. We will discuss the implications of this simple biological realization in some detail.) We learned that virtually everyone benefits from reestablishing healthy bowel flora after removing grains. We learned that iodine deficiency is making a comeback and can impair weight loss and health improvement efforts. Many removed wheat and enjoyed increased energy but didn't experience the full return of youthful vigor because synthetic perchlorate fertilizer residues and brominated flour whiteners from bagels and pizza impaired thyroid function, leaving them with less-than-perfect ability to control weight, a head of prematurely thinning hair, and sluggish bowel function. As more and more people have said no to grains, we have recognized that, while grain elimination is powerful, there may be metabolic derangements that block weight loss and must therefore be addressed, no matter how meticulous the diet. We gained a better understanding that autoimmune, inflammatory, and neurological conditions require additional efforts to maximize the potential for a rebound to total health. We've come to appreciate that the entire package of benefits from grain elimination goes beyond, say, weight loss, and adds up to an astoundingly powerful collection of health-restoring, anti-aging, youth preserving, performance-enhancing, and life-prolonging practices.

Even if you've already enjoyed a major health success by eliminating wheat, understanding the strategies articulated in *Wheat Belly Total Health* and putting them to use can take your health efforts several steps further. If you are among the many people who have shed 30, 50, 100, or even more pounds of wheat-induced visceral fat and reversed one or more health conditions, there are still many more steps you can take to further improve your health.

Or you may be among those who, minus wheat, failed to enjoy a full return to health. You may find yourself still struggling with 60 or more pounds of weight you want to shed, plus joint pains, skin rashes, and other health problems; you may be left wondering if there is something you can do, short of prescription medications and procedures, to restore your health. Or perhaps you now realize just how good you feel minus wheat and are motivated to achieve total health in as many ways as possible to ensure long-term ideal health. Or you may be brand new to the wheat-free message. If so, this is your ultimate guide to going grain-free. Regardless of which category you fall into, you have come to the right place for answers.

We are reminded that humans are truly adaptable, resilient, fit, and vigorous, and have a natural, innate capacity to be healthy, slender, and happy—provided that no grains are permitted entry into our bodies and all health disruptions are corrected in their wake.

LIFE UNGRAINED: UNRESTRAINED HIGH PERFORMANCE

Despotic governments oppress their people. Burdensome health-care costs weigh down our economy. One hundred extra pounds of body fat overtax hips, knees, and feet that are ill-equipped to bear such loads, and they groan, creak, and erode away under the burden. Likewise, the mix of components in grains undermines human functioning from head to toe. Unload such crushing burdens and people are freed, the economy is boosted, joints are relieved, and human functioning is liberated.

Minus the health- and life-impairing effects of grains, we venture into discussions about *performance*: How well you perform emotionally, mentally, professionally, and physically once the major impediments have been removed. This applies to accomplishments in school, at work, in relationships, in sports—in virtually every setting we encounter in life. It means aiming to maximize how good you feel and look to get that extra boost of mojo that can make the difference between *getting through* your day or *blasting* through your day. Total health is outwardly evident; you see it in smoother skin, a flatter tummy, freedom from leg swelling, an easy gait, and ease and vigor of motion in all directions. It's also reflected internally through deeper sleep, less-turbulent menstrual cycles, freedom from headaches, and problem-free digestion.

In addition to less-disruptive menstrual cycles, women can enjoy improved fertility and reductions in perversely high estrogen levels, and they get reacquainted with the concept of feeling good most or all of the time, rather than just once in a while or not at all. Male sexual performance improves as men enjoy lower levels of estrogen, higher levels of testosterone, and reductions of embarrassingly large breasts.

Total health can, in many instances, be measured. You can aim for perfect metabolic health as it's reflected in triglycerides and cholesterol panels, blood sugars, hemoglobin A1c (long-term blood sugar), thyroid tests, and screenings to determine levels of various nutrients. It can also be reflected in measures such as blood pressure and body fat percentage.

While you may be able to walk, run, or jump more easily, faster, farther, and higher minus the aches, pains, and energy impairment of grains, high-performance competitors enjoy similar benefits, and a growing number of professional athletes are embracing the grain-free lifestyle. In this book, we discuss how to gain an even greater competitive edge with strategies that go beyond eliminating grains. Sometimes the additional steps are wonderfully simple, such as correcting iodine and iron deficiencies; other times the solutions are more elaborate, such as the strategies required to restore and maintain bowel health and undo the effects of endocrine disruption. But the goal is to unmask your individual potential and achieve the highest levels of performance in health and life in as many ways as reasonably possible. We aren't trying to create a race of superhuman grain-free men and women, but we can achieve levels of life performance that we previously enjoyed only fleetingly, if at all.

Many of these efforts may not have been necessary had we not been blindsided by these nutritional blunders in the first place. Had we grown up without exposure to Frankengrains with unique, health-disruptive effects, or without thyroid and sex hormone disruption from grains that are compounded by the ocean of endocrine gland–impairing industrial chemicals we swim in, things might be different. Had we also enjoyed the luxury of living outdoors in a semitropical climate and getting a full night of restorative sleep each and every night and had we not been exposed to the chronic, unrelenting stress of modern life, well, maybe we would have enjoyed peak functioning all along. But that is simply not the case for the majority of people. Thankfully, once we understand what went wrong, we can right the situation and, in most cases, fully restore your innate capacity for high levels of life performance.

ACHIEVING UNGRAINED TOTAL HEALTH IN THREE STEPS: NO MORE, NO LESS

Wheat Belly Total Health is presented in three parts that are a logical and necessary sequence that *must* occur if your goal is total health. Like learning to crawl before you walk or studying algebra before cracking the code on calculus, total health unfolds in a natural progression.

You cannot, for instance, regain health as long as grains remain a part of your diet: Health *cannot* be perfect as long as multigrain buns, rye toast, or tacos made from genetically modified corn flour remain a part of your dietary experience. You might not even be aware that grains are exerting their harmful effects while you go about your business working, sleeping, sitting in the drive-thru, or watching *Keeping Up with the Kardashians*. You might be unaware, for instance, that an abnormally increased degree of intestinal permeability is boiling away beneath the surface, waiting to eventually trigger an autoimmune condition in your body that will result, for instance, in the stumbling speech, incoordination, and muscle weakness of multiple sclerosis. Or opacities may be accumulating in the lenses of your eyes, obscuring your vision with milky blurriness, waiting to be diagnosed as cataracts when you're 53, despite the "balanced diet" and exercise program you've been following for the last 30 years. Or a gradual impairment of mind function may develop beneath your awareness until one day you find that you can't remember where you parked your car, your way home, or who that unfamiliar stranger is that you share your bed with. Just because you fail to perceive it doesn't mean it isn't there. It's there regardless of how good you feel, and it needs to be corrected before you can even begin to hope for total health.

In Part I, I discuss why the elimination of *all* grains, wheat and otherwise, is essential if you are to begin your journey back to total health. It is essential because no amount of other healthy foods, nutritional supplements, exercise, or drugs can fully overcome the health-thwarting effects of grains should they remain in your diet. Grain elimination is evolutionarily appropriate for a member of the species *Homo sapiens*; it is consistent with your physiology and metabolism, and it begins—but does not complete—your journey back to total health.

In Part II, we deal with just how to accomplish this journey, including how you can survive the process of withdrawal from the opiates in grains—probably the most challenging hurdle to overcome in your journey back to health and the one that, if you are not properly coached and equipped, can backfire and set you back to your former grain-consuming ways. I teach you how to know when you've been reexposed to closely related proteins that force your body to revisit the havoc you thought you'd eliminated and threaten to undo everything you've accomplished. I also discuss how your body adapts to this new situation in life without grains and why and how adaptation may not be complete until you take the reins and *make* it complete.

In Part III, I discuss how to pursue health as far as possible once you have removed all the health destruction of grains: how to achieve new heights of energy, sleep, mental clarity, mood, bowel function, endocrine health, metabolic health, exercise, and physical functioning. We'll apply all of the lessons we've learned along the way as we discover that, minus grains, life and health are actually quite wonderful.

Too many of us, forced to accept this mantra of "healthy whole grains," have never been shown the path to easily and effortlessly accomplish total health. Once the health disruptions of grains are exorcised from your life and you recognize their purported health benefits for the fictional notions they are, everything gets so much better. Without grains, wondrous things begin to happen in just about every way. *That* is what "total health" means.

PART I

NO GRAIN
IS A
GOOD GRAIN

Grazed,
Grass-Fed,
and Fattened

CHAPTER 1

LIBERATE YOUR INNER COW:
LIFE UNGRAINED

Goldfish do not eat sausages.
—John Cleese, "How to Feed a Goldfish," *Monty Python's Flying Circus*

SINCE YOU ARE reading this book, I take it that you are a member of the species *Homo sapiens*. You are likely not a giraffe, toad, or woodpecker. Nor are you a ruminant, those taciturn creatures that graze on grass.

Ruminants, such as goats and cows, and their ancient, wild counterparts, ibex and aurochs, enjoy evolutionary adaptations that allow them to consume grasses. They have continuously growing teeth to compensate for the wear generated by coarse, sandlike phytolith particles in grass blades; produce in excess of 100 quarts of saliva per day; have four-compartment stomachs that host unique microorganisms to digest grass components, including a compartment that grinds and then regurgitates its contents up as a cud to rechew; and a long, spiral colon that's also host to microorganisms that further digest grassy remains. In other words, ruminants have a gastrointestinal system uniquely specialized to consume grasses.

You don't look, smell, or act like a ruminant. Then why would you eat like one?

Those of you who have already forgone wheat do not, of course. But if you remain of the "healthy whole grain"–consuming persuasion, you have fallen victim to believing that grasses should be your primary source of calories. Just as Kentucky bluegrass and ryegrass in your backyard are grasses from the biological family Poaceae, so are wheat, rye, barley, corn, rice, bulgur, sorghum, triticale, millet, teff, and oats. You grow teeth twice in your life, then stop, leaving you to make do for a lifetime with a prepubertal set that erupted around age 10; produce a meager quart of saliva per day; have three fewer stomach compartments unpopulated by foreign organisms and without grinding action; don't chew a cud; and have a relatively uninteresting, linear, nonspiral colon. These adaptations allow you to be omnivorous—but *not* to consume grasses.

Early members of our species found nourishment through scavenging, and then hunting, animals such as gazelles, turtles, birds, and fish, and consuming the edible parts of plants, including fruit and roots, as well as mushrooms, nuts, and seeds. Hungry humans instinctively regarded all of these as food. About 10,000 years ago, during a period of increasing temperature and dryness in the Fertile Crescent, humans observed the ibex and aurochs grazing on einkorn, the ancient predecessor of modern wheat. Our hungry, omnivorous ancestors asked, "Can we eat that, too?" They did, and surely got sick: vomiting, cramps, and diarrhea. At the very least they simply passed wheat plants out undigested, since humans lack the ruminant digestive apparatus. Grass plants in their intact form are unquestionably unappetizing. We somehow figured out that for humans, the *only* edible part of the einkorn plant was the seed—not the roots, not the stem, not the leaves, not the entire seed head—just the seed, and even that was only edible after the outer husk was removed and the seed was chewed or crushed with rocks and then heated in crude pottery over fire. Only then could we consume the seeds of this grass as porridge, a practice that served us well in times of desperation when ibex meat, bird eggs, and figs were in short supply.

Similar grass-consuming adventures occurred with teosinte and maize (the ancestors of modern corn) in the Americas; rice from the swamps of Asia; and sorghum and millet in sub-Saharan Africa, all requiring similar manipulations to allow the edible part—the seed—to be consumed by humans. Some grasses, such as sorghum, posed other obstacles; its content of poisons (such as hydrocyanic acid, or cyanide) results in sudden death when the plant is consumed before maturity. Natural evolution of grasses led to wheat strains such as emmer, spelt, and kamut as wheat exchanged genes from other wild grasses, while humans selected strains of corn with larger seeds and seed heads (cobs).

What happened to those first humans, hungry and desperate, who figured out how to make this one component of grasses—the seed—edible? Incredibly, anthropologists have known this for years. The first humans to consume the grassy food of the ibex and aurochs experienced explosive tooth decay; shrinkage of the maxillary bone and mandible, resulting in tooth crowding; iron deficiency; and scurvy. They also experienced a reduction in bone diameter and length, resulting in a loss of as much as 5 inches in height for men and 3 inches for women.[1]

The deterioration of dental health is especially interesting, as dental decay was uncommon prior to the consumption of the seeds of grasses, affecting less than 1 percent of all teeth recovered, despite the lack of toothbrushes, toothpaste, fluoridated water, dental floss, and dentists. Even though they lacked any notion of dental hygiene (aside from possibly using a twig to pick the fibers of wild boar from between their teeth), dental decay was simply not a problem that beset many members of our species prior to the consumption of grains. The notion of toothless savages is all wrong; they enjoyed sturdy, intact teeth for their entire lives. It was only after humans began to resort to the seeds of grasses for calories that mouths of rotten and crooked teeth began to appear in children and adults. From that point on, decay was evident in 16 to 49 percent of all teeth recovered, along with tooth loss and abscesses, making tooth decay as commonplace as bad hair among humans of the agricultural Neolithic Age.[2]

In short, when we started consuming the seeds of grasses 10,000 years ago, this food source may have allowed us to survive another day, week, or month during times when foods we had instinctively consumed during the preceding 2.5 million years fell into short supply. But this expedient represents a dietary pattern that constitutes only 0.4 percent—less than one-half of 1 percent—of our time on earth. This change in dietary fortunes was accompanied by a substantial price. From the standpoint of oral health, humans remained in the Dental Dark Ages from their first taste of porridge all the way up until recent times. History is rich with descriptions of toothaches, oral abscesses, and stumbling and painful efforts to extract tainted teeth. Remember George Washington and his mouthful of wooden false teeth? It wasn't until the 20th century that modern dental hygiene was born and we finally managed to keep most of our teeth through adulthood.

Fast-forward to the 21st century: Modern wheat now accounts for 20 percent of all calories consumed by humans; the seeds of wheat, corn, and rice combined make up 50 percent.[3] Yes, the seeds of grasses provide half of all human calories. We have become a grass seed–consuming species, a development enthusiastically applauded by agencies such as the USDA, which advises us that increasing our consumption to 60 percent of calories or higher is a laudable dietary goal. It's also a situation celebrated by all of those people who trade grain on an international scale, since the seeds of grasses have a prolonged shelf life (months to years) that allows transoceanic shipment, they're easy to store, they don't require refrigeration, and they're in demand worldwide—all the traits desirable in a commoditized version of food. The transformation of foodstuff into that of a commodity that's tradeable on a global scale allows financial manipulations, such as buying and selling futures, hedges, and complex derivative instruments—the tools of mega-commerce—to emerge. You can't do that with organic blueberries or Atlantic salmon.

Examine the anatomy of a member of the species *Homo sapiens* and you cannot escape the conclusion that you are *not* a ruminant, have none of the adaptive digestive traits of such creatures, and can only consume the seeds of grasses—the food of desperation—by accepting a decline in your health. But the seeds of grasses *can* be used to feed the masses cheaply, quickly, and on a massive scale, all while generating huge profits for those who control the flow of these commoditized foods.

MUTANT NINJA GRASSES

The seeds of grasses, known to us more familiarly as "grains" or "cereals," have always been a problem for us nonruminant creatures. But then busy geneticists and agribusiness got into the act. That's when grains went from bad to worse.

Readers of the original *Wheat Belly* know that modern wheat is no longer the 4½-foot-tall traditional plant we all remember; it is now an 18-inch-tall plant with a short, thick stalk; long seed head; and larger seeds. It has a much greater yield per acre than its traditional predecessors. This high-yield strain of wheat, now the darling of agribusiness, was not created through genetic modification, but through repetitive hybridizations, mating wheat with non-wheat grasses to introduce new genes (wheat is a grass, after all) and through *mutagenesis,* the use of high-dose x-rays, gamma rays, and chemicals to induce mutations. Yes: Modern wheat is, to a considerable degree, a grass that contains an array of mutations, some of which have been mapped and identified, many of which have not. Such uncertainties never faze agribusiness, however. Unique mutated proteins? No problem. The USDA and FDA say they're okay, too—perfectly fine for public consumption.

Over the years, there have been many efforts to genetically modify wheat, such as by using gene-splicing technology to insert or delete a gene. However, public resistance has dampened efforts to bring genetically modified (GM) wheat to market, so no wheat currently sold is, in the terminology of genetics, "genetically modified." (There have been recent industry rumblings, however, that make the prospect of true GM wheat a probable reality in the near future.) All of the changes introduced into modern wheat are the results of methods that predate the technology to create GM foods. This does not mean that the methods used to change wheat were benign; in fact, the crude and imprecise methods used to change wheat, such as chemical mutagenesis, have the potential to be *worse* than genetic modification, yielding a *greater* number of unanticipated changes in genetic code than the handful introduced through gene-splicing.[4]

Corn and rice, on the other hand, have been genetically modified, in addition to undergoing other changes. For instance, scientists introduced genes to make corn resistant to the herbicide glyphosate and to express *Bacillus thurigiensis* (Bt), a toxin that kills insects, while rice has been genetically modified to make it resistant to the herbicide glufosinate and to express beta-carotene (a variety called Golden Rice). Problem: While, in theory, the notion of just inserting one silly gene seems simple and straightforward, it is anything but. The methods of gene insertion remain crude. The site of insertion—which chromosome, within or alongside other genes, within or without various control elements—not to mention disruption of epigenetic effects that control gene expression, cannot be controlled with current technology. And it's misleading to say that only one gene is inserted, as the methods used usually require *several* genes to be inserted. (We discuss the nature of specific changes in GM grains in Chapter 2.)

The wheat, corn, and rice that make up 50 percent of the human diet in the 21st century are not the wheat, corn, and rice of the 20th century. They're not the wheat, corn, and rice of the Middle Ages, nor of the Bible, nor of the Egyptian empire. And they are definitely not the same wheat, corn, and rice that was harvested by those early hungry humans. They are what I call "Frankengrains": hybridized, mutated, genetically modified to suit the desires of agribusiness, and now available at a supermarket, convenience store, or school near you.

Wheat: What Changed . . . and Why Are the Changes So Bad?

All strains of wheat, including traditional strains like spelt and emmer, are problems for nonruminant humans who consume them. But modern wheat is the worst.

Modern wheat *looks* different: shorter, thicker shaft, larger seeds. The reduction in height is due to mutations in Rh (reduced height) genes that code for the protein gibberellin, which controls stalk length. This one mutant gene is accompanied by other mutations. Changes in Rh genes are thereby accompanied by *other* changes in the genetic code of the wheat plant.[5] There's more here than meets the eye.

Gliadin

While gluten is often fingered as the source of wheat's problems, it's really gliadin, a protein within gluten, that is the culprit behind many destructive health effects of modern wheat. There are more than 200 forms of gliadin proteins, all incompletely digestible.[6] One important change that has emerged over the past 50 years, for example, is increased expression of a gene called Glia-α9, which yields a gliadin protein that is the most potent trigger for celiac disease. While the Glia-α9 gene was *absent* from most strains of wheat from the early 20th century, it is now present in nearly *all* modern varieties,[7] likely accounting for the 400 percent increase in celiac disease witnessed since 1948.[8]

New gliadin variants are partially digested into small peptides that enter the bloodstream and then bind to *opiate receptors* in the human brain—the same receptors activated by heroin and morphine.[9] Researchers call these peptides "exorphins," or exogenous morphine-like compounds. Gliadin-derived peptides, however, generate no "high," but they do trigger increased appetite and increased calorie consumption, with studies demonstrating consistent increases of 400 calories per day, mostly from carbohydrates.

Gluten

Gluten (gliadin + glutenins) is the stuff that confers the stretchiness unique to wheat dough. Gluten is a popular additive in processed foods such as sauces, instant soups, and frozen foods, which means the average person ingests between 15 and 20 grams (g) per day.[10] Gluten has been genetically manipulated to improve the baking characteristics of its glutenin. Geneticists have therefore crossbred wheat strains repeatedly, bred wheat with non-wheat grasses to introduce new genes, and used chemicals and radiation to induce mutations. Breeding methods used to alter gluten quality do not result in predictable changes. Hybridizing two different wheat plants yields as many as 14 unique glutenin proteins never before encountered by humans.[11]

Wheat Germ Agglutinin

The genetic changes inflicted on wheat have altered the structure of wheat germ agglutinin (WGA), a protein in wheat that provides protection against molds and insects. The structure of WGA in modern wheat, for instance, differs from that of ancient wheat strains.[12] WGA is indigestible and toxic, resistant to *any* breakdown in the human body, and unchanged by cooking, baking, and sourdough fermentation. Unlike gluten and gliadin, which require genetic susceptibility to exert some of their negative effects, WGA does its damage directly. WGA *alone* is sufficient to generate celiac disease–like intestinal damage by disrupting microvilli, the absorptive "hairs" of intestinal cells.[13]

Phytates

Phytic acid (phytates) is a storage form of phosphorus in wheat and other grains. Because phytates also provide resistance to pests, grain-breeding efforts over the past 50 years have selected strains with increased phytate content. Modern wheat, maize, and millet, for instance, each contain 800 milligrams (mg) of phytates per 100 g (3½ ounces) of flour. Phytate content increases with fiber content, so advice to increase fiber in your diet by consuming more "healthy whole grains" also increases the phytate content of your diet. As little as 50 mg of phytates can turn off absorption of minerals, especially iron and zinc.[14] Children who consume grains ingest 600 to 1,900 mg of phytates per day, while enthusiastic grain-consuming cultures, such as modern Mexicans, ingest 4,000 to 5,000 mg of phytates per day. These levels are associated with nutrient deficiencies.[15]

Alpha-Amylase Inhibitors and Other Allergens

Wheat allergies are becoming more prevalent. Numerous allergens have been identified in modern wheat that are not present in ancient or traditional forms of the plant.[16] The most common are *alpha-amylase inhibitors,* which are responsible for causing hives, asthma, cramps, diarrhea, and eczema. Compared to older strains, the structure of modern alpha-amylase inhibitors differs by 10 percent, meaning it may have as many as several dozen amino acid differences. As any allergist will tell you, just a few amino acids can spell the difference between no allergic reaction and a severe allergic reaction, or even anaphylactic shock. People in the baking industry frequently develop a condition called *baker's asthma.* There is also a peculiar condition called *wheat-derived exercise-induced anaphylaxis* (WDEIA), a severe and life-threatening allergy induced by exercising after eating wheat. Both conditions are caused by an allergy to gliadin proteins.[17] Many other proteins have undergone changes over the last 40 years: lipid transfer proteins, omega-gliadins, gamma-gliadins, trypsin inhibitors, serpins, and glutenins. All trigger allergic reactions.

LIFE OUTSIDE THE GRAIN MOOOVEMENT

The start of grain consumption for humans coincides with the dawn of the domestication of livestock. We learned that some herbivorous species, such as aurochs and ibex, when confined and allowed to reproduce in captivity, could be put into the service of the human diet. While we were domesticating these creatures into cows and goats, they showed us that their diet of grasses was also something we could try to mimic. They also contributed to human diseases by giving us smallpox, measles, tuberculosis, and rhinoviruses that cause the common cold.

While much of the world followed the lead of grazing ruminants and adopted a diet increasingly reliant on the seeds of grasses, not all cultures took this 10,000-year dietary detour. A number of hunter-gatherer societies throughout the world never embraced grains, relying instead on traditional omnivorous menus. The diets followed by such societies therefore largely reflect the diets of pre-Neolithic humans, i.e., diets that predate the development of agriculture. The modern world has, over the past few hundred years, encroached on these primitive societies, particularly if their land or other resources were prized. (Think Native Americans and Canadians of the Pacific Northwest or Aboriginal populations of Australia.) Each instance provides a virtual laboratory to observe what happens to health when there is a shift from a traditional grain-free to a modern grain-filled diet.

We have cultural anthropologists and field-working physicians to thank for such insights. Scientists have studied, for instance, the San of southern Africa, Kitavan Islanders of Papua New Guinea, and the Xingu peoples of the Brazilian rain forest, all of whom consume foods obtained from their unique habitats. None consume modern processed foods, of course, meaning no grains, no added sugars, no hydrogenated oils, no preservatives, and no artificial food coloring. People following their ancestral diets consistently demonstrate low body weight and body mass index (BMI); freedom from obesity; normal blood pressure; normal blood sugar and insulin responses; lower leptin levels (the hormone of satiety); and better bone health.[18] Body mass index, reflecting a ratio of weight to height, is typically 22 or less, compared to our growing ranks of people with BMIs of 30 or more, with 30 representing the widely accepted cutoff for obesity. The average blood pressure of a Xingu woman is 102/66 mmHg, compared to our typical blood pressures of 130/80 or higher. The Xingu experience less osteoporosis and fewer fractures.

The Hadza of northern Tanzania are a good example of a hunter-gatherer society that, despite contact with Westerners, has clung to traditional methods of procuring food.[19] The women dig for roots and gather edible parts of plants, while the men hunt with bows and poison-tipped arrows and gather honey from bees. The average BMI of this population? Around 20, with vigor maintained into later life, as grandparents help rear grandchildren while mothers gather and prepare food. Despite a lifestyle that appears physically demanding on the surface, the total energy expenditure of the Hadza is *no different* than that of modern people—not greater or less than, say, an average accountant or school-teacher.[20] Activity is parceled a bit differently, of course, with hunter-gatherers tending to experience bursts of intense activity, followed by prolonged rest, and modern cultures gradually playing out activity throughout the day, but detailed analyses of energy expenditure among primitive people show virtually *no difference*. This challenges the notion that modern excess weight gain can be blamed on increasingly sedentary lifestyles.[21] (Note that this is not true for all hunter-gatherer cultures; the Luo and Kamba of rural Kenya, for instance, exhibit high levels of energy expenditure. The point is that differences in weight are not solely explained by differences in energy expenditure.)

Humans are adaptable creatures, as the wide variety of diets consumed worldwide attest. Some rely almost exclusively on the flesh, organs, and fat of animals, such as that of the traditional Inuits of the northern-most Pacific Northwest of North America. Some diets are high in starches from roots (such as yams, sweet potatoes, taro, and tapioca) and fruit, as with the Kitavans of Papua New Guinea or the Yanomami of the Brazilian rain forest.

The incorporation of foods from the mammary glands of bovines has provoked expression of a lactase-persistence gene that allows some adults to consume milk, cheese, and other products that contain the sugar lactase after the first few years of life—an advantage for survival. The semino-madic Maasai people of central Africa are a notable example. Largely herders of goats, sheep, and cattle, they traditionally consume plentiful raw meat and the blood of cows mixed with milk, and they've done so for thousands of years. This lifestyle allows them to enjoy freedom from cardiovascular disease, hypertension, diabetes, and excess weight.[22]

This is the recurring theme throughout primitive societies: A traditional diet, varied in composition and high in nutrient content but containing no grains or added sugars, allows people to enjoy freedom from all the chronic "diseases of affluence." Even cancer is rare.[23] This is not to say that people following traditional lifestyles don't succumb to disease; of course they do. But the range of ailments is entirely different. They suffer infections such as malaria, dengue fever, and nematode infestations of the gastrointestinal tract, as well as traumatic injuries from falls, battles with humans and animals, and lacerations, reflecting the hazards of living without modern tools, conveniences, central governments, or modern health care.

What happens when a culture that has avoided the adoption of agriculture and grain consumption is confronted with modern breads, cookies, and chips? This invasion by modern foods has played out countless times on a worldwide stage, with the same results each and every time: weight gain and obesity to an astounding degree, tooth decay, gingivitis and periodontitis, tooth loss, arthritis, hypertension, diabetes, and depression and other psychiatric conditions—all the modern diseases of affluence. Like a broken record, this same refrain has played over and over again in varied populations, on every continent.

It has been observed in Pima Indians of the American Southwest, where 40 to 50 percent of adults are obese and diabetic, many toothless.[24] It has been observed in native tribes of Arizona, Oklahoma, and the Dakotas, resulting in 54 to 67 percent of the population being overweight or obese.[25] Peoples inhabiting circumpolar regions of Canada and Greenland have all experienced dramatic increases in obesity and diabetes.[26] In Pacific Islanders, such as the Micronesian Nauru, 40 percent of adults are obese with diabetes.[27] Modernized diets have put Australian Aboriginal populations in especially desperate health straits, with 22 times the risk of complications of diabetes, 8 times higher cardiovascular mortality, and 6 times greater mortality from stroke compared to non-Aboriginal Australians.[28]

Until recently, the Maasai of central Africa, Samburu of Kenya, and Fulani of Nigeria showed virtually no overweight or obesity, no hypertension, and low total cholesterol values (125 mg/dl). When relocated to urban settings, hypertension and obesity explode, with 55 percent overweight or obese.[29] Former hunter-gatherers develop iron deficiency anemia and folate deficiency as they transition away from hunting game and gathering wild vegetation and rely on purchased foods, especially corn.[30] Dr. Roberto Baruzzi, a Brazilian physician, studied hunter-gatherers of the Xingu region of Brazil in the 1960s and 1970s and found slender people with no discernible excess body fat, no diabetes, no cardiovascular disease, no ulcers, and no appendicitis. A repeat survey in 2009, following 30 years of contact with modern food, found 46 percent of the people overweight or obese, 25 percent of the men hypertensive, and most with abnormalities of cholesterol panels (such as low HDL cholesterol or high triglycerides), and rampant dental decay.[31] Another recent assessment of Aruák natives of the Xingu region documented 66.8 percent of men and women as overweight or obese, 52.1 percent of women with abdominal obesity, and 37.7 percent of men with hypertension.[32]

All of these groups represent humans who have not developed the *partial* tolerances agricultural societies evolved over 10,000 years that allow them to consume the seeds of grasses. Consequently they, more so than us, show exaggerated responses to consumption of grains and sugars.

The diseases of modernization are unfortunately intertwined with the diseases of poverty, given the disrupted and marginalized lives indigenous people often endure at the heavy-handed ways of modern society. Typically, an overreliance on cheap grains and sugars characterizes the diets of these latecomers to the modern world, replacing gathered vegetation, for instance, with flours, convenience foods, and sweets. And if Western aid is required due to starvation and maldistribution (which is common when former hunter-gatherers are disconnected from their traditional lifestyles), do we fly in beef, salmon, coconuts, or cucumbers? Nope: We send in the grain—wheat, maize, rice—which feeds humans as well as their livestock.

Type 2 diabetes, in particular, is the defining disease acquired when hunter-gatherer populations join the modern world in dietary and health habits—so much so that anthropologists have labeled diabetes "the price of civilization." And, of course, all of us modern humans, being hunter-gatherers at our genetic core, are experiencing diabetes at an unprecedented rate. This modern disease is expected to afflict a third of all adults in coming years, as well as a growing proportion of children and teenagers.[33] The world of humans now obtains 50 percent of its calories from the seeds of grasses and is increasing consumption of sucrose and fructose. Meanwhile, we're being urged to further *increase* our reliance on "healthy whole grains" in the developed world while we resort to cheap, accessible grains of any sort in the less-developed world. Under these circumstances, we can expect no relief from this global man-made pandemic—unless we reject the notion of consuming the seeds of grasses outright.

Dr. Weston Price: Snapshots of Westernization

Dr. Weston Price was a dentist practicing in Cleveland, Ohio, during the early 20th century. He was troubled by the amount of tooth decay he witnessed in his patients, particularly children, and intrigued by reports that "savages" (people living in primitive settings) were virtually free of tooth problems. So Dr. Price did something extraordinary: He left his home and, along with his wife, Florence, began a 10-year worldwide journey to chronicle the dietary habits of primitive cultures, documenting his findings with careful examinations of teeth, facial structure, and more than 15,000 photographs. His efforts provide a remarkable visual record of what primitive cultures looked like and what happens to primitive humans when they begin to consume modern foods.

His travels took him to the Inuits of Alaska, the native Americans of the Pacific Northwest and central Canada, Melanesians and Polynesians, Aborigines of Australia, the Maori of New Zealand, descendants of the ancient Chimú culture in coastal Peru, and tribes of Africa, including Maasai, Kikuyu, Wakamba, Jalou, Muhima, Pygmies, Baitu, and Dinkas. In each locale, he examined and photographed teeth, faces, and other features he found interesting. In short, Dr. Price produced a fascinating record of people living their traditional lifestyles at a moment in time when it was all about to end.

In every culture of the dozens he studied—without exception—he found tooth decay, tooth loss, and dental abscesses or infections to be uncommon, typically affecting no more than 1 to 3 percent (and sometimes none) of the teeth he examined. He also noted the absence of gingivitis and periodontitis, and few to no crooked or crowded teeth. While a keeper of meticulous records, he also observed that facial structure was different, with primitive people enjoying what he called "fully formed facial and dental arches" and a lack of narrowed nasal passages.

Even more remarkably, Dr. Price specifically sought out members of these cultures who had recently transitioned to consuming "white man's food"—people who were bartering for the breads, pastries, and candies of Westerners visiting or bordering their land. In every instance, he observed an astounding increase in tooth decay, affecting 25 to 50 percent of teeth examined, along with gingivitis, periodontitis, tooth loss, infectious abscesses, crooked and crowded teeth, and reductions in the size of the maxillary (midfacial) bone and mandible (jawbone). Nearly toothless mouths in teenagers and young adults were not uncommon.

The traditional diets of these societies were typically fish, shellfish, and kelp among coastal cultures and animal flesh and organs, raw dairy products, edible plants, nuts, mushrooms, and insects among inland cultures. With only two exceptions (the Lötschental Valley Swiss, isolated by the Alps, who consumed a coarse rye bread, and the Gaelic people of the islands of the Outer Hebrides, who consumed crude oats), grains, sugars, and processed foods were notably absent. (The Swiss had an intermediate number of dental caries, more than other cultures studied, while the Gaelic population did not.)

What is even more startling about Dr. Price's observations of the rarity of tooth decay and deformity is that none of these cultures practiced any sort of dental hygiene: no toothbrushes, no toothpaste, no fluoridated water, no dental floss, and no dentists or orthodontists. While Dr. Price's observations cannot be used to precisely pinpoint the nutritional distinctions between modern and traditional cultures, they nonetheless make a powerful point. Anyone wishing to read Dr. Price's account can find it reproduced in a recent reprint.[34]

This social "experiment" has also occurred in the opposite direction: a *return* to traditional diet and lifestyle after a period of Westernization. In 1980, Kerin O'Dea, MD, while at the Royal Children's Hospital in Melbourne, conducted an extraordinary experiment: She asked 10 diabetic, overweight Aboriginal individuals living Western lifestyles, all of whom retained memories of prior lifestyles, to move back to their origins in the wilds of northwestern Australia and follow their previous hunter-gatherer diet of kangaroo, freshwater fish, and yams. They began their adventure with high blood glucose levels of (on average) 209 mg/dl, high triglycerides of 357 mg/dl, as well as abnormal insulin levels. After 7 weeks of living in the wild, killing animals, and eating familiar gathered foods, the 10 lost an average of 17.6 pounds of body weight and dropped their blood glucose to 119 mg/dl and triglycerides to 106 mg/dl.[35] Of the original 10, five returned nondiabetic. In a 2005 lecture, Dr. O'Dea remarked: "I was struck by the change in people when they were back in their own country: They were confident and assertive, and proud of their local knowledge and skills. At the time we were not able to measure markers of psychosocial state, however observation suggested a very positive change."[36]

Search the four corners of the earth today and you will find that the only surviving hunter-gatherer population that's untouched by modern diet is the Sentinelese of the North Sentinel Island in the Indian Ocean. Because their language is strikingly different from all languages in neighboring lands, it is thought that the Sentinelese have been isolated since anatomically modern humans first migrated to this part of the world 60,000 years ago.[37] Attempts to visit their island have been met with volleys of arrows, spears, and rocks, so observations are limited. From what has been observed, however, they are lean and healthy, hunting, fishing, and gathering foods without the "benefit" of agriculture.

We have to be careful not to regard the life of the hunter-gatherer human as idyllic or problem-free: They had plenty of problems. While it is widely believed that stress is a modern phenomenon, this is absurd. Which is more stressful: struggling to pay your bills or having a marauding, bloodthirsty tribe of humans slaughter your friends, seize the women, and enslave the children? We need to observe some of the practices of primitive cultures, such as head shrinking by the Jivaro Indians of the Amazon or cannibalism by the Carib of the Lesser Antilles and Venezuela, to remind ourselves that the world of humans can be an inhospitable place. Violence inflicted by and upon humans has characterized our existence from the start. While violence is certainly still a part of modern life, legal and political constraints that became necessary as human populations developed greater reliance on the practice of agriculture make it far less a part of day-to-day life than it was, say, 50,000 years ago. Yes, there is a bright side to agriculture and civilization.

The development of civilization and the cultivation of the seeds of grasses: two processes that ran parallel over the past 10,000 years that led to concepts such as sedentary non-nomadic life, land ownership, centralized government, and many other phenomena we now accept as part of modern life. But when we observe what happens to cultures unexposed to the seeds of grasses who are then compelled to consume them, we observe an exaggerated microcosm of what the rest of the world is now experiencing.

EAT LIKE AN EGYPTIAN

Tooth decay, dental infections, crooked teeth, iron and folate deficiencies, diabetes, degenerated joints, weight gain, obesity: I've just described the average modern person. Take a member of a primitive culture following their traditional diet and feed them the processed foods of modern man—complete with the enticing products of the seeds of grasses—and within a few years, we've given them all the same problems we have, or worse. Yes, without "modern civilization" they might succumb to the greedy ambitions of a violent neighboring clan, but with grain in their lives, they'll have to engage in battle while sporting a 44-inch waist, two bad knees, and a mouth that's missing half its teeth.

While obesity and the diseases associated with it are virtually absent from hunter-gatherer cultures, neither are they entirely new. Diseases of affluence developed even before geneticists introduced changes into grains. Hippocrates, a Greek physician in the 3rd century BC, and Galen, a Roman physician of the 2nd century AD, both made detailed studies of obese people. William Wadd, an early-19th-century London physician and a lifelong observer of the "corpulent," made this observation after the autopsy of an obese man:

> The heart itself was a mass of fat. The omentum [a component of the intestines] was a thick fat apron. The whole of the intestinal canal was imbedded in fat, as if melted tallow had been poured into the cavity of the abdomen; and the diaphragm and the parietes [walls of organs] of the abdomen must have

been strained to their very utmost extent, to have sustained the extreme and constant pressure of such a weighty mass. So great was the mechanical obstruction to the functions of an organ essential to life, that the wonder is, not that he should die, but that he should live.[38]

What is new is that overweight and obesity have been transformed from that of *curiosity* to that of *epidemic*. The situation we confront in the 21st century is all the more astounding because modern epidemiologists and health officials declare that the causes of the epidemic of overweight, obesity, and their accompanying diseases are either unclear or that the burden of blame should be placed on the gluttonous and sedentary shoulders of the public. But the answers can be discerned through observations of primitive societies plagued by *none* of the issues plaguing us.

More than the presence of grains distinguishes primitive from modern life, of course. Hunter-gatherers also drank no soft drinks; consumed no processed foods laced with hydrogenated fats, food preservatives, or food colorings; and consumed no high-fructose corn syrup or sucrose. They were not exposed to endocrine disruptive chemicals released by industry into our groundwater and soil, and which taint our food. Civilizations of ancient Greece and Rome and of 19th-century Europe also did not consume these components of the modern diet (except for increasing consumption of sucrose beginning in the 19th century). No Coca-Cola, Crisco, brightly colored candies lit up by FD&C Red No. 3, or polychlorinated biphenyl (PCB)–laced water graced their tables. But they did consume the seeds of grasses.

So just *how much* can we blame on the adoption of the seeds of grasses into the human diet? Let's consider that question next. Each variety of seeds of grasses poses its own unique set of challenges to nonruminants who consume them. Before we get under way in our discussion of regaining health in the absence of grains, let's talk about just how they ruin the health of every human who allows them to adorn his or her plate.

CHAPTER 2

LET THEM EAT GRASS

I asked the waiter, "Is this milk fresh?"
He said, "Lady, 3 hours ago it was grass."
—Phyllis Diller

GRASSES ARE EVERYWHERE.

They grow on mountains, along rivers and lakes, in valleys, vast steppes, savannahs, prairies, golf courses, even your backyard. And they now reign supreme in the human diet.

Grasses are wonderfully successful life forms. They are geographically diverse, inhabiting every continent, including Antarctica. They are a study of how life can adapt to extremes, from the tundra to the tropics. Grasses are prolific and hardy, and they evolve rapidly to survive. Even with the explosive growth of the human population, worldwide expansion of cities and suburbs, and asphalt spanning coast-to-coast, grasses still cover 20 percent of the earth's surface area. Just as insects are the most successful form of animal life on the planet, grasses are among the most successful of plants. Given their ubiquity, perhaps it's not unexpected that we would try to eat them. Humans have experimented with feasting on just about every plant and creature that ever inhabited the earth. After all, we are creatures who make food out of tarantulas and poisonous puffer fish.

While grasses have served as food for many creatures (they've even been recovered from fossilized dinosaur feces), they were not a food item on our dietary menu during our millions of years of adaptation to life on this planet. Pre-*Homo* hominids, chimpanzee-like australopithecines that date back more than 4 million years, did not consume grasses in any form or variety, nor has any species of *Homo* prior to *sapiens*. Grasses were simply not instinctively regarded as food. Much as you'd never spot an herbivorous giraffe eating the carcass of a hyena or a great white shark munching on sea kelp, humans did not consume any part of this group of plants, no matter how evolutionarily successful, until the relatively recent past.

The seeds of grasses are a form of "food" added just a moment ago in archaeological time. For the first 2,390,000 years of our existence on earth, or about 8,000 generations, we consumed things that hungry humans instinctively regarded as food. Then, 10,000 years or just over 300 generations ago, in times of desperation, we turned to those darned seeds of grasses. They were something we hoped could serve as food, since they were growing from every conceivable environmental nook and cranny.

So let us consider what this stuff is, the grasses that have populated our world, as common as ants and earthworms, and been subverted into the service of the human diet. Not *all* grasses, of course, have come to grace your dinner plate—you don't save and eat the clippings from cutting your lawn, do you?—so we'll confine our discussion to the grasses and seeds that humans have chosen to include on our dinner plates. I discuss this issue at some length, because it's important for you to understand that consumption of the seeds of grasses underlies a substantial proportion of the chronic problems of human health. Accordingly, removing them yields unexpected and often astounding relief from these issues and is therefore an absolutely necessary first step toward regaining health, the ultimate goal of this book. We will spend a lot of time talking about how recovering full health as a non-grass-consuming *Homo sapiens* of the 21st century— that means you—also means having to compensate for all of the destruction that has occurred in your body during your unwitting grain-consuming years. You've consumed what amounts to a dietary poison for 20, 30, or 50 years, a habit that your non-grain-accustomed body partially—but never completely—adapts to, endures, or succumbs to. You then remove that poison and, much as a chronic alcoholic needs to recover and heal his liver, heart, brain, and emotional health after the flow of alcohol ceases, so your body needs a bit of help to readjust and regain health minus the destructive seeds of grasses.

So what makes the grasses of the world a food appropriate for the ruminants of the earth, but not *Homo sapiens?* There is no single factor within grains responsible for its wide array of bowel-destroying effects— there is an *arsenal.*

NONWHEAT GRAINS: YOU MIGHT AS WELL EAT JELLY BEANS

There is no question that, in this barrel of rotten apples, wheat is the rottenest. But you still may not want to make cider with those other apples.

What I call "nonwheat grains," such as oats, barley, rye, millet, teff, sorghum, corn, and rice, are nonetheless seeds of grasses with potential for curious effects in nonruminant creatures not adapted to their consumption. I would classify nonwheat grains as *less bad* than the worst—modern wheat—but *less bad* is not necessarily *good*. (That extraordinarily simple insight—that less bad is not necessarily good—is one that will serve you well over and over as you learn to question conventional nutritional advice. You will realize that much of what we have been told by the dietary community, the food industry, and even government agencies violates this basic principle of logic again and again.) Less bad can mean that a variety of undesirable health effects can still occur with that seed's consumption—those effects will just not be as bad as those provoked by modern wheat.

So what's the problem with the seeds of nonwheat grasses? While none achieve the nastiness of the seeds of modern wheat, they each have their own unique issues. For starters, they're all high in carbohydrates. Typically, 60 to 85 percent of the calories from the seeds of grasses are in the form of carbohydrates. This makes sense, since the carbohydrate stored in the seed was meant to provide nutrition to the sprouting plant as it germinates. But the carbohydrate in seeds, called amylopectin A, is rapidly digested by humans and raises blood sugar, gram for gram, *higher than table sugar does*.

For instance, a 1-cup serving of cooked organic, stoneground oatmeal has nearly 50 grams of net carbohydrates (total carbohydrates minus fiber, which we subtract because it has no glycemic potential), or the equivalent of slightly more than 11 teaspoons of sugar, representing 61 percent of the calories in oatmeal. This gives it a glycemic index (GI, an index of blood sugar–raising potential) of 55, which is enough to send blood sugar through the roof and provoke all the phenomena of glycation, i.e., glucose modification of proteins that essentially acts as biological debris in various organs. This irreversible process leads to conditions such as cataracts, hypertension, the destruction of joint cartilage that results in arthritis, kidney disease, heart disease, and dementia. (Note that a glycemic index of 55 falls into what dietitians call the "low" glycemic index range, despite the potential to generate high blood sugars. We discuss this common fallacy in Chapter 5.) *All* nonwheat grasses, without exception, raise blood sugar and provoke glycation to similar degrees.

Human manipulation makes it worse. If corn is not consumed as intact kernels but instead is pulverized into fine cornstarch or cornmeal, the surface area for digestion increases exponentially and accounts for the highest blood sugars possible from any food. This is why the glycemic index of cornstarch is 90 to 100, compared to 60 for corn on the cob and 59 to 65 for sucrose or table sugar.

For years, we've been told that "complex" carbohydrates are better for us than "simple" sugars because the lengthy carbohydrate molecules of amylopectin A and amylose in grains don't raise blood sugar as high as sugars with one or two sugar molecules, such as glucose (one sugar) or sucrose (two sugars: glucose and fructose), do. But this is simply wrong, and this silly distinction is therefore being abandoned: The GI of complex carbohydrates is the same as or higher than that of simple sugars. The GI of whole wheat bread: 72; the GI of millet as a hot cereal: 67. Neither are any better than the GI of sucrose: 59 to 65. (Similar relationships hold for the glycemic load, a value that factors in typical portion size.) The World Health Organization (WHO) and the Food and Agriculture Organization of the United Nations have both advised dropping the complex versus simple distinction, and rightly so, as grains, from a blood sugar viewpoint, are the same as or worse than sugar.

And the problems with nonwheat grains don't end with blood sugar issues.

LECTINS: GOOD ENOUGH FOR THE KGB

The lectin proteins of grains are, by design, toxins. Lectins discourage creatures, such as molds, fungi, and insects, from eating the seeds of a plant by sickening or killing them. After all, the seed is the means by which plants continue their species. When we consume plants, we consume defensive lectins. Lectin proteins' effects on humans vary widely, from harmless to fatal. Most plant lectins are benign, such as those in spinach and white mushrooms, which cause no adverse effects when consumed as a spinach salad. The lectin of castor beans is an entirely different story; its lectin, ricin, is highly toxic and is fatal even in small quantities. Ricin has been used by terrorists around the world. Gyorgy Markov, Bulgarian dissident and critic of the Soviet government, was murdered by KGB agents in 1978 when he was poked with the tip of an umbrella laced with ricin.

The lectin of the seed of wheat is wheat germ agglutinin (WGA). It is neither as benign as the lectin of spinach nor as toxic as the lectin of ricin; it is somewhere in between. WGA wreaks ill effects on everyone, regardless of whether you have celiac disease, gluten sensitivity, or no digestive issues at all. The lectins of rye, barley, and rice are structurally identical to WGA and share all of its properties and are also called "WGA." (The only substantial difference is that rye, barley, and rice express a single form of lectin, while genetically more complex wheat expresses up to three different forms.) Interestingly, 21 percent of the amino acid structure of WGA lectins overlaps with ricin, including the active site responsible for shutting down protein synthesis, the site that accounts for ricin's exceptional toxicity.[1]

Lectin proteins have the specific ability to recognize glycoproteins (proteins with a sugar side chain). This makes plant lectins effective in recognizing common glycoproteins on, say, the surface of a fungal cell. But that same process can occur in humans. When a minute quantity, such as 1 milligram, of WGA is purified and intestinal tissue is exposed to it, intestinal glycoproteins are bound and severe damage that resembles the effects of celiac disease results.[2] We also know that WGA compounds the destructive intestinal effects of celiac disease started by gliadin and other grain prolamin proteins.[3] If you have inflammatory bowel disease, ulcerative colitis, or Crohn's disease, grain lectins intensify the inflammation, making cramps, diarrhea, bleeding, and poor nutrient absorption worse.

WGA is oddly indestructible. It is unaffected by cooking, boiling, baking, or frying. WGA is also untouched by stomach acid. Though the acid produced in the human stomach is powerfully corrosive (dip your finger in a glass full of stomach acid and you won't have a finger for very long), WGA is impervious to it, entering the stomach and passing through the entire gastrointestinal tract unscathed, undigested, and free to do what it likes to any glycoproteins exposed along the way.

While most WGA remains confined to the intestine, doing its damage along the 30-foot length of this organ, we know that a small quantity gets into your bloodstream. (We know this because people commonly develop antibodies to this protein.) Once WGA enters the bloodstream, odd things happen: Red blood cells clump (or "agglutinate," the basis for WGA's name), which can, under certain circumstances (obesity, smoking, sedentary living, dehydration, etc.), increase the tendency of blood to clot—the process that leads to heart attack and stroke. WGA is often called a *mitogen* because it activates cell division, or *mitosis* (a concept familiar to anyone who studies cancer, a disease characterized by unrestrained mitosis). WGA has indeed been demonstrated to cause mitosis in lymphocytes (immune system cells) and cells lining the intestine.[4] We know that such phenomena underlie cancer, such as the intestinal lymphoma that afflicts people with celiac disease.[5] WGA also mimics the effects of insulin on fat cells. When WGA encounters a fat cell, it acts just as if it were insulin, inhibiting activation of fat release and blocking weight loss while making the body more reliant on sugar sources for energy.[6] WGA also blocks the hormone leptin, which is meant to shut off appetite when the physical need to eat has been satisfied. In the presence of WGA, appetite is not suppressed, even when you're full.[7]

All in all, grain lectins are part of a potent collection of inflammatory factors. Indigestible or only partially digestible, they fool receptors and thwart hormonal signals after gaining entry to our bodies through the seeds of grasses.

VIP: Very Important Peptide

The lectin found in wheat, rye, barley, and rice (WGA) also blocks the action of another very important hormone called *vasoactive intestinal peptide*, or VIP.[8] While studies have been confined mostly to experimental models, not humans, the blocking of VIP has the potential to explain many of the peculiar phenomena that develop in people who consume grains but do not have celiac disease or gluten sensitivity.

VIP plays a role in dozens of processes. It is partly responsible for:

- Activating the release of cortisol from the adrenal glands[9]

- Modulating immune defenses against bacteria and parasites in the intestine[10]

- Protecting against the immune destruction of multiple sclerosis[11]

- Reducing phenomena that can lead to asthma and pulmonary hypertension (increased pressure in the lungs)[12]

- Maintaining healthy balance of the immune system that prevents inflammatory bowel diseases, Crohn's disease, and ulcerative colitis[13]

- Promoting sleep and maintaining circadian rhythms (day-night cycles)[14]

- Participating in determining taste in the tongue[15]

- Modulating the immune and inflammatory response in skin that protects us from psoriasis[16]

In other words, the diseases that are at least partially explained by blocking VIP sure look and sound like the collection of conditions that we witness, day in, day out, in wheat-consuming people: low cortisol levels responsible for low energy, worsening of asthma and pulmonary hypertension, worsening of Crohn's disease and ulcerative colitis, disruption of sleep, distortions of taste such as the reduced sensitivity to sweetness (meaning you need more sugar for sweetness), and psoriasis. The VIP pathway may prove to be one of the important means by which grains disrupt numerous aspects of health.

GRAINS AND A MOUTHFUL OF BACTERIA

Grains affect the microorganisms that inhabit our bodies. These *microbiota* live on your skin and in your mouth, vagina, and gastrointestinal tract.

Over the last few years, there has been a new scientific appreciation for the composition of human microbiota. We know, for instance, that experimental animals raised in an artificial sterile environment and thereby raised with a gastrointestinal tract that contains no microorganisms have impaired immunity, are prone to infections, are less efficient at digestion, and even develop structural changes of the gastrointestinal tract that differ from creatures that harbor plentiful microorganisms. The microorganisms that inhabit our bodies are not only helpful; they are *essential* for health.

The bacteria that share in this symbiotic relationship with our bodies today are not the same as those carried by our ancestors. Human microorganisms underwent a shift 10,000 years ago when we began to consume the seeds of grasses. DNA analyses of dental plaque from ancient human teeth demonstrate that oral flora of primitive non-grain-consuming humans was different from that of later grain-consuming humans. Alan Cooper, PhD, of Australia's University of Adelaide Centre for Ancient DNA, and Keith Dobney, PhD, of the United Kingdom's University of Aberdeen, analyzed bacterial DNA from teeth of hunter-gatherers before grains. They then compared it to early grain-adopting humans and later Neolithic, Bronze Age, and medieval populations—periods when agriculture flourished. Pregrain hunter-gatherers demonstrated wide diversity of oral bacterial species, predominant in species unassociated with dental decay. Grain-consuming humans, in contrast, demonstrated reduced diversity, with what the researchers called a "more disease causing configuration," a pattern that worsened the longer humans consumed grains.[17] Mouth bacteria underwent another substantial shift 150 years ago during the Industrial Revolution, with the proliferation of even greater disease-causing species, such as *Streptococcus mutans*, coinciding perfectly with the mechanical milling of flours. Disease-causing species of oral flora are now ubiquitous and dominate the mouths of modern humans, sustained by modern consumption of grains and sugars.[18] Dr. Dobney comments: "Over the past few hundred years, our mouths have clearly become a substantially less diverse ecosystem, reducing our resilience to invasions by disease-causing bacteria."[19]

This study rounds out what anthropologists have been telling us for years: When humans first incorporated grains into our diets, we experienced an explosion of tooth decay, tooth loss, and tooth abscesses.[20] We now know that grains, from einkorn and barley to maize and millet, were responsible for this marked shift in dental health, because they caused disturbances in oral microorganisms.

Insights into oral flora do not necessarily tell us what happened to bowel flora, though there is some overlap. Even though we all begin our lives with sterile gastrointestinal tracts ripe to be populated with organisms provided at birth from the vaginal canals of our mothers, many events occur during our development that lead to divergences between the organisms in our mouths and those in our bowels—such as the appearance of teeth, stomach acidification, the hormonal surge of puberty, and antibiotics. Nonetheless, we can still take some lessons about human diet and bowel flora by studying . . .

THE SCIENCE OF SCATOLOGY

In addition to knowing that the oral flora of humans changed once we chose to consume grains, we also know that primitive humans had different bowel flora than modern humans. The ancient remains of human feces, or *coprolites*, have been recovered from caves and other locations where humans congregated, ate, slept, died, and, of course, moved their bowels.

Though we have to make allowances for the inevitable degeneration of fecal material over time, we can make observations on the varieties of bacterial species present in coprolites and thereby primitive human intestinal tracts. We know, for instance, that some *Treponema*, a species of bacteria important for digestion of fibrous foods and anti-inflammatory effects, are widely present in coprolites of pregrain cultures but are nearly absent from modern humans.[21]

These observations are important because we know that abnormal conditions of the gastrointestinal tract, such as irritable bowel syndrome, peptic ulcers, and ulcerative colitis, are associated with changes in bowel flora composition.[22] We may uncover a connection between these changes in flora and autoimmune diseases, weight control, cancer, and other conditions.

We don't know how many of these changes are due to diet and how many are due to the diseases themselves, but we do know with certainty that the composition of human oral and bowel flora underwent changes over time. And the facts are clear: When humans began to consume the seeds of grasses, the microorganisms cohabiting our bodies changed, and they changed in ways that affect our health.

Let's now discuss each nonwheat grain individually and explain why, like wheat, they do your health no favors.

Maybe We'll Chew a Cud: Adaptations to Consuming the Seeds of Grasses

It would be wrong to argue that *no* human adaptations have evolved over the several thousand years we've consumed the seeds of grasses. There have indeed been several changes in the human genetic code that have developed in grain-consuming societies and that are thereby notably *absent* in nonagricultural native North and South American, South Pacific, and Australian populations.

- Genes for increased expression of the salivary enzyme amylase, determined by the AMY1 gene, allow increased digestion of the amylopectin starches of grains.[23]

- The gene for hemochromatosis, a condition of excessive iron storage that increases the number of red blood cells in the bloodstream, is believed to be an adaptation to iron deficiency that developed in grain-consuming humans. Because it is a relatively recent mutation, genes for enhanced iron absorption are carried by less than 10 percent of people of northern European descent.

- Variations in genes that determine diabetes susceptibility are believed to have evolved with the consumption of the seeds of grasses, with recent variants providing partial protection from the disease.[24] Judging by the worldwide explosion of diabetes, though, these attempts at genetic adaptation are inadequate.

Yes, as a species, we are *trying* to adapt to a diet dominated by the seeds of grasses and their adverse health effects, but such adaptations are not enough. We haven't had sufficient time to adapt to the many effects of prolamin proteins, lectins, and changes in oral and bowel flora, or the mental, emotional, or autoimmune effects of grain consumption (all of which I discuss in later chapters). These continue at a high level across all populations that enthusiastically consume the seeds of grasses. Perhaps, in another few hundred thousand years, we will fully adapt and thrive without disease while consuming the seeds of grasses. The *Homo sapiens* of a grain-dominated future may chew a cud, grow some extra stomach compartments, and add "moo" to the dictionary.

50 SHADES OF GRAIN

This man, whom I once thought of as a romantic hero, a brave shining white knight—or the dark knight, as he said. He's not a hero; he's a man with serious, deep emotional flaws, and he's dragging me into the dark.

—E. L. James, *Fifty Shades of Grey*

All of the grains that fill the modern diet to bursting are grasses. Ground, baked, roasted, toasted, and popped, they come in an astounding variety of forms, colors, and flavors, as they are among the most popular ingredients in modern processed food. Who would have guessed that popcorn and pretzels are closely related, or that tortillas and Cinnabon are kissing cousins? Beneath those comforting smells and flavors, however, are buried dark secrets, undisclosed confidences, and demons ready to engulf you in their embrace, enfolding your mind and body in their effects. As wheat is a grass, its bewitching effects are shared to various degrees by the seeds of other grasses.

The problems posed by the tortured relationship between wheat and humans are largely shared by other wheat-derived grains, including triticale (a cross between wheat and rye), bulgur, and traditional strains of wheat such as spelt and kamut. When discussing "wheat," I therefore am referring to all the closely related grains in the wheat family. Let's consider several of the most popular nonwheat grains in all their lurid glory.

Rye

The history of rye consumption dates back to the early days of wheat consumption, when humans first experimented with consuming einkorn. Rye, another grass, grew as a weed in fields of wheat, an example of *Vavilovian mimicry,* or the ability of a weed to mimic a cultivated plant. This weed came to be recognized by humans as yet another seed of a grass that could be consumed, and farmers often harvested both wheat and rye with the same sickle or thresher without bothering to separate them.

Rye has gained some blessings in nutritional circles because compared to wheat, it has less potential to trigger insulin, despite identical potential for raising blood sugar.[25] (To be fair, just about *anything* compared to *Triticum aestivum*, our favorite grain to bash, comes up smelling like roses.)

Rye and wheat share a high content of gliadin protein, with all its potentially toxic effects. (Rye gliadin is called *secalin*, although the structures are nearly identical.) The secalin protein has similar potential to do bad things as its gliadin counterpart.[26] Likewise, the lectin of rye is nearly identical to wheat's destructive lectin, wheat germ agglutinin, and therefore shares its potential for causing intestinal toxicity, clumping red blood cells, provoking abnormal growth of immune system lymphocytes, and mimicking insulin.[27] Rye shares with wheat a peculiar and only recently recognized phenomenon: the formation of acrylamide, a compound believed to be a carcinogen and neurotoxin.[28] Rye and wheat contain a high content of the amino acid asparagine, which, when heated at high temperatures during baking or deep-frying, reacts with the plentiful carbohydrates present to form acrylamide. (It also forms in French fries.) Modern reliance on nitrogen-rich synthetic fertilizers also boosts the asparagine content of rye and wheat, increasing acrylamide formation further.

For all practical purposes, given the crossbreeding that has occurred via natural Vavilovian means as well as the breeding efforts of humans, the differences are minor, meaning that they are virtually one and the same. Being wheat-free should also mean being rye-free.

Rye and the Work of the Devil

Rye has the unique potential to be infected with a parasitic fungus, *Claviceps purpurea,* that produces a human toxin called ergotamine. When ingested in, say, a loaf of rye bread, it exerts a range of hallucinogenic effects on humans, partly because it is converted to lysergic acid diethylamide, commonly known as LSD.

History is filled with fascinating and terrifying stories of humans exposed to rye and ergotamine. Because some victims afflicted with contaminated rye experienced an intense dermatitis (skin inflammation), the condition became known as St. Anthony's Fire, named after the early 11th-century sanctuary operated by monks to treat victims of ergot poisoning. During the Middle Ages, writers described hysterical outbursts afflicting previously normal people, including thrashing and writhing while shouting, "I'm burning!" The afflicted would eventually collapse, after which their bodies would blacken. And at least one observer has ascribed the madness of the Salem witch trials to ergotamine poisoning after determining that many of the 19 young women accused of being witches lived near a rye field. A "witch cake" made of rye flour was fed to a dog to confirm a "bewitching" effect.[29]

The rye itself was, of course, entirely innocent, since it was the common parasitic infestation of the grass that was to blame. But, as with so many other matters surrounding the relationship between the seeds of grasses and the hapless humans who try to consume them, it should come as no surprise that it is a relationship fraught with danger.

Barley

The origins of barley consumption parallel that of einkorn and emmer wheat in the Fertile Crescent, which is now Iraq, Iran, and Turkey. For many years, barley was the preferred grain among ancient people of Greece and Egypt, spreading to Europe 7,000 years ago. Barley has largely been demoted to animal fodder, with most human exposure nowadays coming in the form of the barley malt used to make beer. As with rye, barley also shares many characteristics with its close grass relative, wheat. People with celiac disease, for instance, who avoid wheat because it's a source of gluten (and thereby gliadin), must also avoid barley due to gliadin's similarities with barley's equivalent protein, hordein. Gliadin and hordein overlap extensively, suggesting that the peculiar human effects of wheat are shared by barley.[30] The lectin of barley is also virtually identical to wheat germ agglutinin, thereby sharing its potential for gastrointestinal toxicity. Barley's allergic effects also overlap with those of wheat, meaning that the same asthma, sinus drainage and congestion, skin rashes, and gastrointestinal distress provoked by a wheat allergy can also be provoked by barley.[31]

Corn

After modern wheat and its problematic closest brethren, rye, barley, bulgur, and triticale, corn is the next problem grass. (For the sake of clarity, I will call maize by its North American colloquial name, "corn." While corn outside the United States and Canada can mean wheat or be a nonspecific term for any grain, here it will be used to refer to maize.)

Like einkorn wheat, corn is among the oldest of cultivated grains, dating back 10,000 years to pre-Mayan times in South America, but corn didn't make it onto European menus until 1493, when Christopher Columbus brought seeds to Spain. Corn was rapidly embraced, largely replacing barley and millet due to its spectacular yield per acre. Widespread, habitual consumption of cornbread and polenta resulted in deficiencies of niacin (vitamin B_3) and the amino acids lysine and tryptophan, causing widespread epidemics of pellagra, evidenced as what physicians of the age called "The Four Ds": dermatitis, diarrhea, dementia, and death. Even today, pellagra is a significant public health issue in rural South America, Africa, and China. Meanwhile, in coastal Peru, Ecuador, Mexico, and the Andes mountain highlands, increased corn consumption led to increased tooth decay, tooth loss, anemia, and iron deficiency, as well as loss of height in children and adults.[32]

Today, farmers fatten livestock by feeding them intact corn kernels. But much of the corn consumed by humans is in the form of cornmeal or cornstarch, or derivatives of corn such as high-fructose corn syrup. This concentrated source of fructose is a form of sugar that fails to signal satiety—you don't know when to stop. Corn and wheat jockey for inclusion in just about every processed food, many of which contain both. Corn in some form is therefore found in obvious sources, such as corn chips, cornbread, breakfast cereals, soft drinks with high-fructose corn syrup, tacos, tortillas, and corn dogs, but also in some not-so-obvious foods, including hamburger meat, ketchup, salad dressings, yogurt, soup mixes, candy, seasoning mixes, mayonnaise, marinara sauce, fruit drinks, and peanut butter.

Corn strains with the highest proportion of rapidly digested amylopectin, rather than the less efficiently digested amylose, are chosen to grind into cornstarch. Given the exponential increase in surface area that results when corn is reduced to granules or powder, these products are responsible for extravagant rises in blood sugar. With a glycemic index of 90 to 100, the highest of any food, they are perfectly crafted to contribute to diabetes.[33]

Corn allergies are on the rise, likely due to changes in alpha-amylase inhibitor proteins, lipid transfer proteins, and others. Because the various grasses that we call "grains" are genetically related, there can be *overlapping* grain allergies in humans exposed to them.[34] Repeated and prolonged exposure to corn proteins, as in people who work in agriculture, food production, or the pharmaceutical industry (cornstarch is found in pills and capsules), can lead to as many as 90 percent of workers developing a corn allergy.[35] Such extravagant levels of allergy development do not occur in people working with apples, beef, kale, or olives—only grains.

The *zein* protein of corn triggers antibodies reactive to wheat gliadin, which can lead to gastrointestinal distress, diarrhea, bloating, bowel urgency, and acid reflux after corn consumption.[36] The immune response responsible for the destruction of the small intestine that occurs in people with celiac disease can also be triggered, though less severely, by the zein protein of corn. Nevertheless, cornstarch is—wrongly—used in gluten-free foods.[37]

Though they look quite different and the modern processed products that emerge from them look, smell, and taste quite different, wheat and corn are too closely related for comfort. Minimal to no exposure is the desired strategy for nonruminant *Homo sapiens*.

Genetic Modification: Don't Look, Don't Tell

Since gene-splicing technology made it possible to insert or remove specific genes in plants and animals, we have been reassured repeatedly by the FDA, the USDA, and by agribusiness that the products of this technology are safe for the environment and for human consumption. And they have 90-day animal testing data to prove it.

While wheat was manipulated with methods that predate genetic modification and therefore didn't raise many eyebrows, other genetically modified (GM) grains, especially corn and rice, have somehow escaped public scrutiny, and strains have made it onto supermarket shelves in North America and other parts of the world. Recent studies have raised questions about the safety of GM crops, as well as the herbicides and pesticides that go with them. One French research group, for instance, obtained internal proprietary research data from Monsanto that were used to justify claims of safety for both glyphosate-resistant corn and Bt toxin corn, the two most prevalent GM crops. (This information was not relinquished voluntarily, but rather was obtained by a court order.) When they tried to reproduce the Monsanto data but applied more detailed tissue analyses, they failed to reproduce the same benign findings, instead observing evidence for kidney, liver, heart, spleen, and adrenal toxicity with both forms of GM corn.[38] The first effort to extend the period of observation beyond 90 days raised more disturbing questions. Over 2 years of observation, increased mortality, breast tumors, liver damage, and pituitary disruption from both glyphosate-resistant corn and glyphosate itself were reported, in contrast to Monsanto's benign 90-day findings.[39]

Further questions have been raised regarding the safety of Bt toxin corn. This strain of corn has a gene for a protein that's toxic to insects inserted right into it, so it kills pests who try to eat the plant. While Bt toxin–expressing bacteria have been sprayed on crops by organic farmers for 40 years with apparent safety, critics have pointed out that GM corn now expresses Bt toxin within the seed (the corn kernels) directly ingested by consumers. One study in mice demonstrated toxic effects on blood cell formation,[40] while another observed prediabetic patterns.[41] Genetically modified rice has also been demonstrated to change the composition of bowel flora in mice, with decreased healthy *Lactobacillus* and increased unhealthy *Escherichia coli* species.[42]

Glyphosate itself, the world's most widely used herbicide, is applied to glyphosate-resistant corn. It has estrogenic activity, promoting the growth of breast cancer cells; disrupts male fertility; and disrupts endocrine function in a number of other ways.[43] There is also the issue of the environmental impact of glyphosate on wildlife, including aquatic bacteria and amphibians, such as frogs, which experience toxic effects.[44]

Interestingly, one strain of rice—Golden Rice, which has been genetically modified to express beta-carotene to alleviate the vitamin A deficiency that plagues rice-consuming societies—has been at the forefront of the biotechnology effort to paint genetic modification as something beautiful to behold and safe for consumption. Agribusiness giant Syngenta has been promoting Golden Rice as an example of what the science of genetic modification can accomplish, despite the vigorous opposition of many farmers who wish to avoid using GM grains. Critics have also accused its promoters of trying to capitalize on a common nutrient deficiency by a more profitable route than, say, just having vitamin A–deficient populations eat an occasional sweet potato, which would match or exceed the benefits provided by Golden Rice. (But you can't trademark a regular, nutritious sweet potato.)

Much of the science purporting to explore the safety of GM crops reads more like marketing than science, with researchers gushing about the safety and nutrition of the crop, herbicide, or pesticide in question, rather than impartially reporting the science. This brings us to the fundamental problem when deep-pocketed influences such as agribusiness or the pharmaceutical industry are involved: How much can we believe when much of the positive "science" is generated by those who stand to benefit from it?

Rice

Despite sharing a genetic heritage with other grasses, rice is among the more benign of grains, though it's far from harmless. Viewed from the perspective of the ancient human experience that reveals the destructive health effects of other grasses, ancient rice is the only grain that was *not* associated with effects such as increased tooth decay, facial malformations, and iron deficiency.[45] The less-harmful nature of rice can be partly explained by the very low content (less than 1 percent) of prolamin proteins in rice.[46]

The history of rice as yet another seed of grasses consumed by humans dates back 8,000 years to the foothills of the Himalayas, followed by evidence for human cultivation in southern China 4,000 years ago. Rice is the ideal commodity food, as it can be stored for many years without degrading. Health problems from rice, unlike other grains, are less common. Nonetheless, overreliance on rice with the husk removed (i.e., white or polished rice) led to widespread problems with beriberi, a condition that results in partial paralysis and heart failure due to a lack of the B vitamin thiamin—conditions that, I believe you would agree, are beriberi bad. This condition can develop within a few weeks, and it became a problem that plagued Asian sailors and soldiers given rations largely consisting of rice.

As with the seeds of all other grasses, rice shares the potential for excessive glycemic effects. Carbs account for 85 percent of the calories in rice, among the highest of all seeds of grasses. Rice-consuming cultures, for instance, can still experience plenty of diabetes. But the comforting notion that rice is among the most benign of grains is being challenged, as it has been the recipient of extensive genetic modification. This includes efforts to make it glyphosate resistant and able to express the Bt toxin, posing the same safety questions as for glyphosate-resistant and Bt toxin–containing corn.

And there's another issue looming over this particular seed of a grass: Rice is unique among grasses in its natural ability to concentrate inorganic arsenic from soil and water. (We can't blame agribusiness for this effect.) Rice has a high arsenic content, according to reports confirmed by FDA analyses, though the FDA reassures us that no acute toxicity develops from such exposure.[47] Substantial research, however, has associated chronic arsenic exposure with multiple forms of cancer, as well as cardio-vascular and neurological diseases.[48] In Bangladesh, where arsenic exposure is a major public health problem, increasing chronic arsenic exposure, starting at low levels, is associated with premalignant skin lesions, high blood pressure, neurological dysfunction, and increased mortality.[49] This analysis suggests that adverse health effects can manifest with chronic exposure provided by as little as one serving (approximately 1 cup cooked) of rice per day. The FDA had previously established an upper limit for arsenic in apple juice of 10 parts per billion; analyses of rice have found many rice products approaching or exceeding this cutoff.

The data that already exist linking low-level exposure of arsenic-contaminated water with increases in many chronic diseases is, in my mind, all the information we need. Makes you shudder to think about the old Rice Diet. Though at the more benign end of the spectrum as far as seeds of grasses go, enthusiastic consumption of rice in any form (white, brown, or wild) is clearly not a good idea for health. Occasional consumption of small quantities (around ¼ cup) is likely all a healthy human can tolerate before triggering such concerns.

Oats

Oats are relative newcomers to the human dietary grass experience, having been first consumed only about 3,000 years ago. Few cultures embraced this grain, often regarding it as fodder for livestock or the food of barbarians, until the Welsh and Scottish became avid oat consumers.

Yet another close relative of wheat and member of the grass family, its gliadin-like protein, avenin, shares less overlap in its structure than its counterparts in rye and barley do. For this reason, the role of oats in the diet of people with celiac disease has been debated for 50 years. The avenin protein is clearly more benign, though some oat varieties can mimic the immune effects of gliadin.[50] (The notion of "gluten-free oats" is therefore a fiction, as they still have a protein that can overlap in structure and effect.) Oats lack a lectin protein, so they do not contribute to the intestinal damage and inflammation inflicted by wheat germ agglutinin.[51] This focus on the relatively benign nature of oats by comparison to the worst grain of all, though, falsely lulls people into thinking that just because it doesn't have gluten-like properties, it must be good for you. Once again, overly simplistic nutritional thinking can get us into trouble.

There is plenty of talk about oats being "heart healthy" and a rich source of soluble fiber, referring to the beta-glucan in oats that has been shown to reduce total and LDL cholesterol. All of that is true—except for the heart-healthy part. Although the beta-glucan fiber does indeed have some healthy effects on cholesterol values, the plentiful amylopectin starch of oats raises blood sugar to high levels and therefore provokes extravagant glycation—the irreversible process of modifying proteins when blood glucose rises. Oats provide an example of something that contains a mixture of good things and bad. The good effects are transient, such as the beta-glucan allowing healthier bowel movements and lower LDL cholesterol, or the B vitamins providing nutrition. But the bad effects are irreversible, especially those of glycation. Consumption of oats, like rice, is best kept to a minimum.

Sorghum

Sorghum was, until sucrose and high-fructose corn syrup became dominant, a popular source for sugar. Until the early 20th century, sorghum syrup was poured over pancakes and used to make candy. Like all grains, sorghum is largely carbohydrate, with approximately 75 percent of its calories coming from starch, triggering glycation as enthusiastically as the starchy seed of any other grass. It remains popular as fodder for livestock because it's as useful for rapid fattening as wheat and corn are.

Sorghum is an especially interesting grass, as it is toxic, and even fatal, when consumed before it's fully mature; its high cyanide content has been known to decimate herds of livestock, causing death by cardiac arrest. This grass grows wild in much of Africa and is believed to have been first domesticated in the savannahs around 4,000 years ago. While it is a "true grass" from the family Poaceae, sorghum is less closely related to the grasses discussed above. The gliadin protein counterpart in sorghum, kafirin, is only distantly related and therefore does not trigger celiac or other undesirable gliadin responses. Despite the more benign nature of kafirin proteins, sorghum is still the seed of a grass and is therefore largely indigestible. Accordingly, the proteins in sorghum are poorly digested; about half of them pass right through the human gastrointestinal tract undisturbed.[52] This has prompted manipulations to increase digestibility, including mutating the plant's genetics with gamma radiation and chemicals, genetically modifying it by inserting genes for more digestible proteins, and mechanically or enzymatically processing the flour, all to enhance digestibility.

It is not clear what would happen to humans who relied too much on sorghum as a calorie source. But given its problematic indigestible proteins and high starch content, it is worth minimizing exposure, as with rice and oats.

There's a Snake in the Grass

To complete our discussion of the seeds of grasses, I should mention that bulgur is simply a combination of different strains of wheat, though often of the durum variety, such as that used in pasta. But it is still wheat, with virtually all the same problems. Triticale is the result of mating wheat with rye; as you would predict, it also shares all of the same issues due to its parentage.

Millet, teff, and amaranth, all added to our diets over the last few thousand years, are among several other less-common seeds of grasses that humans consume. None cause the range of health difficulties that wheat, rye, barley, corn, bulgur, triticale, or sorghum are responsible for, nor have they been the recipients of enthusiastic genetic modification. However, they're still high in carbohydrates given their amylopectin content. In France, ortolan songbirds made morbidly obese on a diet of millet and oats, then drowned in Armagnac, set on fire, and consumed whole were considered a delicacy that was savored for its rich, dripping fat. (This is now outlawed.) Just like corn and wheat, grains whose only known problem is their amylopectin starch are still quite effective at fattening up pigs, cows, songbirds, and humans.

Some people feel that they can consume a small quantity of these glycemically challenging grains now and then without paying a health price, but bear in mind that each time you consume these starchy seeds you invite greater and greater health compromises, just as you do when you eat a bag of jelly beans.

THE HUMAN DIET: A GRASS-FREE ZONE

You may want your beef to be grass-fed, but *you* shouldn't be that way.

You may have come to recognize that the deeper we dig into this thing called grains or, more properly, the seeds of grasses, the worse it gets. We uncover more and more reasons why nonruminant *Homo sapiens* are just not equipped to handle the components of these plants: lectins in wheat, rye, barley, and rice; the prolamin proteins gliadin, secalin, hordein, zein, and kafirin; acrylamides; cyanide; and arsenic—not to mention that we suffer deficiencies like pellagra and beriberi when we come to overrely on these seeds. Ironically, the world's calories are *most concentrated* in the calories of the *most destructive* grains—wheat and corn—and some serious questions have now been raised about the safety of rice.

Funny how this just doesn't happen with broccoli, celery, walnuts, olives, eggs, or salmon—foods we can consume ad lib and digest easily, without triggering blood sugar, glycation, autoimmunity, dementia, or other disease-related effects. As you might predict from the stories I've related so far, eliminating the seeds of grasses that were not on the instinctive menu for *Homo sapiens* frees us of many of the health conditions that plague modern humans, including rampant tooth decay, hypertension, diabetes, depression, and a wide range of neurological and gastrointestinal disorders—conditions notably absent or rare in humans following traditional diets. So I urge you to release your inner ruminant; recognize grains for the indigestible, often toxic seeds of grasses that they are; and allow your struggling *Homo sapiens* to fully express itself. I predict that you will rediscover health at a level you may not have known was possible.

In the next chapter, we consider just *why*—beyond desperation, beyond convenience, beyond appeal—grains have managed to dominate the human diet over a relatively short period of time. Why have grains gone from an occasional food of hungry, desperate humans, to the dominant food supply for mankind?

CHAPTER 3

THE REIGN OF GRAIN

It takes two people to make a lie work: the person who tells it,
and the one who believes it.
—Jodi Picoult, *Vanishing Acts*

"HEALTHY WHOLE GRAINS."

It's the dietary battle cry of the 21st century, echoed by all official providers of nutritional advice, the dietary community, and a trillion-dollar food industry. It's the guiding principle of academic curricula in nutrition, embraced by makers of processed food who produce, along with sugar, mind-boggling quantities of foods from wheat, corn, and rice. Is it all based on the purported health benefits of grains—or are there other motivations at work?

Remember family farms, those places idealized or satirized by TV shows such as *The Big Valley*, *The Waltons*, and *Green Acres*? It was only 60 years ago that, in the United States, we had more than 6 million of them, mostly near small towns like Walton's Mountain or Hooterville. These were places where a family typically owned a few dozen acres to grow tomatoes, cucumbers, and lettuce, along with some chickens, pigs, and a cow or two. They grew food for themselves and sold the surplus. Today, small family farms, along with John-Boy and Arnold Ziffel, are largely relics of the past, with the few that remain run by aging part-time farmers whose primary jobs are off the farm. The food on your table is much more likely to come from a large operation of thousands of acres growing huge tracts of single crops (a farming method called *monoculture*) like wheat and corn. Parallel transformations from small farm to big business have occurred in the dairy and meat industries.

Farmers, family and otherwise, are stepping up to meet the demands of a worldwide public that has made grains 50 percent of their calories.

That's direct human consumption of grains. Grains, now favored in place of forage and grass, are also the preferred feed for livestock. This trend began in the 1960s, and livestock now consumes the bulk of the grain produced in the world, outstripping human consumption sevenfold. And we haven't even discussed how much corn is cultivated for ethanol.[1] Grains are, by anyone's definition, big business.

Whenever there's a peculiar situation, we have to ask: Who benefits? Is agribusiness simply responding to consumer demand by providing, for instance, $300 billion in snacks worldwide? Or are there forces at work that quietly cultivate this situation for other reasons? Answering these questions takes us a bit off course from the discussion of why and how forgoing grains gets you closer to total health. But I'm going to ask you to indulge this digression, as understanding this irksome situation will arm you better in the fight against reliance on the seeds of grasses for nutrition.

So let us digress.

THE ART OF THE COMMODITY

Pretend you are a businessman with ambitions to create a system that will generate millions, or perhaps billions, of dollars. And say you'd like to accomplish it through the world of food, rather than crude oil, iron ore, or gold. You're not all that concerned with environmental issues, long-term sustainability, or the health of the consuming public. Your goals are elegantly simple: You'd like to conduct your venture on a worldwide scale for maximum profit.

You certainly cannot achieve such ambitious goals by doing something as pedestrian as growing kale or cultivating an organic farm. You can't do it by selling fresh foods to a local market: too small, too little room for growth, too much darned hard work. Conquering the world shouldn't be so hard! Throw me a frickin' bone here, people. How about manufacturing processed foods on a large scale using low-cost inputs, such as high-fructose corn syrup, cornstarch, wheat flour, sucrose, and the odd food coloring or two, and then creating the illusion of value-added convenience, health, weight management, and sexiness? Well now we're talking, Mr. Bigglesworth!

But food can be hard work and dirty business. Moreover, most foods, such as eggs, pork, and produce, have finite shelf lives measured in just days—a shipping delay of just a few days could mean that your entire inventory becomes a worthless pile of rot. Lots of foods require refrigeration, adding another layer of cost and risk. Then you have to meet all sorts of regulatory requirements issued by agencies such as the FDA, USDA, and federal, state, county, and local health departments. What if you are the sort of businessman who doesn't care to get his hands dirty? You don't want to actually *handle* the food; you just want to make large transactions on paper or electronically. Buy low, sell high, bank your profit. No dirty hands, no messy, rotten food.

You therefore want to transact millions or billions of dollars worth of food, but you don't want to touch the stuff, deal with logistics, worry about risks, or contend with endless regulatory hassles. In other words, you want to *arbitrage* your way to profits, i.e., take advantage of the different prices paid for a product in wide demand from every level of society and that sells as easily in Spokane as it does in London or Brisbane. And you want to do it with something that passes for food and enjoys extended, perhaps limitless, shelf life and can be transported over long distances to take maximum advantage of worldwide price differentials.

What we're talking about buying and selling is called a *commodity*. This is a good or collection of goods—whether iron ore, crude oil, gold, tin, or aluminum—that is relatively indistinguishable from source to source and by different consumers. Commodities leave little or no room for variety, for boutique versions, for uniqueness. It's all the same everywhere, for everyone.

Grains are on the short list of foods consumed by humans that conform perfectly to a commodity market. (Coffee beans, tea, sugar, and soybeans are among the handful of others.) You won't find heirloom tomatoes, radishes, garlic, or grass-fed beef on any commodity exchange. Karl Marx observed that "From the taste of wheat it is not possible to tell who produced it: a Russian serf, a French peasant, or an English capitalist." When a loaf of multigrain bread is purchased, how many people are concerned with whether the wheat flour, oats, millet, or rye came from Iowa, Saskatchewan, or the Ukraine? There is little difference between corn from Brazil and corn from Kansas, and the consumer can't tell the difference.

Of course, you can pretend that there is some enticing appeal to your San Francisco sourdough bread or "authentic" Mexican tortillas. But it's all created from the same commodity grains.

FOOD: THE ULTIMATE COMMODITY EXCHANGE

Beginning in the late 19th century and for many years afterward, high-volume grains—wheat, corn, and rice—were handled as commodities, all under the control of relatively few individuals and private companies. The Kansas City Board of Trade and the Chicago Board of Trade were founded to facilitate the trading of futures contracts for wheat, corn, and oats in the 1870s. These were the very first products to trade on a commodities market, preceding even crude oil and iron ore.

This was not about grain farmers laboring to grow their crops, then carting them to the mill and hoping to sell for a favorable price. This was about a financial system with rules written by a select few who were intent on trading and profiting from large transactions that are only possible with foods that can be traded as commodities on a worldwide scale. More recently, large companies that trade in grain contracts have found it even more profitable to extend their businesses outside of just paper transactions and have worked toward vertical integration, getting their hands dirty in the messy business of the grains themselves. Today, companies that trade grains are also likely to own grain storage facilities, milling operations, trucking and railroad companies, and myriad other operations involved in the production, distribution, shipping, milling, and sale of grains.

Large-scale demand, long shelf life, long-distance transportability, and worldwide price differences: These are the criteria that must be met to allow a grain trader to purchase a million tons of hard winter wheat from a grain cooperative in Kansas and ship it by train, and then ocean tanker, to a port in Vladivostok. That wheat will serve a population that desires the product due to a poorer-than-usual yield—a situation that increased the price per bushel to a level the trader finds desirable. That single transaction can net many millions of dollars.

Commodity traders also prefer to deal in markets that are growing, not stagnant or shrinking. Although people enlightened by books like

Wheat Belly, as well as those who are jumping on the gluten-free band-wagon, have caused a drop in grain sales for food production, the net effect will likely be *increased* grain sales, since grains are also used to feed the livestock that will provide calories increasingly obtained from beef, pork, poultry, eggs, and farmed seafood. For every ton of grain consumed by humans in the United States, 7 tons are consumed by livestock.[2] From the perspective of the grain trade, this is called a win-win situation.

Welcome to the world of Cargill, Archer Daniels Midland Company (ADM), Louis Dreyfus, Bunge, and Continental Grain Company: multi-billion-dollar companies that make the grain world go round, trading, arbitraging, and cashing in on the millions of tons of grains the world's consumers now demand. In the world of large grain trades, not a lot has changed in the 35 years since journalist Dan Morgan, a 30-year veteran of the *Washington Post*, wrote his detailed exposé of the grain-trading indus-try, *Merchants of Grain*: "[T]here they are, in the late 1970s, one of the most remarkable phenomenons in the whole business world: the Hirsches, Borns, Louis-Dreyfuses, Andrés, Fribourgs, Cargills, and MacMillans, all survivors and all still in control . . . [I]n no other major industry in the world are *all* the leading companies private, family-owned, family-operated concerns right down to the last few issues of voting stock."[3]

Despite the enormity of their economic sway over world markets, most of these companies were, until recently, private corporations that did not have an obligation to publicly disclose their financial dealings to the US Securities and Exchange Commission. (ADM is an exception, having been publicly traded since the mid-20th century; Bunge became a publicly traded company as recently as 2001, after 183 years of operating privately.) As a result, the billions of dollars of grain trading that occurred during much of the 20th century operated largely in the shadows of business—elusive, mysterious, and often represented by large paper trades made before any actual grain was shipped or changed hands.

Although the dealings of these companies are generally outside the radar of public scrutiny, federal agencies are indeed aware. In the United States, the federal government relied on the Central Intelligence Agency (CIA) to track the dealings of grain traders, as well as grain production and agricultural policy in places such as the former Soviet Union—issues they viewed as important to the health of US agribusiness and food security.

(Due to the recent push for transparency from the federal government in the United States, such redacted reports are available for anyone to read online from the CIA's files at http://www.foia.cia.gov/collection/princeton-collection.)

While this near monopoly on food commodities prevailed throughout the 20th century, it continues to a substantial degree in our era. The worldwide grain market is still dominated by a handful of commodity traders, all intent on gaining a larger and larger stake in the diet of the world, human or otherwise. Of course, their intent is not to cultivate locally grown vegetables or humanely raised, pasture-fed beef grazing on clover and grass, nor is it to follow sustainable practices that generate the smallest carbon footprint while making their fortunes. It is, as much as possible, to convert the diets of humans and livestock into a commodity-dominated process, with maximum reliance on products with a long shelf-life that are open to price variation worldwide. This creates the perfect situation for profiting from the inequities of an expanding marketplace. Yes: Expanding profits on a massive scale underlie much of the push for increased human consumption of grains.

Over the last nearly 20 years, we've also witnessed the increasing push toward genetically modified grains, which now provide the added financial advantage of patent protection: Seeds must be purchased from the patent holder (Monsanto, Dow AgroSciences, or Syngenta) every year, since farmers are prohibited from saving seed, as they have done every year since the dawn of agriculture 10,000 years ago. While wheat has not yet been converted to genetically modified strains, corn, rice, and other crops have. But GM wheat is surely coming, public outcry be damned. The seed market now stands at around $22 billion worldwide. Agribusiness sees this as a great opportunity to cash in on the world's diet by selling GM seed and then strictly and aggressively enforcing patents. We've already seen this in Monsanto's courtroom tactics in prosecuting the "unauthorized" use of GM seed that inadvertently gets mixed into a field of non-GM crops.[4]

The enemy of large-scale, commoditized grains-as-food is small-scale, locally produced food, since such relatively tiny and disparate operations cannot be controlled by one centralized corporate entity and are beyond the financial reach of the big players. If domination of the world market for food is your goal, then the seeds of grasses are your game.

THE BLURRED LINE BETWEEN
GOVERNMENT AND AGRIBUSINESS

The agribusiness multinationals of our time that control the flow of commodity crops around the world wield an astonishing amount of clout in government circles. Staggering sums are spent, year in and year out, by agribusiness companies to influence public policy in their favor. Recent efforts to oppose labeling of GM foods show us just how badly these companies want to keep the public in the dark about which foods contain GM ingredients. Opposition to Proposition 37 in California, which would have required labels on products containing GM foods, drew $45 million in financial support from Monsanto, Syngenta, Coca-Cola, PepsiCo, General Mills, Kraft, Nestle, the Corn Refiners Association, and the American Bakers Association—a virtual Who's Who in agribusiness and food processing. Those who opposed the bill outspent proponents (mostly supporters of organic farming) five to one, resulting in defeat of the legislation in 2012.

One typical tactic of agribusiness over the past century has been to employ players who know how to play both sides of the game, as regulators and as the regulated. Consequently, high-level executives and attorneys have seamlessly bounced between, for instance, a post at the USDA, an executive position at Cargill, and another post at the USDA. To a surprising degree, the rosters of key personnel in government regulatory agencies and those of key personnel in agribusiness overlap over time. I believe there is a saying about foxes and henhouses that applies to this sort of situation.

There is some logical justification for such "golden revolving doors," as they are known, between government and industry. After all, these are experts in specific fields that often require deep knowledge that's held by relatively few people. But with virtually no checks and balances over the process, it also means that such appointments can potentially be used to manipulate policy.

The list of questionable appointments is too long to recount in full, but among the many agribusiness executives who've held high-level positions in government was Charles Conner, appointed by President George W. Bush. Conner, former head of the Corn Refiners Association, was appointed Special Assistant to the President for Agriculture, Trade, and Food Assistance and then, in 2005, became Deputy Secretary of Agriculture. In an especially notorious instance of these "henhouse" appointments, Michael R. Taylor, an attorney for agribusiness giant Monsanto and the firm's vice president for public policy, became the FDA's Deputy Commissioner for Policy and helped draft the FDA's policy for bovine growth hormone, the Monsanto product given to cows to stimulate milk production. This policy not only paved the way for unrestricted use of the drug, but also prohibited any producer from labeling dairy products as *not* containing bovine growth hormone. And in one of the most recent golden revolving door exchanges, Carol Browner, who led the EPA under President Bill Clinton and then served as director of the White House Office of Energy and Climate Change Policy under President Barack Obama, left her post for a high-level position at Bunge, a company whose history has been marred over the years by a number of convictions over environmental crimes.

Lobbyists on the agribusiness payroll working at the federal and state government levels supplement the golden revolving door of agribusiness-friendly key executives. The agribusiness lobby is among the most powerful and well-funded of all lobbying groups, making the automotive and education industries look like mom-and-pop businesses. Agribusiness rivals the spending of lobbying giants that include oil, gas, defense, and communications. The Center for Responsive Politics reports that in 2012, agribusiness spent $139,726,313 on its lobbying efforts—nearly double the amount spent a decade earlier. Similar sums are spent year in, year out, to wine, dine, and curry favor with politicians and policymakers to make sure that government policy remains friendly to agribusiness. One hundred million dollars can buy an awful lot of favorable treatment. Similar vigorous lobbying efforts are focused on the USDA, which is among the most lobbied of government agencies. The USDA receives more than three times the lobbying aimed at the US Securities and Exchange Commission and more than 20 times that aimed at the Social Security Administration.

Political contributions are another way agribusiness influences policy, donating millions of dollars every year to congressmen, senators, and other elected politicians friendly to the agribusiness agenda. In 2011, agribusiness contributed nearly $92 million.[5] In 2012, more than $60 million was donated to the 435 members of Congress alone. Perhaps all of this should come as no surprise, given the impressive size of these companies: Syngenta's 2012 revenue was $14.2 billion, Monsanto's was $13.5 billion, and General Mills's was $17.8 billion. Other operations of similar magnitude populate the agribusiness and processed food landscape, as well, commanding considerable financial power that can be used to muscle public opinion, legislation, and marketing in their favor.

Grains are therefore the darlings of agribusiness, as they are the favorites of government agencies that provide dietary advice, such as the USDA, which emphasizes grains in its MyPlate and (previously) MyPyramid recommendations. "Eat more healthy whole grains" is therefore not just advice purported to increase health, but advice that increases the commoditization of the human diet. Combine this with the growing worldwide appetite for inexpensive meat that is increasingly a grain-derived product, and you understand how the human diet has become a virtual grainfest.

YOUR ASS IS GRASS

When viewed from the perspective of governments and big agribusiness, the current dietary status quo makes perfect sense: This is how to make a lot of money on a gargantuan scale by shifting the worldwide diet toward high-yield, commoditized grain products, while ensuring that the government will offer advice and policies favorable to this system.

So what's wrong with a situation that allows more people to eat, reduces starvation, and happens to allow some enterprising companies to profit, all while allowing congressmen to have an occasional nice dinner or all-expenses-paid weekend in Barbados? Well, what's wrong is that it ruins your health.

Let's shift our discussion toward that line of thinking. In Chapter 4, we'll talk about what happens to humans who have been encouraged to obtain 50 percent or more of their calories from the seeds of grasses.

CHAPTER 4

YOUR BOWELS HAVE BEEN FOULED: INTESTINAL INDIGNITIES FROM GRAINS

There is nothing more frightful than ignorance in action.
—Johann Wolfgang von Goethe

IF YOU'RE LIKE most people, you were persuaded that grains, in all their processed or whole grain glory—flaked, puffed, dried, sugar coated, sprouted, or crisped—were perfect human foods. Like a widget on a factory production line, you and your life have been assembled, stamped, approved, and molded by forces that stand to profit from the commoditization of the human diet.

But you weren't given the whole story. You were told that "healthy whole grains" were the ticket to nutritional heaven, not the most destructive choices on your plate. You weren't informed that this cheap, convenient way of eating was also the most expedient way to feed the world's booming population while profiting those who are properly positioned to benefit. The "healthy whole grains" yarn enjoys the company of other marketing fictions, such as "children in Third World countries will be healthier on soy infant formula than on breast milk" and "e-cigarettes are safer than cigarettes."

It didn't start as deception. It began as an act of desperation, when humans first consumed the seeds of grasses strictly because they needed the calories. But desperation took a detour when taste and the physiology of grain-derived opiates took over, revealing the unexpected appeal of tasty foods crafted from the seeds of grasses. Our acute need caused us to ignore chronic consequences, even while our teeth rotted and fell out. From the 20th century on, though, economic opportunism and dietary misinterpretation have been largely responsible for establishing the current grains-as-food-for-every-meal lifestyle.

But before we get to all the ways you can regain health by removing grains from your diet, let's discuss how to recognize what the destruction of health from grains looks like. This will help you understand what can be blamed on grains and what should not. While we might be able to blame grains, for instance, for a tumultuous marriage plagued by irrational behavior that ends badly, or for years of unexplained diarrhea prompting repeated unnecessary endoscopies and colonoscopies and bewildered, glazed looks from doctors, we should *not* blame grains for the chronic health impact of Lyme disease acquired from a tick bite 12 years ago or the despair caused by chronic lead exposure. Understanding these issues will help you more capably craft a program for health, avoid unrealistic expectations (although expectations should indeed be high), and better recognize related problems when they appear. But I can assure you that there is probably *no* aspect of life, physical or emotional, untouched by your consumption of grains.

In *Wheat Belly*, I was guilty of oversimplification. I knew that just persuading the world that modern wheat was not the dietary angel it was portrayed to be, but rather the most awful Frankengrain, was a huge enough undertaking for one book. For readers of the original *Wheat Belly*, I will cover some familiar ground in this and the next chapter, but I will expand the discussion, relate new lessons, and include the latest science.

When you read what happens to typical grain-consuming people, you can't help but be struck by the realization that we are describing nearly everyone around us. The range of destructive health effects wrought by grain consumption is so far-reaching that, by the end of this chapter, and certainly by the end of this book, you will come to understand that the wide-ranging and myriad chronic health conditions that afflict humans can, to an astounding degree, be blamed on grain consumption. Accordingly, when we remove this collection of things called "healthy whole grains," we regain health in ways that, even today, continue to astound all of us engaged in this adventure.

I'll begin the discussion of the adverse health effects of grains at the first place your body has waged its battle against grains. This is dietary ground zero: your gastrointestinal tract.

Grains wreak an astonishing array of digestive havoc. People struggle for years, dealing with the turmoil of bloating, abdominal pain, and diarrhea, many of them eventually ending up in the emergency room, endoscoped top and bottom, typically with no cause identified, only to be prescribed one of the few catchall drugs: acid-suppressing medication, laxatives, or antibiotics. A particularly common complaint of the grain consumer is disruptive and embarrassing bowel urgency that keeps people from leaving their homes or traveling or that forces them to dash to the bathroom with barely a warning. Some of the worst constipation you could imagine, called *obstipation*, with bowel movements happening as infrequently as every several weeks, is silently endured, as fiber and laxatives are ineffective against it. The range and frequency of bowel disruption by grains is all the more astounding when we hear just how much they are supposed to be good for gastrointestinal health.

Grains are not only *not* good for gastrointestinal health, but they are actually poisonous when consumed chronically. Diarrhea, constipation, obstipation, malabsorption, and inflammatory bowel disease should come as no surprise to those who consume the collection of toxins contained in the seeds of grasses. Let's quickly map out the digestive system to give you a greater appreciation for just how grains upset the entire system and to help you understand why additional efforts are often required to regain health after grains are removed.

IT STARTS WITH A GULP

Digestion is the miraculous process of converting things ingested, animate or inanimate, into the components of your body. The human gastrointestinal tract starts at your lips and teeth, which begin the process of tearing food into fragments. Your tongue and sense of smell serve testing functions, distinguishing the distasteful and foul-smelling (and thereby potentially unsafe) from the tasty (which is our main criterion for determining what should or should not be eaten). Salivary glands provide lubricant and are the first source of digestive enzymes. The oropharynx at the back of your throat divides and protects your respiratory from your digestive system and is lined with lymph tissue to respond to foreign invaders. Then comes your esophagus, the muscular passageway to your stomach. In your stomach, powerful hydrochloric acid degrades food and provides an environment inhospitable to microorganisms. Protein breakdown is initiated by the stomach enzymes pepsin and gastric lipase, followed by a soup of digestive enzymes (including pancreatic lipase, trypsin, chymotrypsin, collagenase, and others) released by your pancreas to further digest proteins, fats, and carbohydrates.

Your liver then joins the process by producing bile, a green-colored liquid synthesized from discarded hemoglobin from aged red blood cells—an example of the incredible efficiency of nature. Bile is stored in your gallbladder, neutralizes the acidity from your stomach acid, and is secreted into your small intestine to further digest fats. Your liver also receives nutrients absorbed via your small intestine, converting them into forms transportable through the bloodstream and usable by various organs. Partially digested food and liquids proceed through your duodenum, then jejunum and ileum, segments of the small intestine responsible for nutrient absorption. Though labeled "small" because of its narrow diameter, your small intestine is the longest part of your gastrointestinal tract, typically measuring 24 feet in length. This adaptation makes us efficient digesters of protein compared to ruminants, who have shorter small intestines.

After passing through your small intestine, food finally gets to your colon, the organ charged with the function of completing unfinished digestion. It does so by housing trillions of microorganisms that digest any remaining polysaccharides, even those indigestible by humans, and absorbing any residual nutrients while also helping maintain hydration by absorbing water from its semi-liquid contents and converting those contents into semisolid form. Lower down, your rectum serves a storage function that allows the elimination of its contents to occur at opportune moments, rather than in the middle of a business meeting or during jumping jacks.

I recount this amazingly elaborate process to highlight just how many steps along the way can be disrupted. In fact, given its complexity, it almost seems a wonder that digestion *ever* occurs smoothly. Safety mechanisms and redundancies built into the system through evolutionary adaptation maximize the likelihood that what you've ingested will be safely converted into the nutrients you require, while the undigested remains will be passed out quietly and without fanfare. The complexity of your digestive system is part of its beauty, but also part of its vulnerability. Disruption of this multistep process can come in many forms, including pinpoint disruption of intestinal permeability by poisons such as cholera toxin, autoimmune attacks against layers of small intestinal tissue characteristic of Crohn's disease, and factors that alter the composition of microorganisms.

GRAINS: A DISEMBOWELING EXPERIENCE

Let's put it all together and describe what happens when us nonruminants choose to eat the seeds of grasses in multigrain bread, cornstarch, puffed rice in a rice cake, or a bowl of oatmeal. It should come as no surprise that disruptions of this otherwise marvelous system develop. We don't fatally succumb to our first or second bite, of course, but over an extended period of time our health declines and we wonder why, though we're eating what we thought were healthy foods in moderation, exercising, and heeding conventional health advice, we end up with disastrous health consequences. These are the gastrointestinal effects of consuming the seeds of grasses.

Acid Reflux and Reflux Esophagitis

Millions of people are plagued by the discomfort of acid reflux and esophageal inflammation and are prescribed acid-suppressing medications such as Prilosec, Prevacid, Pepcid, and Protonix, which they take every day for years. Treatment for acid reflux and reflux esophagitis has proven to be enormously profitable. Annual revenues for these drugs for one company alone, AstraZeneca, exceeded $23 billion in 2011.[1] More than one billion people—one out of every seven people on the planet—have been prescribed these drugs since their appearance on the market 35 years ago.

These drugs are not without health consequences. They have been associated with vitamin B_{12} and magnesium deficiency; impaired calcium absorption, osteoporosis, and increased bone fracture risk; and increased risk of pneumonia.[2] Use of such prescription drugs has been associated with changes in bowel flora resulting in dysbiosis (disrupted bowel flora) and increased potential for intestinal infection with *Clostridium difficile*.[3] The dysbiosis provoked by such drugs is believed to explain the deterioration of multiple sclerosis symptoms that often develops with their use.[4] Because the drugs are often ineffective and result in their own collection of health problems, physicians increasingly advise patients to undergo surgical procedures, such as fundoplication (surgically wrapping the stomach around the esophagus) to avoid using the drugs. But for the majority of people taking these drugs for acid reflux and reflux esophagitis, the real solution is as simple as saying "no" to all grains.

Bowel Urgency and Irritable Bowel Syndrome

I am astounded by the number of people who relate tales of explosive bowel urgency, often with just seconds of warning, that cause their lives to be filled with anxiety during social situations, travel, or a simple trip to the store. While grains are commonly painted as good for bowel health because of the fiber they contain, the other components of grains create feelings of urgency, the symptoms of which are often labeled irritable bowel syndrome (IBS). Gliadin and related prolamins, glutenins, wheat germ agglutinin (WGA), alpha amylase, and trypsin inhibitors are bowel toxins, and bowel urgency is your body's way of telling you that it is trying to get rid of some toxin causing irritation. It is wise to listen to your bowels, and they are saying, "stop the grains."

IBS, particularly if diarrhea is present, is also proving to be more celiac disease–like than previously suspected in that it is associated with increased intestinal permeability and a high likelihood of dysbiosis.[5] IBS and/or "gluten sensitivity" are therefore not as benign as previously advertised, given that increased intestinal permeability has the potential to initiate autoimmune processes, among other issues.

Dysbiosis

Grains and other factors cause changes in bowel flora, allowing unhealthy species of bacteria to proliferate while suppressing or entirely knocking off healthy species, a condition called dysbiosis or small intestinal bacterial overgrowth (SIBO). Abnormal bacteria can also migrate into the upper small intestine and stomach, where they don't belong, rather than being confined to the lowest end of the small intestine and the large intestine. In its most severe form, dysbiosis is experienced as nausea, abdominal distress, diarrhea or constipation (typically diagnosed as irritable bowel syndrome), fatigue and low energy, inflammation of the skin and joints, diffuse muscle pain (often called fibromyalgia), nutrient deficiencies, and autoimmune diseases.

One of the ways grains can trigger dysbiosis involves your gallbladder and pancreas, which are normally part of a wonderfully orchestrated system. When oils or fats are sensed in the duodenum, the hormone cholecystokinin (CCK) is released, stimulating the gallbladder to release bile and the pancreas to release a mix of digestive enzymes, all of which work to digest food. Funny thing, though: CCK receptors in the gallbladder and pancreas are glycoproteins, the kind of protein that WGA loves to bind.[6] This blocks the CCK signal received by the gallbladder to release bile and the pancreas to release digestive enzymes. The result is inefficient, incomplete digestion. Undigested food ferments and decays in the presence of bacteria, effects you experience as bloating, gas, and changes in stool character, including lighter color and floating (due to undigested oils and fats). Over time, dysbiosis sets in, as the rotting food encourages growth of decay-causing bacteria. To top it all off, the failed release of bile by the gallbladder leads to bile stasis, which allows formation of gallstones.

Dysbiosis can also exacerbate existing conditions. Some people, genetically predisposed, develop inflammatory bowel diseases, ulcerative colitis, and Crohn's disease after exposure to the bowel toxins of grains. Should dysbiosis develop, these conditions are made even worse, as sufferers may experience diarrhea, bleeding in the stool, poor nutrient absorption, pain, and a long-term risk for complications, such as colon cancer for those with ulcerative colitis or small intestinal lymphoma and fissures for those with Crohn's disease.

Constipation

A condition as pedestrian as constipation serves to perfectly illustrate many of the ways in which grains mess with normal body functions, as well as just how wrong conventional "solutions" can be. Constipation remedies are like the Keystone Kops of health: They stumble, fumble, and bump into each other, but never quite put out the fire.

Drop a rock from the top of a building and it predictably hits the ground—not sometimes, not half the time, but every time. That's how the bowels are programmed to work, as well: Put food in your mouth, and it should come out the other end, preferably that same day and certainly no later than the following day. People living primitive lives without grains, sugars, and soft drinks enjoy such predictable bowel behavior: Eat some turtle, fish, clams, mushrooms, coconut, or mongongo nuts for breakfast, and out it all comes that afternoon or evening—large, steamy, filled with undigested remains and prolific quantities of bacteria, no straining, laxatives, or stack of magazines required. Live a modern life and have pancakes with maple syrup for breakfast, instead. You'll be lucky to pass that out by tomorrow or the next day. Or perhaps you will be constipated, not passing out your pancakes and syrup for days or passing it incompletely in hard, painful bits and pieces. In constipation's most extreme forms, the remains of pancakes can stay in your colon for weeks. The combined effects of impaired CCK signaling, reduced bile release, insufficient pancreatic enzymes, and changes in bowel flora disrupt the orderly passage of digested foods.

We are given advice to include more fiber, especially insoluble cellulose (wood) fibers from grains, in our diets. We then eat breakfast cereals or other grain-based foods rich in cellulose fibers and, lo and behold, it does work for some, as indigestible cellulose fibers, undigested by our own digestive apparatus as well as undigested by bowel flora, yield bulk that people mistake for a healthy bowel movement. Never mind that all of the other disruptions of digestion, from your mouth on down, are not addressed by loading up your diet with wood fibers. What if sluggish bowel movements prove unresponsive to such fibers? That's when health care comes to the rescue with laxatives in a variety of forms, some irritative (phenolphthalein and senna), some lubricating (dioctyl sodium sulfosuccinate), some osmotic (polyethylene glycol), some no different than spraying you down with a hose (enemas).

The methods of modern health care build on the problem. Perhaps you develop iron deficiency from grain phytates, necessitating prescription iron tablets that cause constipation. You also develop high blood pressure and are prescribed thiazide diuretics and beta-blockers, both of which increase constipation. Autoimmune thyroid disruption that can develop from prolamin proteins of grains also slows bowel function. When joints hurt from grain consumption, nonsteroidal anti-inflammatory agents are taken, resulting in slowed stool passage. If you're emotionally depressed due to grain consumption, antidepressants are prescribed that slow normal bowel reflexes that maintain motility. The constant message is to get more fiber, drink more fluids, take a laxative.

The longer stool-in-progress stays in the lower small intestine and colon, the longer it has to putrefy. Just as food sitting out in the open air rots, so can stool sitting too long in the bacteria-rich environment of the intestinal tract. Slowed passage of putrefied stool has been linked to increased cancer risk, especially of the rectum.[7] Over time, constipation and the straining it causes lead to hemorrhoids; anal fissures; prolapse of the uterus, vagina, and rectum; and even bowel obstruction, a surgical emergency. Once again, the health-care system, with its enthusiasm for procedures, has solutions. As banal, uninspiring, and ordinary as it is, constipation has a world of important lessons to teach us about our relationship with the seeds of grasses. Yes, there is order and justice in the digestive world, but you won't find it in that box of fiber-rich cereal.

Note that I barely mention celiac disease or gluten sensitivity, as most of the gastrointestinal disruptions caused by grains are of neither variety. When those diseases are removed from the discussion, you can appreciate just how much gastrointestinal distress and disruption is due to the various toxic components of grains. You can also appreciate why defenders of grains, such as the Whole Grains Council, try to minimize the problem by arguing that gluten is the only problem component in grains and that gluten is a problem for a relative few. Nope: Grains are simply the innocent seeds of grasses, incompletely digestible just like the rest of grass plants. This indigestibility allows toxins to persist, intact and ready to block, irritate, and inflame the gastrointestinal tract of *Homo sapiens* who never should have eaten the stuff in the first place. This results in insufficient bile and pancreatic enzymes, impaired digestion, gallstones, and dysbiosis, coupled with intestinal inflammation—the human gastrointestinal tract doesn't stand a chance.

The Celiac Concession and the Clash over Gluten Sensitivity

Defenders of grains would have us believe that the only problem with consuming the seeds of grasses is celiac disease, the destruction of the lining of the small intestine that occurs in people with genetic susceptibility from carrying HLA-DQ2 or HLA-DQ8 genes, coupled with positive tests for transglutaminase or endomysial antibodies and an abnormal biopsy of the small intestine. Celiac disease affects around 1 percent of the population and the gliadin, secalin, and hordein proteins of wheat, rye, and barley are issues only for these people, they argue. Just a few years ago, this represented a major concession from the defenders of grains.

More recently, this notion has crumbled like stale bread as consensus has grown for the idea that there is another form of intolerance to these same proteins. Labeled *non-celiac gluten sensitivity* (NCGS), it is believed to cause many of the same symptoms experienced by celiac sufferers. Bloating, diarrhea, abdominal pain, fatigue, and headache are experienced by these people in the absence of the markers for celiac disease, yet they have symptoms reliably triggered by reexposure to grains. Because of differences in how this condition is defined, anywhere from a few percent to 30 percent of the population are estimated to have NCGS.[8] Some celiac disease experts have proposed that irritable bowel syndrome, a condition that affects 25 percent of the population, should be regarded as the *same condition* as NCGS. People with NCGS have a greater likelihood of antibodies to gliadin; 56 percent showed such antibodies in one analysis, suggesting that an autoimmune process is at work.[9] The possibility that NCGS represents reactions to other components of grains, such as WGA or trypsin or amylase inhibitors, has not yet been fully explored. Nonetheless, the expanding world of grain intolerances has kept grain's defenders busy, and they've had to concede that there may indeed be problems with grain consumption in more than the 1 percent of people with celiac disease.

I don't envy those in the position of having to defend grains. More recently, they have tried to put a positive spin on "gluten-free grains," such as amaranth, rice, and millet, hoping to maintain their market presence but deflect growing antigluten criticism. Defend the seeds of grasses as dietary staple, and it should come as no surprise that you find yourself in an increasingly lonely corner.

FORTIFICATION: NOT GOOD ENOUGH

It should come as no surprise that, given the gastrointestinal disruption caused by grains, nutrient absorption can be impaired enough to create several common deficiencies. Of course, this is contrary to what we're told will happen if we consume more "healthy whole grains." Grains like whole wheat bread, stoneground oatmeal, and multigrain muffins do indeed have a respectable profile of B vitamins, fiber, and phytonutrients. But the nutrients of grains are accompanied by factors that impair the absorption of nutrients, which then cause nutritional deficiencies. This vicious cycle only ends when you remove grains from your diet and seek other sources of nutrients.

IRON DEFICIENCY began when early humans first consumed the seeds of grasses. Iron deficiency can impair the ability to run, hunt, gather food, or tolerate weather extremes, so it has a potential impact on survival. Because of this, it has exerted an evolutionary pressure over the last 10,000 years that led to the appearance of the gene for hemochromatosis, which partially counteracts the iron-impairing effects of grains.[10] All grains contain high quantities of phytates, the component of grains responsible for impaired iron absorption. Ironically, many grain breeders select high-phytate strains of grains because they have improved pest resistance. Whole wheat, corn, and millet, for instance, contain 800 milligrams (mg) of phytates per 100 grams (approximately 3½ ounces) of flour. It takes as little as 50 mg of phytates to slash iron absorption by 80 to 90 percent.[11]

Because phytates essentially turn off the human capacity for iron absorption and most of us do not have hemochromatosis, consumption of grains is the most common explanation for iron deficiency anemia in situations in which blood loss is not the cause.[12] Iron deficiency is a worldwide problem; it's the most common cause of anemia. In Egypt, for example, iron deficiency doubled between 2000 and 2005 as grain consumption of baladi bread increased.[13] The "solution"? Fortify the bread with iron. It should come as no surprise that 46 percent of people with celiac disease show decreased iron stores (low ferritin levels) and anemia from iron deficiency, though, because the effect is not mediated by gluten but by phytates, and grain-induced iron deficiency is exceptionally common in those who don't have celiac disease, as well.[14] People who have Crohn's disease, malabsorption, and dysbiosis are also more prone to iron deficiency. Grains cause iron-deficiency anemia with its associated symptoms of fatigue, light-headedness, and breathlessness. Grains contain iron, but it is the less well-absorbed "non-heme" form, rather than the more efficiently absorbed "heme" form found in hemoglobin and myoglobin from animal products. Despite the fact that grains contain iron, the net effect of grain consumption is reduced iron status. Iron deficiency is therefore a common health price we pay when we consume the seeds of grasses.

ZINC DEFICIENCY also develops in populations dependent on grain consumption.[15] Deficiency of zinc was thought to be rare until 1958, when a severe case was diagnosed in an Iranian man who appeared to be around 10 years old at age 22. He had an enlarged liver and spleen, heart failure, and an appetite for eating dirt. Characteristic of his culture, 50 to 90 percent of his diet consisted of unleavened tanok bread, along with potatoes, fruit, vegetables, and occasional meat. Zinc supplementation corrected his health problems.[16] The component in wheat responsible for the deficiency was not clear, however, until chickens and pigs were diagnosed with zinc deficiency due to the phytate content of wheat fed to them. Zinc deficiency has since proven to be widespread.

The phytates that block iron absorption are also responsible for blocking zinc absorption. The phytates contained in just 2 ounces of grain flour are sufficient to nearly completely block intestinal zinc absorption.[17] And in the seemingly endless string of breeding blunders, here's one more: Modern breeding efforts have selected plants with higher quantities of phytates because of their pest resistance. The ever-resourceful grain industry has, not unexpectedly, manipulated grain crops to increase zinc content to compensate. (One method includes using fertilizers supplemented with zinc.)

Zinc deficiency correlates with grain consumption: The more that's consumed, the more likely zinc deficiency is to develop.[18] This is a nutritional problem of growing worldwide significance, as increasing reliance on grains, especially wheat, corn, and rice, has worsened zinc status in an estimated two billion people.[19] Between 35 and 45 percent of older adults are zinc deficient, and 67 percent of people with untreated celiac disease have zinc deficiency.[20]

Because zinc is essential for hundreds of different body processes, deficiency can manifest in varied ways. Mild deficiency typically shows as rashes, diarrhea, and hair loss. Vegans, vegetarians, and people who limit consumption of animal products are especially prone to zinc deficiency, since plant products contain minimal zinc compared to the higher zinc content of meats, poultry, shellfish, and organ meats.[21] Combine the poor zinc content of plant products with the impaired absorption caused by grain phytates, and it's not uncommon for vegans and vegetarians to develop difficulties even mounting a normal immune response. Additionally, fertility and reproduction are adversely impacted, children and adolescents can experience impaired growth, and neurological maturation is impaired, among other diverse effects of moderate to severe zinc deficiency. For this reason, the Institute of Medicine has estimated that vegans and vegetarians require 50 percent more zinc than omnivores do.[22] Removing grains from the diet improves zinc status, and if lost grain calories are compensated for with an increase in zinc-rich foods, such as meats, there is a net increase in zinc intake and absorption. (Also, see page 172 for more information on how to correct zinc deficiency.)

VITAMIN B_{12} DEFICIENCY is also common, affecting 19 percent of people with celiac disease and 16.6 percent of people without celiac disease.[23] B_{12} deficiency is another signature deficiency of grain consumption, as several grain components collaborate to impair its absorption. Wheat germ agglutinin (WGA) blocks the intrinsic factor protein produced in the stomach and essential for B_{12} absorption in the small intestine, the means by which 60 percent of all B_{12} is absorbed.[24] Grain consumption can also trigger antibodies against the intrinsic factor or against the stomach parietal cells that produce intrinsic factor.[25]

Severe B_{12} deficiency has serious implications, including pernicious anemia (fatal if untreated) or macrocytic anemia, describing the abnormally large red blood cells that develop as a result of this condition. Abdominal pain, an enlarged liver, and a characteristic cherry red tongue develop with B_{12} deficiency. Lesser degrees of deficiency have health and performance implications, too, as they can lead to diminished concentration and learning ability. Typical of the silliness of modern nutritional thinking, the solution often offered is increased B_{12} supplementation in grains to compensate for these effects.[26]

Because dietary B_{12} is obtained mostly from animal-sourced products, such as meat, liver, and eggs, vegans and vegetarians who consume grains are especially likely to develop a deficiency. People with inflammatory bowel diseases (Crohn's disease and ulcerative colitis) are also especially prone to vitamin B_{12} deficiency.

FOLATE DEFICIENCY is less common than deficiencies of iron, zinc, and vitamin B_{12}. It is, however, known to occur in people with celiac disease and gluten intolerance.[27] People with inflammatory bowel diseases also suffer from impaired folate absorption sufficient to cause deficiency. Also, situations in which greater folate needs develop, especially pregnancy, can magnify the severity of deficiency. In all these situations, assessment of folate levels should be performed and supplementation instituted. (See page 184 for more information.) Folate deficiency has serious implications, including birth defects in children born from folate-deficient mothers and increased potential for gastrointestinal cancers. Many of the same phenomena that develop with vitamin B_{12} deficiency are caused by folate deficiency, since folate and B_{12} participate in many similar processes.

Folate is the form that occurs naturally in foods, while folic acid is the synthetic form added to foods or taken in supplement form. Because modern diets dependent on processed grains and sugar are potentially deficient in folate, manufacturers in the United States and Canada have been required to add synthetic folic acid to grain products since 1998 to decrease the incidence of birth defects. This has indeed improved the folate status of most people, but it is proving to be a double-edged sword: Folate levels increased more than intended, and increased reliance on synthetic folic acid has also been associated with increased colon and prostate cancers.[28]

VITAMIN D DEFICIENCY is a widespread phenomenon with significant implications for health. Vitamin D deficiency is the rule, rather than the exception. While we can blame more severe cases of deficiency on grains, it also commonly occurs independent of grain consumption. Various other modern habits have served to worsen our vitamin D status, including inhabiting cold climates deprived of year-round sunlight, wearing clothes that cover skin surface area (since vitamin D is activated in our skin by sunlight), increasingly indoor lifestyles, aversion to organ consumption, especially liver (they contain vitamin D), and aging, which is associated with a progressive loss of the ability to activate vitamin D in the skin.[29] Living in the tropics is no guarantee of adequate vitamin D status, though; a recent assessment of elderly males living in a tropical climate, for instance, revealed that 66.7 percent were deficient.[30] Vitamin D status is such a crucial factor for health that we discuss it at greater length later in the book (see page 175).

People with celiac disease are especially prone to vitamin D deficiency, which also contributes to low bone mineral density. In one clinical study, only 25 percent of people showed normal bone density at the time of their celiac disease diagnosis.[31] Bone demineralization (loss of calcium) that weakens bones is worsened by the impaired calcium absorption characteristic of celiac disease, also.

GUT FLORA: DON'T GET YOUR BOWELS IN AN UPROAR

You can view bacterial flora that inhabit the intestinal tract like a garden: If you fertilize it properly, provide sufficient water and nutrients, and avoid herbicides and pesticides that disrupt the natural balance, your garden will yield a bounty of vigorous, healthy crops. If you fail to water or fertilize it properly, you will likely have a lousy yield of stunted crops, not to mention lots of weeds. Bowel flora operate on similar principles.

We know that diet plays an important role in shaping the composition of bowel flora, even in the absence of disease. For example, bowel flora of children living in rural Africa and eating traditional diets, when compared to European children eating a modern diet, demonstrate striking differences. The African children have higher than expected numbers of Bacteroidetes, an adaptation theorized to enhance efficiency in digesting plant matter.[32] I've discussed how the adoption of grains changed the composition of mouth and gut flora in humans. Changes in oral flora have clear implications for dental disease; changes in gastrointestinal flora have less clear implications, but it should come as no surprise that there could be such changes, given the toxic effects grains have on the intestines. The composition of bacteria in the gastrointestinal tract, concentrated in the colon, varies from individual to individual, shifts with age and hormonal status, and is modified by exposure to antibiotics and components of diet. When factors that allow healthy bacteria to survive are altered, bowel flora species change and microorganisms can extend above the normal furthest segment of the small intestine, a situation called small intestinal bacterial overgrowth, or SIBO. That's when nasty things can happen: bloating, diarrhea, nutritional deficiencies, and inflammation. (See "Small Intestinal Bacterial Overgrowth: The Case of the Human Petri Dish," on page 66.)

It is estimated that more than 1,000 different species of bacteria dwell in our intestines. Unfortunately, most of our understanding of the composition of bowel flora involves comparing people with various diseases, such as ulcerative colitis, to people without the same disease. It is not clear whether the changes in bowel flora composition are part of the cause or simply a consequence of the disease. People without disease are also assumed to be normal, but this may not be true, since "normal" ignores potentially disruptive factors such as prior antibiotic use, emotional stress, and unnatural distortions of diet, such as grain and sugar consumption. Nobody quite knows what normal or ideal bowel flora looks like yet.

A number of health conditions have been associated with changes of bowel flora, including multiple sclerosis, fibromyalgia, diabetes (both type 1 and type 2), irritable bowel syndrome, gallstones, acid reflux and esophagitis, irritable bowel syndrome, ulcerative colitis, Crohn's disease, and food allergies.[33] Funny thing: Each and every one of these conditions has also been associated with grain consumption, especially consumption of wheat, rye, and barley.

Changes in the composition of our bacteria develop as quickly as days to weeks after a change in diet.[34] Right now, our understanding of bowel flora remains limited, but it is rapidly yielding to study. I believe that in the next few years we will know with confidence how to assess an individual's bowel flora status and how to know when it has been fully corrected. In the meantime, the steps required to reestablish what we currently believe represents an ideal composition of bowel flora will be discussed in Chapter 9.

Small Intestinal Bacterial Overgrowth: The Case of the Human Petri Dish

Put a petri dish out in the open air and, over just a few days, it will be ripe with bacteria and fungi. Likewise, mess up the health of the human intestine by allowing undesirable bacteria and fungi to gain an advantage and reducing normal bacterial species, and you have the equivalent of a human petri dish. Such a situation is common, and it's called small intestinal bacterial overgrowth (SIBO), or dysbiosis, an abnormal overabundance of bacteria in the normally sparsely populated upper small intestine, or jejunum, along with changed species in other parts of the intestinal tract. (Changed bowel flora also occurs in the large intestine and even the stomach and duodenum, but a SIBO or dysbiosis diagnosis is often made by sampling the contents of the jejunum of the small intestine, which is why we have the somewhat misleading "small intestine" label of the condition.)

SIBO has been associated with a number of conditions, including fibromyalgia, irritable bowel syndrome, Crohn's disease, ulcerative colitis, and anatomical distortions introduced by prior bowel surgery.[35] SIBO is common in people with celiac disease, and when "normal" people are assessed for SIBO, up to 35 percent demonstrate evidence for abnormal intestinal infestations, even if no symptoms are present.[36] When SIBO is diagnosed in people with bothersome symptoms, the conventional treatment is to prescribe an antibiotic, such as rifaximin, to wipe out bowel flora, both good and bad. And it works, though it ignores the question of why the SIBO developed in the first place. And, of course, wiping out bowel flora does not guarantee that your intestines will repopulate with healthy bacteria, particularly if the cause of the SIBO remains uncorrected.

The Difficulties of *C. difficile*

One disturbing trend in the world of SIBO is the increasing incidence of infection by *Clostridium difficile,* a strain of bacteria capable of inflicting severe damage on the colon. Called pseudomembranous colitis, in its worst form it can involve sepsis (entry of bacteria into the bloodstream) and death.

Ordinarily, *C. difficile* quietly inhabits the colons of healthy people (or at least what is commonly regarded as healthy) in low numbers, as it competes with other bacteria for nutrients and is suppressed by factors expressed by other species. We know that *C. difficile* can emerge following the use of antibiotics that indiscriminately knock off bowel flora, good and bad, which of course requires even more antibiotics. More recently, though,

C. difficile has proven to be a source of trouble even without a preceding course of antibiotics. Drugs that are widely prescribed to suppress stomach acid, such as Prilosec, Protonix, and Prevacid, have been associated with distortions of bowel flora that allow populations of *C. difficile* to thrive.[37] But the reasons why this organism is becoming increasingly aggressive are unclear. Might the distortions of bowel flora caused by grains, changed by agribusiness, play a role? There are no answers at present, but it sure would add up as cleanly as 2 + 2 = 4.

YOUR GUT IS LEAKING

Leakiness is a condition that plagues roofs and bathroom faucets or is suffered by spy agencies when errant contractors leak classified US security information, but hopefully your seafaring ship, microwave, and intestinal tract are free from leaks. For many years, it has been suspected that an abnormally increased degree of intestinal permeability is responsible for triggering diseases such as type 1 diabetes, Crohn's disease, ankylosing spondylitis, multiple sclerosis, and celiac disease.[38] Every day, your gastrointestinal tract must contend with bacteria, fungi and other organisms, bacterial toxins, and even larger critters, such as protozoa and insects. It must therefore make millions of "decisions" every day, with each and every meal: What should be allowed passage into the lymph system and bloodstream? What should not?

This tightly controlled system can go haywire. Fragments of gliadin and related prolamin proteins exert *direct* toxic inflammatory effects on the intestinal lining in anyone foolish enough to ingest grains—effects that can result in abnormally increased intestinal permeability.[39] No genetic susceptibility is required for this effect; all testing for celiac disease or "gluten sensitivity" may be negative in those with intestinal permeability.

In addition to these direct effects, gliadin can also *indirectly* increase intestinal permeability. While at the University of Maryland, Alessio Fasano, MD, discovered that the zonulin protein in the lining of the gastrointestinal tract is a target for the gliadin protein of wheat.[40] Once activated, the zonulin protein triggers increased leakiness of the barriers ("tight junctions") between intestinal cells, permitting molecules that should be confined within the intestinal tract to gain access to the rest of the body. While the intensity of the effect is variable (depending on the genetically determined form of zonulin), everyone is subject to this effect to one degree or another. Given their structural similarities, the prolamin proteins of other grains exert similar effects.[41] The implications of Dr. Fasano's work are huge. His findings mean that the abnormally increased intestinal permeability induced by gliadin and related proteins is the first step leading to autoimmunity, as the body's immune system is tricked into attacking its own organs in those with genetic susceptibility. In other words, even if you have a genetic susceptibility to rheumatoid arthritis, joint swelling, inflammation, and disfigurement may never show unless the process is initiated by consumption of grain proteins. Or, if you have a genetic susceptibility to multiple sclerosis, fatigue, numbness, inco-ordination, and bladder or bowel dysfunction may never appear unless grain proteins cause increased intestinal permeability that allows the genetic susceptibility to manifest. We discuss this distinct pathway that relates autoimmune diseases with grain consumption in Chapter 13.

VENOMOUS, DEBAUCHED, AND DEPRAVED

If, at the end of this discussion of the gastrointestinal effects of grains, you conclude that grains are not only harmful for bowel health and nutrition but are also a dreadful, nasty, trouble-making collection of bowel toxins, you are empowered with the key to understanding why so many people are plagued by chronic gastrointestinal complaints, regardless of how "bal-anced" their diet, how vigorously they exercise, or how many nutritional supplements they take.

While the gastrointestinal system is ground zero for the human body's battle against grains, it is by no means the only battleground. We'll discuss the rest of the battered, barren, land mine–strewn health land-scape in Chapter 5.

CHAPTER 5

GRAINS, BRAINS, AND CHEST PAINS

I couldn't repair your brakes, so I made your horn louder.
—Stephen Wright

IN THE CONFRONTATION between grains and the human body, the gastrointestinal tract is directly in the line of fire—but the war certainly doesn't end there. Let's penetrate deeper and examine the wounds and scars left by grains as they disrupt, agitate, and discombobulate the finely balanced machinations of the human body—joints, skin, glands, respiratory system, and brain—leaving no organ untouched. It's a long chapter with lots of detail meant to show you the astounding scope and frightening severity of the unhealthy human experience that exists because, as a species, we made this terrible decision to consume the seeds of grasses.

GRAINS AND AUTOIMMUNITY: DASTARDLY DUO

Mutt and Jeff. Abbott and Costello. Cheech and Chong. Garlic and bad breath. Where you find one, you find the other, and so it is with grains and autoimmune conditions in humans.

When the human immune system is unable to distinguish proteins in your colon, thyroid gland, pancreas, or brain from foreign organisms invading your body, it recruits B and T lymphocytes into an army to wage war on your own organs. We call this *autoimmunity*. It's a process that, in an astounding proportion of cases, begins with the muffins you have for breakfast or the slice of pizza you ate for dinner. The complex pathways worked out by Alessio Fasano, MD, of the University of Maryland, and his colleagues (see page 67) open up an entirely new perspective on diseases that involve autoimmunity. Recall that the gliadin protein of wheat and the nearly identical proteins of rye and barley can remain undigested. Intact gliadin proteins provoke increased permeability of the intestinal tract, which allows foreign substances access to the bloodstream. The mis-recognition process of autoimmunity can begin with a bacterial protein that gets into the bloodstream, but it can also start with a grain protein. The gliadin protein and the transglutaminase enzyme of the liver or pancreas bear a strong resemblance to one another, so the presence of gliadin in the bloodstream can trick the immune system into causing autoimmune hepatitis or autoimmune pancreatitis.

This is *big*. This is as big as identifying and capturing the Mafia don responsible for dozens of gangland-style murders and millions of dollars of contraband, convicting him, and putting him away for life. It means that we now have a direct path linking gliadin and related grain prolamin proteins with autoimmune conditions. This sequence of events is not limited to people with celiac disease or gluten sensitivity; this applies to *everyone*. Susceptibility will vary based on genetic factors, but it is separate and distinct from the gastrointestinal disruption caused by celiac disease. It means that a person with no abdominal symptoms from wheat consumption—no heartburn, bowel urgency, colitis, etc.—and who tests negative for celiac disease or gluten sensitivity can still develop the joint deformity of rheumatoid arthritis years later or the neurological impairment of multiple sclerosis at age 45.

Prolamins and Transglutaminase: Dead Ringers

Remember the 1964 Bette Davis movie *Dead Ringer*, in which one sister, Edith, estranged and angered with her twin, Margaret, shoots her in the head and then covers up her crime by assuming the killed twin's identity? I don't think any better allegorical description for autoimmunity could be crafted, right down to Ms. Davis's talent for portraying unpopular characters.

The human body relies on a class of enzymes called transglutaminases, which are found in the intestinal lining, pancreas, joints, brain, skin, and other organs. Transglutaminase enzymes are responsible for the simple task of removing a nitrogen-containing (amine) group from the amino acid glutamine in the proteins that you consume. In an odd twist of fate, human transglutaminase enzymes resemble the gliadin protein of wheat, as well as the related prolamin proteins of rye, barley, corn, and oats. In other words, if their structures are laid out side-by-side, there is an eerie overlap in sequence among all of them, such that the body's immune response can't tell the difference: They are immune dead ringers.[1] This has been called "molecular mimicry": two unrelated and different proteins with different purposes, but with sections of shared structure that fool the immune system.

Antibodies expressed against grain prolamins—and thereby against transglutaminase—are associated with inflammatory bowel diseases, pancreatitis, joint and muscle inflammation, skin rashes, and other autoimmune and inflammatory conditions.[2] This explains how and why grain consumption causes so many autoimmune and inflammatory diseases other than celiac disease. For example, children with type 1 diabetes (an autoimmune condition of the pancreas) are more likely to express antibodies against the transglutaminase enzyme, also associated with increased potential for autoimmune conditions outside of the pancreas.[3]

It is as unsettling as one twin shooting the other, this relationship between something plant and something human that's close enough to fool even the finely tuned discriminating powers of the human immune system. But such is the unnatural relationship between humans and the seeds of grasses.

Even before the details of increased intestinal permeability were sorted out by Dr. Fasano's team, it had been known for many years that the list of autoimmune conditions attributable to wheat, rye, and barley is formidable. These dangerous and sometimes fatal conditions are enough to make you spit out your last bite of raisin bread.

Addison's disease

Alopecia areata

Ankylosing spondylitis

Antiphospholipid antibody
   syndrome

Autoimmune hemolytic anemia

Autoimmune hepatitis

Autoimmune inner ear disease

Autoimmune
   lymphoproliferative syndrome

Autoimmune
   thrombocytopenic purpura

Behcet's disease
Bullous pemphigoid
Cardiomyopathy (dilated, or congestive)
Celiac disease
Chronic fatigue syndrome
Chronic inflammatory demyelinating polyneuropathy
Cold agglutinin disease
CREST syndrome
Crohn's disease
Dermatomyositis
Discoid lupus
Essential mixed cryoglobulinemia
Food protein-induced enterocolitis syndrome
Graves' disease
Guillain-Barré syndrome
Hashimoto's thyroiditis
Idiopathic pulmonary fibrosis
Idiopathic thrombocytopenic purpura
IgA nephropathy
Insulin-dependent diabetes (type I)
Juvenile arthritis
Ménière's disease
Mixed connective tissue disease
Multiple sclerosis
Myasthenia gravis
Myocarditis
Pemphigus vulgaris
Pernicious anemia
Polyarteritis nodosa
Polychondritis
Polyglandular syndromes
Polymyalgia rheumatica
Polymyositis dermatomyositis
Primary agammaglobulinemia
Primary biliary cirrhosis
Psoriasis
Raynaud's syndrome
Reiter's syndrome
Rheumatoid arthritis
Sarcoidosis
Scleroderma
Sjögren's syndrome
Systemic lupus erythematosus
Takayasu's arteritis
Temporal arteritis
Ulcerative colitis
Uveitis
Vasculitis
Vitiligo
Wegener's granulomatosis

This list shows that the misrecognition process that leads to autoimmunity can involve the joints (rheumatoid arthritis, lupus arthritis), pancreas (autoimmune pancreatitis), small intestine (Crohn's disease), cerebellum (cerebellar ataxia), nerves of the legs and pelvis (peripheral neuropathy), thyroid (Graves' disease and Hashimoto's thyroiditis), skin (psoriasis, alopecia areata), liver (autoimmune hepatitis), and arteries (polyarteritis nodosa)—and it doesn't end there. There's no organ that has *not* been associated with autoimmune attack triggered by grains. This is not to say that every case of, say, autoimmune pancreatitis can be blamed on grains, as other factors may trigger a similar immune response gone awry in susceptible people. But these are all conditions triggered or unmasked by a component of diet, specifically a component of diet that we are urged to eat in greater quantities.

Corn and oats have been associated with a more limited panel of auto-immune conditions. Corn, for instance, has been associated with increased potential for type 1 diabetes.[4] Rice causes a dangerous condition in infants called food protein-induced enterocolitis syndrome, a disordered immune condition that results in lethargy, diarrhea, malnutrition, and dehydration that disappears completely with rice avoidance.[5]

No other food or food group has such a list of diseases, autoimmune or otherwise, associated with its consumption—not sugar, high-fructose corn syrup, soft drinks, or poisonous toadstools. Only grains, the largely indigestible seeds of grasses, are associated with such a frightening list of ways to misguide your immune system.

Type-1 Diabetes: A Disease of Grains?

It's pretty easy to argue that plentiful consumption of the amylopectin A from grains is associated with increased blood sugars and thereby increased potential for type 2 diabetes. But how about type 1 diabetes, in which delicate insulin-producing beta cells of the pancreas are destroyed for a lifetime? There are several lines of evidence that strongly link grain consumption and the changes that lead to type 1 diabetes in genetically susceptible children and adults. Some of the evidence originates with experimental animal models, some comes from observations in humans.

- In experimental mouse and rat models, 64 percent of mice fed wheat-containing chow develop type 1 diabetes, compared to 15 percent of mice fed wheat-free chow.[6] Likewise, feeding corn to diabetes-prone mice increases the percentage that develops type 1 diabetes from 37 to 57 percent.[7]

- Children with celiac disease triggered by the gliadin proteins of wheat, rye, and barley are 10 times more likely to develop type 1 diabetes than children without celiac disease.[8]

- Children with type 1 diabetes are 10 to 20 times more likely to develop celiac disease and/or antibodies to wheat components than children without diabetes.[9]

- Children with type 1 diabetes launch an abnormal (T-lymphocyte) immune response when exposed to gliadin.[10]

I've discussed how gliadin increases intestinal damage and permeability that can lead to increased autoimmunity, but don't forget that grain lectins also damage intestinal tissue, as do partially digested gliadin-derived peptides. And don't forget to throw in a little pancreatic beta cell glucotoxicity (irreversible damage to beta cells caused by the high blood sugars resulting from amylopectin A in grains). In other words, when grains are consumed, the stage is set for an onslaught of autoimmunity and pancreatic damage, which appear to be closely related to intestinal diseases of gliadin proteins, such as celiac disease.

And the situation appears to be getting worse. The National Institutes of Health (NIH) and Centers for Disease Control and Prevention (CDC)–sponsored SEARCH for Diabetes in Youth study has documented that the incidence of type 1 diabetes in children has been increasing 2.7 percent per year since 1978.[11] This observation has been demonstrated by registries in other countries, as well. What we lack is a clinical trial in infants, half of whom start eating grains early in life, half of whom avoid grains from birth; this would, once and for all, clinch the direct connection between grains and type 1 diabetes. You can imagine the difficulties in conducting such a trial, though, so don't hold your breath waiting for such data.

In the meantime, we've got a smoking gun, fingerprints, motive, and opportunity—enough to bring grain up on charges. Do we have enough to convict? I say hang the bastard.

HYPOTHYROIDISM: AUTOIMMUNITY AT WORK

You may have noticed that two thyroid conditions were on the list of autoimmune conditions associated with grain consumption. Of all the various forms of misdirected immunity ignited by grains, thyroid dysfunction is by far the most common.

Let's start with describing what thyroid dysfunction looks like. The thyroid gland, positioned like a bow tie on the front of your neck, is the gland that regulates metabolic rate. When it's overactive, or *hyper*thyroid, your metabolism is excessively high and you have high levels of the thyroid hormones T4 and T3, rapid heart rate, anxiety, and weight loss. When it's underactive, or *hypo*thyroid, your metabolism is slowed, you have reduced levels of T4 and T3, and higher levels of the pituitary hormone thyroid stimulating hormone (TSH), a response intended to prod the thyroid to work harder and release more T4 and T3. By far the most common situation is hypothyroidism. Hypothyroidism is therefore a state of slowed metabolism that causes symptoms such as low energy; feeling inappropriately cold, especially in the hands and feet (due to low body temperature); constipation; hair loss; and dry skin. Failure to lose weight after grain elimination is a common signal of hypothyroidism. While grain elimination is indeed a powerful strategy for weight loss, it alone cannot overcome the effects of hypothyroidism, which must be specifically addressed.

Autoimmune destruction of the thyroid gland is called Graves' disease or Hashimoto's thyroiditis. Gliadin antibodies can occur in 50 percent or more of people with thyroid disease, making it the most common expression of grain-induced autoimmunity.[12] Some people, especially those with Graves' disease, initially experience a period of hyperthyroidism due to inflammation and destruction of thyroid tissue, which causes excessive quantities of thyroid hormone to be released. With or without this period of hyperthyroidism, though, hypothyroidism develops over time, reflecting injury to thyroid tissue and causing the symptoms of hypothyroidism as production of T4 and T3 hormones wanes. Hypothyroidism is underdiagnosed. In common practice, you often have to be miserable before your doctor makes the diagnosis of an underactive thyroid. Some physicians, for instance, will not consider testing or treatment even if you have depression, weight gain, high cholesterol values, and increased cardiovascular risk attributable to this situation. I believe this is wrong and should not be tolerated. Because thyroid issues are so common, so neglected, and so important to overall health and weight, they will be discussed at greater length in Chapter 11.

CORTISOL: A DIFFERENCE OF NIGHT AND DAY

Cortisol is the primary hormone produced by your adrenal glands, the two little glands that sit atop your kidneys. Cortisol plays a crucial physiologic role in many bodily processes, and it does so in a predictable pattern called a "circadian rhythm," an adaptation to life on earth and its 24-hour cycle of day and night. Once again, grains enter the picture and disrupt this normal cycle of life.

Antibodies triggered by gliadin proteins can damage the adrenal glands, resulting in reduced production of adrenal hormones.[13] Disruption of vasoactive intestinal peptide (or VIP; see page 24) by the lectins of wheat, rye, barley, and rice is another means by which adrenal gland function can be impaired. Most commonly, cortisol disruption results in feelings of low energy in the morning, depression, inappropriate surges in nighttime energy, insomnia, cravings for salt, inability to lose weight, low blood pressure, and light-headedness. One of the difficulties with identifying adrenal dysfunction is that the adrenal glands produce more than cortisol; they also produce hormones such as aldosterone (responsible for sodium and potassium status and blood pressure control); adrenaline (responsible for arousal, energy, and metabolism); and adrenal androgens that overlap with the effects of testosterone. One or all adrenal hormones can be disrupted, though the dominant effect is usually determined by disruptions of cortisol.

Disruptions at the hypothalamic and pituitary levels that result in cortisol disruption can be caused by obesity (via the inflammatory phenomena of visceral fat), diabetes, depression, stress, post-traumatic stress disorder (PTSD), and other conditions.[14] New neuroendocrine research is also uncovering potential *glucocorticoid resistance*, or impaired responsiveness to cortisol, in people showing normal or high cortisol blood levels.[15] This may be related to issues with rheumatoid arthritis, Crohn's disease, ulcerative colitis, multiple sclerosis, asthma, chronic fatigue, fibromyalgia, chronic pain, depression, PTSD, and chronic stress. Note that most of the conditions listed get their start with grain consumption.

While other endocrine glands are also capable of all degrees of dysfunction, from subtle to severe, conventionally minded endocrinologists deny this, arguing that the adrenal gland is the only endocrine gland that is either entirely normal or severely dysfunctional enough to threaten life, causing Addison's disease when underactive and Cushing's disease when overactive. They believe it's all or nothing, with no gray area in between. I reject conventional "wisdom" and follow common sense: Adrenal dysfunction can occur to any degree and may involve one or more adrenal gland hormones, or it can occur at the hypothalamic or pituitary level. Besides, the emerging neuroendocrine scientific and clinical literature strongly argues that such disruptions short of life threatening are not only possible, but are common.

You can appreciate that the issues are complex and tangled, involving several hormones and organs. Thankfully, the majority of issues surrounding cortisol and adrenal dysfunction can be reduced to disrupted cortisol circadian patterns due to (1) damage to the adrenal gland from grain consumption, and (2) disruption of pituitary signaling to the adrenal gland due to inflammation and chronic stress, exaggerated by the presence of visceral fat. Later in the book we consider ways to identify, then correct, cortisol disruptions, which can help you feel more energetic, provide relief from depression, restore the normal day-night cycle of energy and sleep, and help break a weight-loss plateau.

MATTER OVER MIND

The effects of grains on the human brain and nervous system, like those in the gastrointestinal tract, are varied and destructive. Neurologist David Perlmutter, MD, has written a book called *Grain Brain*, which is devoted to the effects of grains on brain health (particularly dementia). It's recommended reading for anyone interested in an extensive discussion of brain health impairment developing due to grain consumption.

In the movie *The Matrix*, Morpheus explains to Neo that, "The Matrix is the world that has been pulled over your eyes to blind you from the truth," when describing the computer-simulated world injected into the minds of people to keep them from knowing that machines control everything. While the world of grains is hardly as visually arresting or imaginative as the one in this movie, both worlds are all about mind control. In the movie, human minds are controlled by computers; in the world we live in, our minds have been under the influence of the mind-active components of grains.

The effects of the gliadin and related prolamin proteins on the human brain fall into two categories: (1) reversible effects exerted on the mind via gliadin-derived opiates and (2) autoimmune inflammatory effects, sometimes reversible, sometimes irreversible, on brain and nervous system tissue.

The mind and brain effects of grains are largely due to wheat, rye, and barley, which share the same gliadin protein. Other nonwheat grains also have brain health implications, but they only work through high blood sugars that lead to dementia.

It's Not Your Imagination: Reversible Mind and Brain Effects of Grains

Reversible mind effects begin with the gliadin proteins of wheat, rye, and barley that undergo digestion to smaller 4- or 5-amino-acid-long peptides, which are small enough to penetrate the brain and bind to opiate receptors.[16] The effects of these peptides, dubbed *exorphins*, or exogenously derived morphinelike compounds, vary depending on individual susceptibility. In some conditions, a reversible autoimmune process has also been documented (positive gliadin antibody). Because structural damage has not been associated with these phenomena, these conditions, despite their potential severity and destructiveness, are reversible with grain elimination. There are several conditions that fall into this category.

APPETITE STIMULATION. Grain-derived exorphins trigger the grain consumer to take in 400 more calories per day, every day. This is an average value; some people consume more, others less. At worst, it can cause calorie intake to be 1,000 or more calories per day and higher and trigger food obsessions or other addictive food behaviors. With grain consumption, your appetite is specifically stimulated for carbohydrates, such as pretzels, corn chips, and cookies, and it's stimulated to a lesser degree for fat. The effect tends to be addictive, with cyclic and recurring desire for such foods driving dietary habits and even dominating thoughts and fantasies. Rid yourself of gliadin-derived opiates and calorie intake drops by 400 calories per day. Food obsessions and addictive food relationships are also typically reduced or completely eliminated.[17]

BINGE EATING DISORDER AND BULIMIA. People with binge eating disorder tend to eat in large binges well beyond their need. They are unresponsive to signals that turn off appetite and feel ashamed at their lack of restraint. Bulimia is a similar condition, with binges typically followed by "purging" the excessive quantity of food by vomiting. People with these eating disorders describe intrusive, 24-hour-a-day food obsessions that occur even after finishing a large meal or during the night, triggering nighttime binges. Both conditions are socially incapacitating, ruin relationships, and are associated with low self-esteem. Additionally, the bulimic sufferer who puts a finger in the back of her throat to bring up food exposes her tooth enamel to corrosive stomach acid, rotting her teeth over time. Both conditions represent exaggerated appetite-stimulating responses to gliadin-derived opiates.

MIND FOG. Disrupted concentration, inability to focus, impaired learning, impaired decision-making ability, and sleepiness are exceptionally common after consuming wheat, rye, and barley. Gliadin-derived opiates are the most likely culprits behind these effects, given their known ability to affect the mind. It's also likely that the blood sugar fluctuations caused by all grains contribute, especially the low blood sugar of hypoglycemia.

ATTENTION DEFICIT HYPERACTIVITY DISORDER AND AUTISTIC SPECTRUM DISORDER. While these disorders are unrelated, they share a similar response to gliadin-derived opiates. Children and adults with these conditions experience behavioral outbursts, such as temper tantrums or emotional "storms" without reason, and they have an impaired capacity to sustain attention. Kids with these conditions already have an impaired ability to learn and pay attention for more than a few seconds or minutes; grain-derived opiates just make it worse.[18] A recent analysis demonstrated that kids with autism lack the markers for celiac disease (such as transglutaminase antibody), but they do have increased levels of antibodies to gliadin, especially if gastrointestinal symptoms like diarrhea are present.[19]

PARANOID SCHIZOPHRENIA. The worsening of paranoia, auditory hallucinations (hearing voices and receiving warnings or commands), and social disengagement were among the first observations made when researchers started studying the effects of wheat consumption on brain health, attributable to the gliadin protein–derived opiates.[20] This effect may be confined to schizophrenics who express an autoimmune response to the gliadin protein, the group most likely to improve with wheat, rye, and barley avoidance.[21]

BIPOLAR ILLNESS. We know that people with bipolar illness express higher levels of antibodies in response to the gliadin protein, similar to the phenomenon observed in schizophrenics.[22] Gliadin-derived opiate peptides likely also play a role in generating the distortions in judgment and reality experienced with this condition.

DEPRESSION. If there is predisposition for depression, grains—especially wheat, rye, barley, and corn—can magnify or unmask that tendency.[23] Depression due to the gliadin- and prolamin protein–derived opiates can be mild, resulting in a pervasive feeling of unhappiness and lack of interest, or it can be incapacitating and life threatening, complete with obsessive thoughts of suicide or self-harm. Both wheat and corn are also responsible for reductions in brain serotonin, which regulates mood.[24]

OBSESSIVE-COMPULSIVE DISORDER. A person who has obsessive-compulsive disorder helplessly gives in to the impulse to obsessively and compulsively perform some action or engage in some thought—behaviors that have been associated with wheat consumption.[25] It might be compulsive hand washing, or housecleaning, or checking and rechecking (and rechecking and rechecking) figures in a ledger. Being locked into such behavioral loops can be debilitating for the sufferer, as these rituals can dominate her thoughts and behaviors, as well as sabotage success at school and work and disrupt the health of relationships.

A world of research still needs to be performed to explore these mind-altering phenomena that develop in people who follow the standard advice to consume more grains. MRI, PET, and other brain-imaging modalities may reveal why and how schizophrenics tend to suffer more auditory hallucinations with grain consumption or why kids with autistic spectrum disorder experience impaired attention span. Notably, while some of these effects are associated with an immune response against one or more grain proteins, many are not. But remember: If you know that grains can worsen or cause deterioration in mental conditions, it also means that you know how to *undo* or lessen the severity of all these effects or, as one of Keanu Reeves's fellow rebels in the *Matrix* remarks, "Buckle your seatbelt, Dorothy, 'cause Kansas is going bye-bye."

Brain Drain: Not-So-Reversible Brain Effects of Grains

I discussed how gliadin proteins contribute to the mania of bipolar illness, the paranoia and auditory hallucinations of schizophrenia, and the impaired learning and behavioral outbursts of children with attention deficit disorder and autistic spectrum disorder, phenomena that are reversible or lessened simply by removing grains from the diet. Let's now discuss how grains can also lead to neurological processes that are more difficult, if not impossible, to reverse, though the reasons for their irreversibility are not yet clear.

Intact gliadin initiates a sequence of events that leads to an immune response against brain tissue (for more information, see page 274). Some researchers propose that this represents a form of molecular mimicry in which the immune system confuses a foreign protein (gliadin) with a similarly constructed protein of the body, in this case the synapsin 1 protein of brain tissue.[26] The part of the brain or nervous system involved determines the way in which the damage manifests. For instance, if the cerebellum is affected, the part of the brain responsible for coordination of movement and control over bladder and bowels, a condition called cerebellar ataxia develops. Sufferers stumble while walking and lose control over urine and stool, and an MRI or CT scan of the brain reveals a shrunken, atrophied cerebellum. People become incapacitated with this condition, typically ending up with walkers or in wheelchairs. Eliminating all gliadin-containing proteins from grains will slowly or incompletely reverse cerebellar ataxia, given the slow and often incomplete capacity of neurological tissue to heal.

A condition called peripheral neuropathy, which affects the nerves to the legs, can also develop. Sufferers lose feeling or develop constant leg pain, which ascends higher up the body and worsens over time, eventually resulting in a total loss of feeling and progressive debilitation. It can also involve the internal nervous system of the circulatory and digestive systems. If the vagus nerve to the stomach is affected, for instance, it results in a condition called *gastroparesis*, in which the stomach loses its capacity to propel food forward. While this might seem like an advantage, in that a single meal yields satiety for many hours, it is actually quite destructive because food that sits in the stomach is subject to putrefaction (rotting), causing distress, excessive belching, foul breath, and distortions of bowel flora. (A parallel situation called diabetic gastroparesis can develop in people with advanced diabetes.) If the nerves to the heart are affected, there is a loss of control over heart rate. This leads to a higher resting heart rate and potential for abnormal heart rhythms, such as premature atrial contractions, supraventricular arrhythmias, and atrial fibrillation.

Grains, especially wheat, rye, and barley, can cause seizures. The most common form are temporal lobe seizures (originating in the temporal lobe of the brain) that involve feelings of déjà vu (familiarity), jamais vu (unfamiliarity), amnesia, inappropriate emotions, or pointless repetitive behaviors or tics.[27] Less commonly, generalized or grand mal seizures can also occur due to grain-induced changes in the brain.

Lastly, dementia can result from the consumption of all grains. Wheat, rye, and barley, as usual, are the worst, as recent research has identified antibodies to gluten proteins in the cerebral cortex of the brains of deceased dementia victims.[28] For this reason, Mayo Clinic researchers named this condition *gluten encephalopathy*: dementia from gluten-containing grains. Dementia is much more common, however, as a result of chronic and repeatedly high blood sugars. These are characteristic of all grains, and are also irreversible. The deterioration of gray matter characteristic of dementia is visible on brain imaging as shrinkage of brain volume and loss of the characteristic furrows (called sulci) of healthy human brains, signaling atrophy. We know that diabetics with chronically high blood sugar have a greater risk for dementia. More recent studies demonstrate that blood sugars at the upper end of "normal" are also associated with greater risk for dementia, which is seen on brain imaging as atrophy of the frontal cortex, hippocampus, and amygdala.[29] Accordingly, foods that raise blood sugar the most are associated with the brain atrophy of dementia.

Whole wheat and white flour products raise blood sugar to high levels—even higher than table sugar. Intact corn kernels raise blood sugar to moderately high levels, while cornmeal and cornstarch raise blood sugar to sky-high levels. Grains such as oats, rice, millet, teff, sorghum, rye, and barley raise blood sugar to intermediate to high levels. While they are often described as having a low glycemic index, they would more properly be described as having a *less high* glycemic index, since blood sugars typically rise to the 130 to 200 mg/dl range in nondiabetics (ranges incredibly regarded as "normal" by most health-care practitioners). According to the latest research findings, blood sugars above 100 mg/dl are sufficient to increase the potential for dementia. Because the world is experiencing a massive rise in blood sugars, evidenced by the staggering numbers of people with prediabetes and diabetes, we should anticipate an increase in the number of people with dementia, and we should expect to see it develop earlier in life. This is yet another awful aspect of the widely embraced notion of "healthy whole grains."

Grains, for Crying Out Loud

Irrational fear, anxiousness over the littlest things, anger that bubbles over—all are provoked by the mind-active components of grains. While we know that big, heavy brain issues, such as major depression, bipolar illness, and schizophrenia, are influenced by grains, we see many lesser, though still quite troublesome, emotions and moods caused or amplified by them. These include:

- Aggression
- Anger
- Anxiety
- Inattention
- Indecisiveness
- Insomnia

- Phobias
- Poor impulse control
- Sleep disruption
- Sleepiness
- Suicidal thoughts
- Unhappiness

This means that many people have been plagued by such emotions and thoughts for years, all the while blaming themselves for being weak or flawed. Many resort to prescription antidepressants, anti-anxiety drugs, sleeping pills, drugs for attention deficit disorder, etc., most of which are only partially effective and have substantial side effects. Many have undergone counseling, psychoanalysis, or cognitive behavioral therapy and have endured, cried, felt defeated, lashed out at others, or turned to alcohol and drugs to dull the suffering. Some of the most illustrative stories of the power of grains come from people who have struggled with suicidal thoughts for years, fighting off the impulse to drive a car into oncoming traffic or swallow a bottle of sleeping pills—thoughts that miraculously disappeared within 5 days of having no grains and then abruptly and powerfully returned with any reexposure. On again, off again; on again, off again—incontrovertible proof of individual cause and effect.

There are several ways grains cause mood and emotional effects. While prolamin protein–derived opiates are the culprits in most of these situations, disruption of neuroendocrine hormones, such as vasoactive intestinal peptide, likely plays a role, as well. In addition, the gluten proteins of wheat, rye, and barley and the zein protein of corn have been shown to reduce brain levels of tryptophan,[30] the amino acid that leads to serotonin. Low brain levels of serotonin are associated with depression.

The next time you find yourself yelling at your spouse or kids, feeling unaccountably anxious over a minor problem, struggling to sleep normally, or experiencing some emotional response out of proportion to the situation, question whether the emotionally disruptive effects of grains are at work.

A BIG BELLYFUL OF GRAINS: WHY GRAINS MAKE US FAT

Feed your dog or cat grains in their kibble, and they get fat. Feed your cows and chickens wheat and corn, and they get fat. Feed humans wheat, corn, rice, and other grains, and they get fat.

This ain't rocket science. Nonetheless, conventionally minded nutritionists insist that whole grains cause weight loss. Not true. What the data *really* show is that white flour products cause people to gain weight, and whole grain products cause people to gain a little less weight than white flour does.[31] Whole grains don't make you lose weight any more than drinking a little less vodka makes an alcoholic a little less alcoholic.

The pathways by which grain consumption leads to weight gain, particularly visceral fat of the abdomen, are manifold.

GLIADIN-DERIVED OPIATES STIMULATE APPETITE. Specifically, they stimulate appetite for more grains and sugars: chips, cookies, cupcakes, breads, bagels, pizza. They drive hunger that is physiologically inappropriate, causing you to eat more than your body needs, more frequently and in larger quantities than is necessary for sustenance. In rats administered gliadin-derived fragments, weight increased by 20 percent over 3 months.[32] Block gliadin-derived opiates with opiate blocking drugs, and calorie intake drops by 400 calories per day, whether or not you have an eating disorder.[33] Although obesity in China is not as advanced as that in the Western world, wheat-consuming Chinese are fatter than Chinese who don't consume wheat.[34] The way this works in rats is the way it works in humans, regardless of ethnic origin, color, or political persuasion.

Susceptibility to this effect can vary from individual to individual. It can range from no effect at all to wild, 24-hour-a-day food obsessions, as experienced by some people with bulimia. The effect is most prominent in response to the opiates that derive from wheat, rye, and barley, though corn seems to achieve a similar, though less intense, effect in many people.

AMYLOPECTIN CARBOHYDRATES OF GRAINS RAISE BLOOD SUGAR TO HIGH LEVELS. Anything made of wheat, of course, raises blood sugar to high levels. While whole wheat bread has a GI of 72 (and sucrose has a GI of 59 to 65), there is nothing higher than the GI of cornstarch and rice flour: 90 to 100. High blood sugars are also followed by *low* blood sugars, a response to the release of insulin. Low blood sugars 90 to 120 minutes after consuming grains are experienced as anxiousness, mental cloudiness, irritability, and *hunger*. The blood sugar highs of grains therefore set you up for an inevitable blood sugar low, a 2-hour cycle of satiety and hunger that sends you back out on a quest to find more food.

High blood sugars also result in high insulin responses, which provoke resistance to insulin, higher blood sugars, higher insulin—around and around in a vicious cycle. This leads to a buildup of visceral fat, the sort of fat that is inflammatory and exudes inflammatory proteins into the bloodstream, adding further to poor insulin response. Grains are among the most potent dietary triggers for growth of visceral fat. That's why I've called it a "wheat belly," but we can also call it a "grain belly." Visceral fat cells also express higher levels of cortisol within each fat cell, a situation that mimics that of people with Cushing's disease or who are taking the drug prednisone, both of which are associated with extravagant weight gain.[35]

GRAIN LECTINS BLOCK LEPTIN. Leptin, the hormone of satiety, which is meant to signal us to stop eating after a meal, is blocked by the lectin of wheat, rye, barley, and rice.[36] Humans, or any other animal, for that matter, should experience satiety once physiological needs have been met. But if grain lectins are in the vicinity, they block the signal to stop.

Can you think of any other food that contains opiates that drive appetite, turns off satiety signals, and causes extravagant hyperglycemia and hypoglycemia? If you're wondering why, after cutting fat and eating more "healthy whole grains," you feel like you can't eat enough, have to knock over the other customers in line at the food buffet, or gain weight by doing everything "right," well, you now understand: Whole, white, sprouted, organic, fresh, or stale, grains make you fat.

DIABETES AND PREDIABETES: ANATOMY OF A BLUNDER

Grains cause diabetes. All the flours and products created from the seeds of grasses play major roles in creating the blood sugar disasters that define diabetes and prediabetes.

I'm sure you have heard all the painful statistics about how Americans and the rest of the world are experiencing an epidemic of diabetes: 26 million in the United States have diabetes, and 35 percent of adults over 20 years old have prediabetes. At this rate, one in three Americans are predicted to be diabetic by 2050.[37] It is an epidemic that dwarfs all other epidemics. The International Diabetes Federation reports that 382 million people had diabetes worldwide in 2013, and that number is expected to increase to 592 million by 2035,[38] numbers that make the 1918 flu pandemic and the bubonic plague seem like minor public health nuisances. But unlike the flu and plague, which involved contagious infectious organisms, the diabetes epidemic is *man-made*: It was not created by rapidly evolving viruses or nasty vermin, but by human blundering.

Public health officials lay blame on the public, of course, claiming that we simply eat too much and move too little. They say that the nearly 500 percent increase in the number of diabetics in the United States, from 5.6 million in 1980 to 26 million in 2011, happened because modern Americans, and now much of the rest of the world, are the most gluttonous and lazy populations that ever walked the earth. We're more gluttonous and lazy than we were in 1980, 1990, or 2000, and we've gotten worse every year since.

I don't think so. Take a look at the graph from National Health Survey data reported by the Centers for Disease Control and Prevention (CDC) showing the number of diagnosed diabetics in the United States.

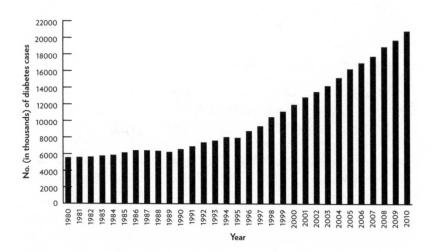

Note that the number of diabetics (represented by vertical bars) began to increase, almost imperceptibly, between 1983 and 1985. This coincides quite nicely with a number of developments.

1. The release of the first Dietary Guidelines for Americans in 1977. Although released in 1977, it took several years of public education before Americans began to adopt advice to cut fat and eat more "healthy whole grains."

2. High-yield, semidwarf strains of wheat, genetically altered by geneticists and agribusiness, were embraced enthusiastically by farmers between 1980 and 1985. By 1985, all wheat products originated with these genetically altered wheats, complete with new gliadin proteins that stimulate appetite. These drove the desire for more food. By the late 1980s, average calorie intake increased by 400 calories per person per day, mostly from snacks and sugary beverages.[39]

3. High-fructose corn syrup, another product of grains, began appearing in processed foods, including many low-fat products.

4. Supermarkets, rather than small neighborhood stores, became the prime retailers of food, particularly products with national brand recognition. Supermarkets stocked shelves with processed foods made with low-cost, commoditized ingredients: wheat flour, cornstarch, high-fructose corn syrup, and sugar. The number of products carried on store shelves ballooned from less than 10,000 before 1980 to 60,000 today.

The Dietary Guidelines for Americans, delivered to us as the USDA MyPyramid and now as MyPlate, tell us that whole grains should comprise a substantial part of our diet, replacing at least half of the processed grains we eat.[40] Based on the flawed notion that replacing something bad (processed white flour products) with something less bad (whole grains) must be good, the essence of their advice is to replace at least some white flour products with whole grains. Of course, not factored into this equation are the high glycemic indexes of *both* white and whole grain products, the changes introduced by agribusiness, and the many people who suffer brain, psychological, and health effects from grain consumption.

When I was in 2nd grade, I started gaining weight.

It wasn't very long before I was the fattest girl in my class. As I got older, I gained more weight. I soon began to hide my eating. I would gulp down big spoonfuls of food out of the pan after I had already eaten the food on my plate. It was a vicious cycle of shame and guilt.

As I reached adulthood, I tried to lose weight. Low-fat, Nutrisystem, a weight-loss clinic: Nothing worked for me because I was starving all the time. I was addicted to wheat- and sugar-based products. Nothing gave me joy like biting into banana nut bread or a doughnut. But then the guilt of not being able to stick with the diet set in. That only made me want to eat more.

Fast-forward to December of 2010. I was 38 years old and I weighed 320 pounds. I had been diabetic since at least 2006. I had the early symptoms of neuropathy. I had hypothyroidism (later diagnosed as Hashimoto's thyroiditis). I had high blood pressure. My face was beet red. People would actually ask me if I had a sunburn. I knew that, if I didn't do something to fix me, I would be dead before I turned 40. Every time I felt a shooting pain in my head or neck, I thought to myself, "Am I getting ready to stroke out? Is this it?" I knew it was coming.

Part of being in denial, especially with diabetes, is that you don't realize what you are doing to your body until you actually feel sick. My diabetes educator told me that I needed 240 grams of carbs a day and to make sure I was eating healthy whole wheat.

I went back to the one thing that I knew had worked for me in the past: low-carb. I was afraid to do it because I had been told it was dangerous, that we needed things like wheat in our diets. It had been so ingrained in me, but I was more afraid of dying.

I removed all grains and sugar from my diet. Within a few days, I was seeing improvements in my blood sugar. The weight was starting to come off. I was feeling really good. But in the back of my mind, I questioned whether this was actually a healthy way of losing weight.

This is where things really clicked in my mind. I set up some accounts with some low-carb support groups. I watched *Fat Head*, read Gary Taubes, and then started reading the *Wheat Belly* blog. I was actually livid. Everything that I had been taught about nutrition was just flat-out wrong! I spent hours a day reading about nutrition, what cholesterol does and what the numbers really mean, and why we actually do not need grain foods in our diets.

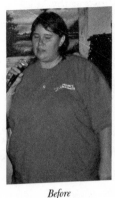
Before

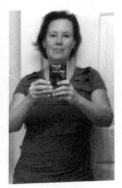
After

There are other things that have cleared up since I've eliminated wheat. I've had irritable bowel syndrome since I was about 5. Gone! I've suffered with acne—gone! Terrible menstrual cycles—I've had regular periods since the first month I was off of wheat. I've always had a really addictive type of personality. My addictions are gone! I've been able to pass this information on to my children. They are all teenagers now: 14, 16, and almost 18. My hope for them is that they won't have to struggle like I have.

Tami, Youngsville, North Carolina

Recall that most of the components of the seeds of grasses are poorly digestible or indigestible—except for amylopectin A. Amylopectin A's unique branching structure makes it highly digestible by the enzyme amylase, found in saliva and your stomach, and yields sharp increases in blood glucose. The amylopectin A of grains is so efficiently digested that, gram for gram, it raises blood sugar higher than table sugar does. This is why two slices of whole wheat bread raise blood sugar higher than 6 teaspoons of table sugar. Other starchy foods, such as tubers (beans, yams, cassava) and legumes, have amylopectins B and C, which are less efficiently digested. Accordingly, grains, refined or whole, are either high GI foods or less-high GI foods. The GI of nearly all grain-based foods ranges from 40 to 100, values that are more than sufficient to raise blood sugar to high levels.[41] (The only exceptions are barley-based breads, which can have a GI as low as 27.)

To be sure, the diabetes and prediabetes epidemics are attributable to more than increasing reliance on the seeds of grasses. The proliferation of sugar, high-fructose corn syrup, sweetened soft drinks, and soft drinks sweetened with aspartame (which, like grain lectins, shuts off leptin),[42] as well as increased exposure to endocrine disruptive industrial chemicals all have played roles. But what other food enjoys the hearty endorsement of all government agencies and dietitians? While agencies such as the USDA and FDA may not condemn products like sugary soft drinks or canned foods containing BPA, they certainly don't tell us to drink or eat as much of these as we can—but they sure do tell us to eat plenty of "healthy whole grains."

The GI potential of grains raises blood sugar, and by a process called *glucotoxicity*, high blood sugars damage the delicate and vulnerable pancreatic beta cells that produce insulin. While type 1 diabetes develops because of an immune reaction that destroys pancreatic beta cells, type 2 (noninsulin dependent) diabetes can be hastened by glucotoxicity. This is why, by the time someone is diagnosed with diabetes, 75 percent or fewer functioning pancreatic beta cells remain, 25 percent or more having succumbed to glucotoxicity.[43] And the effects go even deeper: High blood sugars also result in greater triglyceride production in the liver, the process of *de novo lipogenesis*, or the creation of fats (triglycerides) from sugars. The high levels of blood triglycerides that are typical in grain-consuming people—often 200, 300, 500 or more mg/dl, compared to an ideal level of 60 mg/dl or less seen in primitive cultures and grain-free people—are sufficient to exert a toxic effect on pancreatic beta cells, a process called *lipotoxicity*.[44]

A diet rich in "healthy whole grains" is the perfect formula for creating diabetes. The diabetes epidemic in the United States and world is to be expected; it's developing precisely as you would predict after encouraging *Homo sapiens* to consume as much of the seeds of grasses as possible.

GRAINS: A SEX CRIME

Nothing is out-of-bounds when it comes to the health perturbations inflicted upon humans by grains—not even sex. Sex hormones make women, women and men, men. Grains enter the picture and distinctions begin to blur. It starts with the accumulation of visceral fat, which leads to bizarre shifts in sex hormones.

Visceral fat is peculiar stuff. The recent discovery that the cells of visceral fat express higher levels of cortisol explains why people with accumulated visceral fat look like people who have Cushing's disease (caused by an adrenal gland tumor) or who have taken high doses of the steroid drug prednisone. The difference is that people with Cushing's have high blood levels of cortisol provoking these effects, while people with visceral fat have high levels of cortisol within their fat cells.[45] The excess cortisol of visceral fat can result in testosterone-like effects in women, such as thicker mustache hair, even though cortisol is not a sex hormone. But that's just the start.

Visceral fat in men expresses greater aromatase enzyme activity, which converts testosterone to estradiol, an estrogen. This results in lower testosterone levels and higher estrogen levels,[46] which lead to loss of muscle mass, feminization of body contours, loss of libido, and reduced capacity for achieving erections. Prolactin, a hormone charged with many duties (including breast enlargement; think "pro" plus "lactation"), also increases, worsened by grain exorphins.[47] The combined effects of high estrogen and high prolactin cause breast tissue to grow, causing embarrassing "man breasts."[48] If celiac disease is present, men can experience severely reduced testosterone levels (hypogonadism), failure to develop male characteristics (if the condition is experienced during puberty), and reduced fertility, while others experience increased testosterone but a peculiar unresponsiveness to the hormone.[49]

In women, increases in weight bring even larger increases in the activity of aromatase, which results in dramatically increased blood and tissue levels of estrogens.[50] The higher levels of estrogens in women increase their risk for breast and endometrial cancer by several times.[51] Unlike men, women develop *high* testosterone evidenced by thicker mustaches, acne, and darkening of skinfolds (acanthosis nigricans). Just as in men, women develop higher levels of prolactin that result in more fat deposition in fat cells, stimulate food intake, and make the breasts grow larger.[52] While some may view larger breasts as a desirable trait, this unnatural form of breast enlargement is associated with an increased breast cancer risk.[53] Women with higher blood sugar levels, greater body weight, and the larger waist size associated with visceral fat also experience sexual dysfunction, such as decreased libido and increased difficulty with sexual performance.[54]

Unnatural things happen when you eat something unnatural, and that can have an impact on fertility and pregnancy. You've heard of fertility rites; I call the effect exerted by grains "fertility wrongs." If you thought adolescence was the height of hormonal turmoil, you haven't come to appreciate the effects of grains on fertility. At least puberty, as tumultuous as it can be, is a normal and necessary process we go through to get to reproductive maturity. There's nothing normal or necessary about the havoc wreaked by grain consumption, and people are often surprised to hear just how much it can muck up hormonal status, fertility, and pregnancy.

As in many other aspects of grain consumption, celiac disease serves as a model. (This does not mean that *only* people with celiac disease develop these effects; it means that celiac disease represents one end of a spectrum.) Women with celiac disease experience fivefold more amenorrhea (absence of menstrual cycles) and a higher frequency of miscarriages (often recurrent), infertility, and premature menopause. In pregnant women with celiac disease who are not yet on a corrective diet, there is a high risk for abnormalities of the newborn, especially in utero growth retardation, low birth weight, and premature delivery. But grains can also disrupt pregnancy and fertility in women without celiac disease, usually via an autoimmune response expressed as abnormal antibodies, especially the gliadin antibody.[55] This can result in infertility and repeated miscarriages. Women who experience repeated pregnancy losses can also test positive for antibodies against phospholipids (a condition called antiphospholipid antibody syndrome) and nuclear antigens (antinuclear antibodies), which are expressions of autoimmune diseases such as lupus. We know that the initiating event in many of these instances is grain consumption. Overweight or obese women with the increased visceral fat of habitual grain consumption are threefold as likely as normal weight women to have disrupted menstrual cycles and infertility, and higher risk for miscarriage.[56] Infertility begins to express itself in women with body mass indexes (BMIs) as low as 23.9, with rates of infertility increasing as BMI increases. For a 5-foot, 5-inch woman, the risk would begin at a body weight of 144 pounds or greater.[57] Even children are not spared from visceral fat's effects: Newborns of overweight and obese women are also prone to experience abnormalities such as high birth weight, which leads to a lifetime risk of diabetes and obesity. The entire situation occurs to an exaggerated degree in women with polycystic ovarian syndrome (PCOS), who are more likely to be overweight or obese and have disrupted menstrual cycles, higher levels of testosterone, and reduced fertility.[58] Due to visceral fat, women with PCOS also experience increased levels of testosterone that are often sufficient for a woman to develop masculinizing features, such as facial hair.[59]

So, yes: Your morning ritual of cornflakes or a raisin bran muffin keeps company with other sex crimes, sordid, unsavory, and shameful, but gleefully endorsed by those in the business of handing out conventional dietary advice.

HEART-HEALTHY CIGARETTES, SOFT DRINKS, AND GRAINS

The notion of "heart-healthy grains" makes about as much sense as "heart-healthy cigarettes" or "heart-healthy soft drinks." Stay with me now, as the pathway that leads to increased heart disease risk after consumption of grains is a bit complicated. But once you understand, you will see that "healthy whole grains" should really be called "heart disease–causing grains." Grains are *not* the heart-healthy heroes they are commonly painted to be. (The fallacies of high cholesterol and its relationship to these grains are also discussed in more detail in Chapter 10.)

The heart disease story behind grains begins with the same amylopectin A that not only sends blood sugar through the roof, but is also converted to triglycerides by the liver process of de novo lipogenesis, as discussed above. Some triglycerides are released into the bloodstream, seen as increased very low-density lipoprotein (called VLDL, these are fat-carrying proteins) particles and evident on a cholesterol panel as increased triglyceride levels, while others are retained in the liver, leading over time to nonalcoholic liver disease or fatty liver. Typically, grain consumers have triglyceride levels above the ideal range (60 mg/dl or less) and not uncommonly associated with mild increases in liver enzyme values, AST and ALT, often seen on screening blood tests, reflecting fat accumulation within the liver. Higher triglyceride values also lead to degradation of "good" HDL particles, resulting in lower values for HDL cholesterol on a cholesterol panel.

Excessive quantities of triglyceride-containing VLDL particles that result from plentiful amylopectin A intake from grains are released into the bloodstream and interact with LDL particles, reducing their size—an abnormal situation that is not supposed to occur.[60] Small LDL particles are poorly recognized by the liver and therefore stick around for several *days*, compared to the 24 hours or less of large LDL particles. These small particles are enthusiastically taken up by inflammatory cells that line arteries and are also more prone to glycation (eight times more than large LDL particles) and oxidation. Glycated, oxidized, persistent, and adherent, small LDL particles cause atherosclerotic plaque to grow, increasing heart attack risk and the need for procedures like heart catheterization, angioplasty, and stents.[61]

The wheat germ agglutinin (WGA) protein found in grains also plays a role in cultivating atherosclerosis. Because this highly inflammatory protein can gain access to the bloodstream, WGA activates a growth factor called endothelial growth factor-1, or EGF-1. This growth factor stimulates growth of the cells lining artery walls; stimulates growth of smooth muscle cells of arteries, a fundamental process underlying atherosclerosis; and activates cell adhesion and platelets, which lead to blood clot formation.[62]

The typical profile of someone at greater risk for heart disease from grain consumption therefore includes lower HDL cholesterol values, typically ranging from 30 to 50 mg/dl; triglycerides of 100 mg/dl or higher; and greater quantities of small LDL particles. Susceptibility to glycation can be indirectly gauged by the common HbA1c value used to assess long-term blood sugar fluctuations, as this value reflects the rate of glycation of hemoglobin that parallels the glycation of small LDL particles.

The epidemiologic studies that have attempted to support the argument that whole grains prevent heart disease do no such thing. These studies demonstrate that, as whole grains replace white flour products, there is indeed reduced risk for heart disease, as well as less diabetes, less weight gain, and less colon cancer—no argument. But remember: Less bad is not necessarily good. When we remove grains entirely, however, impressive changes can be observed in the markers that signify heart disease risk: A dramatic reduction in triglycerides and VLDL, increases in HDL, and a plummeting number of small LDL particles are accompanied by reductions in blood pressure and inflammation, loss of inflammatory visceral fat, and reduced glycation. Unfortunately, the flagrant distortions introduced by generous grain consumption do nothing to temper the enthusiasm with which agencies like the American Heart Association and the USDA aggressively push advice to consume whole grains for heart health.

Beyond atherosclerosis and heart attack risk, the prolamin proteins of wheat, rye, and barley have also been shown to impair heart muscle function. Very few factors are capable of seriously impairing heart muscle strength; among such causes are viral infections, extreme alcohol intake, heart attacks with heart muscle damage . . . and grains. In its most extreme expression, grain's destructive effects on heart muscle can be expressed as myocarditis (heart muscle inflammation) that can result in dilated cardiomyopathy, a condition in which the heart muscle is severely impaired, which can cause congestive heart failure and death. One recent analysis of patients with myocarditis showed that 7 percent had abnormal antibodies against wheat.[63] Once it's damaged by, say, a heart attack, the heart muscle is not very good at recovering—unless that damage is caused by grain consumption, in which case it can fully recover.[64]

WHEEZY, ITCHY, SCRATCHY: ASTHMA AND ALLERGIES

Having been an asthma and allergy sufferer for many years, I know all too well the feeling of "air hunger," the breathless desperation of struggling just to walk several feet, as well as the annoyance of an itching, nonstop runny nose and itchy eyes. Since going grain-free, I am free of it all, and I have witnessed similar recoveries in countless people.

Asthma and allergies are largely reactions to various proteins in our environment, foods, cosmetics, toiletries, and other substances we come into contact with. Allergies are common and are increasing worldwide; food allergies, atopic dermatitis and eczema, allergic rhinitis (sinus drainage and congestion), and asthma now affect 6 million American children alone.[65] Since 1985, the frequency of asthma, allergic rhinitis, and eczema has doubled or tripled.[66] How much of this explosion in allergic phenomena can be blamed on grains, and how much can be blamed on agribusiness, which busily fusses with the genetics of grain proteins? Right now, we don't have adequate data to assign blame—just plenty of suspicious associations.

We know that people who come into frequent contact with grains through their work develop allergic and immune reactions with uncommon frequency. Bakers, confectioners, pastry factory workers, people in the milling industry, grain farmers, and cereal handlers in food preparation inhale grain dust and thereby have a high incidence of a form of asthma known as baker's asthma. This condition is caused by the omega gliadins and other proteins in wheat, rye, and barley.[67] Also, 50 percent of grain elevator workers experience allergic phenomena of the skin, sinuses, eyes, and throat when exposed to grains, including oats and barley.[68] If you work with grains, there is a high likelihood that you will develop an abnormal allergic or immune response to one or more of their proteins.

While it is clear that exposure to the allergens in grains causes many, if not most, people to develop some form of allergic response to them, it is not clear just what proportion of *nongrain* allergies are brought on by grains. Based on my experience, I believe it to be a substantial proportion.

Allergic responses to grains can occur in infants and children but can be very difficult to recognize, as they can manifest as vomiting, diarrhea or other changes in bowel movements, colic, change in mood, or failure to thrive (slowed or poor weight gain and growth), none of which point specifically to grains.[69] Diagnostic testing can confidently identify one grain or another as an allergic trigger, as skin testing with the various grains can be performed.

We know that agribusiness has been tweaking the genetics, and thereby changing the protein products, of grains through genetic modification, chemical mutagenesis, and various hybridization methods. What we don't know is whether such changes can be blamed for the widespread surge in allergies and asthma that coincides perfectly with such efforts. But this apple is starting to smell awfully rotten. We discuss the prospects of relief from asthma and allergies further in Chapter 6.

GRAINS GET UNDER YOUR SKIN

Grains are perfect disrupters of skin health. Their prolamins trigger autoimmune skin reactions and turn antibodies against skin enzymes, their lectins fan the fires of inflammation, their proteins provoke allergies, and their amylopectins send blood sugar and insulin sky-high and provoke the skin-disrupting hormone insulin-like growth factor-1 (IGF).[70] The whole grain package adds up to an impressive collection of skin conditions that can take a variety of forms, from simple red, itchy rashes to scaly, oily raised patches to large vesicles to gangrene. Because hair and nails are part of the skin, they, too, can be involved. Among the most common skin conditions attributable to grains are:

ACNE. Acne is a nearly universal problem in modern teenagers—and adults. In contrast, it is virtually unknown in primitive societies. Kitavan Islanders from Papua New Guinea and Aché hunter-gatherers from Paraguay experienced no acne when observed over a period of 3 years.[71] It's believed that acne is provoked by foods that trigger insulin and the hormone IGF.[72] All grains raise blood sugar, and thereby insulin and IGF, to high levels, so they all share the capacity to create facial havoc. Sugary foods, such as soft drinks and candy, also trigger insulin and IGF and can therefore share the blame, as can the whey protein of dairy products that is unique among dairy components in its capacity to trigger insulin and IGF.[73] Repetitive high blood sugars lead to repetitive high insulin and IGF, which causes progressive resistance to insulin, leading to higher levels of insulin and IGF. Round and round, it's the perfect setup for acne.

Just as the bowel flora of someone with, say, irritable bowel syndrome is different, so the skin bacteria of acne sufferers are also different. In acne sufferers, *Propionibacterium acnes* and other species thrive, suggesting that something changed the microbial habitat of their skin and allowed emergence of species that trigger acne.

SEBORRHEA. This common red rash typically occurs along the sides of the nose and on the eyebrows, chest, back, and scalp (where it is called dandruff), and it is caused by the *Malassezia* fungus.[74] Interestingly, the same fungus populates the skin of most humans, even if they don't have seborrhea. The relationship between grains and seborrhea is exceptionally consistent and predictable. Seborrhea is common in grain consumers; it is uncommon for seborrhea to fail to improve or completely disappear with wheat elimination. In fact, I will go so far as to say that seborrhea, especially along both sides of the nose, is *the* signature skin rash of grain consumption, especially wheat, rye, and barley. Typically, seborrheic rashes improve or disappear within a few days of grain elimination.

PSORIASIS. Psoriasis is an annoying and sometimes disfiguring rash that most commonly occurs on the elbows, knees, scalp, and back. Psoriasis typically takes the form of raised red plaques with a white sheen and covers a large area, though a number of other forms can occur. Conventional treatment usually involves steroid creams; the use of drugs typically reserved for cancer, such as methotrexate; immunosuppressive agents, such as cyclosporine; and nasty (and costly) intravenous agents such as etanercept and infliximab. Treatment can go on for years, even decades, and is plagued by incomplete responses. Psoriasis can be yet another form of immune reaction to fragments of gliadin and other grain prolamin proteins, with lesser responses provoked by the amylase inhibitor proteins.[75] While psoriasis has also been associated with celiac disease, it can occur without celiac disease and can be associated with an increased likelihood of a positive (IgA) antibody to gliadin.[76] Wheat germ agglutinin (WGA) blocks vasoactive intestinal peptide (VIP), permitting the skin inflammation of psoriasis to emerge.[77] A diet absent wheat, rye, and barley has been shown to be effective in improving psoriasis, particularly in people with higher levels of the IgA antibody to gliadin.[78] The Wheat Belly experience has provided relief to countless psoriasis sufferers, the majority of whom enjoy improvement or complete relief from their rashes, though it sometimes takes months to achieve (compared to the much more rapid response in cases of seborrhea).

ECZEMA. The term *eczema* is applied to a wide range of rashes that are typically red, itchy, and raised and can occur anywhere on the body. Eczematous rashes are common; one third of the world's population have experienced or will experience an episode at some time in their lives. It is an especially common problem in children, with 30 percent of preschool children and 15 to 20 percent of school kids having eczematous rashes.[79] Eczematous rashes have doubled or tripled between 1995 and 2008.[80] Because eczematous rashes are, to some degree, driven by allergic processes, other allergic phenomena typically accompany eczema, such as asthma, allergic rhinitis and sinus congestion, acid reflux, eosinophilic esophagitis (esophageal inflammation), infantile colic, and allergic enterocolitis (small intestinal and colon inflammation).

People with celiac disease are three times more prone to eczema than people without celiac disease, while relatives of people with celiac disease (who don't have celiac disease themselves) are twice as prone.[81] Because eczema is common outside of celiac disease, there is no shortage of wild theories that blame this chronic, annoying, and sometimes disfiguring condition on everything from dust mites to neurosis to excessive cleanliness. As with any condition that is common and "unexplained," we should always ask whether consumption of the seeds of grasses might be at fault. Eczema has indeed been associated with various foods, including peanuts, dairy, soy, fish, and eggs, as well as grains. Wheat, rye, and barley contain a smorgasbord of proteins that have been associated with eczema, asthma, and other forms of allergies.[82] It remains unclear just what proportion of people with eczema can blame grains. Judging by the number of people who report relief from eczematous rashes within 5 to 7 days of giving up wheat and/or all grains, the effect wheat has upon this condition is substantial.

RECURRENT APHTHOUS STOMATITIS. This mouthful of a disease, known more commonly as mouth ulcers or canker sores, can range from a minor annoyance to a debilitating condition that's sometimes so painful that it interferes with eating and speaking. This condition is really a mixture of responses triggered by different causes, and there is an increased incidence in people with celiac disease. However, the gliadin and related proteins of grains are among the causes, and a surprising proportion of non-celiac sufferers experience relief from adopting a wheat-, rye-, and barley-free diet.[83]

The number of skin conditions caused by grain consumption are simply too numerous to list and detail here, literally numbering in the hundreds and taking on such myriad shapes and forms as bullous pemphigoid, IgA linear dermatosis, prurigo nodularis, atopic dermatitis, palmoplantar pustulosis, generalized acquired cutis laxa, and hundreds more. This is not to say that *all* skin conditions are caused by grains, but an astounding proportion of them are. And what other potential cause is so easy to correct, no nasty oral or intravenous drugs required, while providing an impressive list of other health gains?

LOOK THAT UP IN YOUR *FUNK AND WAGNALLS*

You're not going to find it in any nutrition text, nor in any medical textbook. You won't hear it from the majority of dietitians, physicians, nor mainstream weight-loss programs. But as a society, we've been duped, big-time. We've been persuaded that the foods of desperation, foods that allow large-scale commoditization of the world's diet, foods that impair health in both their worst and their best forms, were meant to serve as the centerpiece of diet. When we strip away the hype, the glamour, the thinly veiled "scientific" arguments, we find the profiteering, market positioning, blundering (at best), and lies (at worst) that have come to dominate nutritional thinking.

It is important to recognize all the health effects of grain consumption because we are really describing the chronic health problems of modern society. Now let's discuss what happens to members of the species *Homo sapiens* who return to our glorious grain-free roots.

PART II

LIVING GRAINLESSLY

Restoring the
Natural State of
Human Life

CHAPTER 6

GRAINLESS LIFE: BEGINNINGS

All great change in America begins at the dinner table.
—Ronald Reagan

IF YOU HAVEN'T already done so, brace yourself for some changes—
big changes. Hitch up your pants, smooth your skirt, tell the kids to keep
quiet, buy the in-laws a round-trip ticket to Sarasota, and strap yourself
firmly into your chair, because you are about to embark on a whirlwind
process that will take your mind and body through changes that will
transform your life.

If you are new to the *Wheat Belly* message, you will learn that grain
elimination ranks right up there with other life-changing events, such as
birth, puberty, marriage, and parenthood. This is not just improvement
in nutrition or a new spin on low-carb dieting meant to help you fit into
the skinny jeans stored in your closet since 1997. Nor is it the equivalent
of crossing sugary soft drinks off your grocery list to shed the sugar
weight. Nope—nothing of the kind. It is no exaggeration to say that for
many, if not most, people, eliminating grains changes their lives.

If you are a seasoned wheat-free enthusiast familiar with the arguments made in *Wheat Belly*, you'll find that in this chapter I expand the
discussion, casting a wider net and explaining why eliminating grains
beyond wheat yields even greater effects and why understanding the
full head-to-toe impact of prior grain consumption is necessary. I will
discuss all the wonderful and empowering strategies that I did not talk
about in *Wheat Belly*—strategies that will give you the best chance of
regaining something as close to total, ideal health as possible. The

benefits begin when you push away your last muffin or bag of pretzels, but they extend further than you can imagine. Yes, grain elimination is the first crucial step, but there are other steps to climb to regain control over as many aspects of your health as humanly possible. This is about diverting your life down a new course that changes the way you think, how you feel, the way you look, how easily and painlessly you move, the drugs you take or don't take, the health conditions you develop or don't develop, the way you age, the way you die, and when it happens. This nutritional path allows you to revert to the lifestyle that your body was intended to follow, unmasking the adaptations of the last 2.5 million years. Yes, as a modern expression of *Homo sapiens*, you may harbor an adaptation or two that are part of the 10,000-year effort to accommodate grain consumption, but even so your body will breathe, digest, move, and think more easily minus the disruptive effects of grains.

The consequences of removing grains from your life are so profound because grains never belonged there in the first place. Put aside the trickery of taste and accept the truth: Humans and grains are incompatible. It's okay to grow a lawn with them, feed them to your goats, use them to thatch a roof, or collect them for compost, but it's not okay to eat them. The seeds of grasses provide sustenance when nothing better is available, but when consumed chronically, they disrupt health at so many levels that it should come as no surprise that health and lives become unrecognizably better when they are removed. When you stop consuming grains, your body will need to readjust. Liberated from the poisonous and destructive effects of grains, however, you will rediscover what health *truly* looks and feels like.

What happens to the body when we remove the seeds of grasses? It starts with a common withdrawal process. Stop eating tomatoes and there is no withdrawal process. Stop eating olives, pork rinds, or eggplant, and there is no nausea, malaise, or headache. Cease the sugary snacks and soft drinks and you might miss them, but there is no withdrawal, no mind and few body readjustments to make. Stop wheat and related grains and all metabolic hell can break loose, including very distinct withdrawal symptoms.

OXYCONTIN, METHADONE, AND BREAKFAST CEREAL

It's important to understand and recognize right from the very start that once you stop consuming the seeds of grasses and their unique components, you may experience a withdrawal process. Someone addicted to heroin, morphine, or Oxycontin will, when their supply of the drug dries up, experience anxiety, nausea, sweating, dysphoria (dark moods), muscle aches, abdominal cramps, vomiting, diarrhea, and headache. It is a predictable and unpleasant process. A similar process occurs after you've bid farewell to your last bit of wheat, rye, barley, and corn, but it is a process that must be endured for you to reclaim health. Like a gangrenous limb, healing can proceed only once it has been removed.

Grain withdrawal has been given a variety of names over the years: detoxification, Atkin's flu, Paleo flu, and low-carb flu, to name a few. Because this only happens with various forms of carbohydrate restriction (there is no corresponding "low-fat flu" or "low-calorie flu"), it has often been attributed to deprivation of sugars from carbohydrates and a temporary inability of the body to convert energy from fat stores. This is indeed partly true and can account for up to several weeks of low energy. This phase of withdrawal is due to the absence of readily digested carbohydrates, the amylopectins of grains, which causes your body to obtain energy from fat stores. This process is called *mitochondrial fatty acid beta oxidation*, which refers to the cellular reaction required to convert fat stores to energy. The cellular apparatus for "burning" fat operated at a low level while a constant flow of grain amylopectins was present, but it now has a high demand placed on it, and it will take 4 to 6 weeks to reach peak capacity. Once this occurs, you'll feel a surge in energy and an ability to engage in vigorous activity, as well as weight loss from fat stores.[1] Your aerobic capacity at this point will *exceed* what it was prior to this shift in energy source—an important performance issue for athletes, in particular.

But how do we explain the depression, emotional outbursts, and dark thoughts that ensue within hours to days of your last bagel? How do we account for the nausea, intensive grain cravings, dehydration, and light-headedness that plague you for days after your last sandwich? What about the muscle cramps, bloating, constipation, headache, and intensification of joint pain—effects not attributable to hypoglycemia or poor mobilization of energy? And why, once withdrawal is over, does an entire constellation of symptoms *recur* with reexposure to wheat, barley, rye, or corn? Whether intentional or inadvertent, ingesting grain after getting through withdrawal will bring on diarrhea, bloating, joint pain, mind fog, ravenous appetite, headaches, depression, and suicidal thoughts—none of which can be blamed on sugar or an inadequate flow of fatty acids.

When the consumption of wheat and its closely related prolamin protein sources (rye, barley, and corn) ceases, there is a withdrawal process from gliadin-, secalin-, hordein-, and zein-derived opiate-like peptides that almost seems to *punish* you for removing them, making your life miserable for a time. Typically, people experience incapacitating fatigue, nausea, headache, and depression that lasts for 5 days, though it can last as little as a day or as long as several weeks. Not everyone experiences withdrawal, though the 40 percent of people who do describe a miserable experience that disrupts lives, annoys family and friends, impairs performance at school and work, and causes them to miss karaoke night at the pub. They report that it's not too different from having a case of self-induced influenza. But everyone survives.

It is important that you recognize grain withdrawal for what it is. Some people will say, "I feel awful. It must mean that I *need* grains." Don't fall into that trap: It is a withdrawal syndrome, a process necessary to undo the effects of addiction. Those awful feelings you have rumbling in your bowels, and those dark thoughts and emotions? Yup: That's how your brain and body say goodbye to the effects of the seeds of grasses. Ignore the advice to "listen to your body," if it's interpreted to mean that grains are somehow necessary for your body to function. This is nonsense. There is nothing beneficial in grains that cannot be readily obtained from other foods.

Because it is a form of opiate withdrawal, the grain withdrawal process cannot be avoided. Similarly, an alcoholic who wishes to rid her life of alcohol can only do so by stopping the flow of bourbon and beer and suffering the withdrawal consequences—there's no way around it. Alcohol withdrawal phenomena, such as hallucinations, disorientation, and seizures, can be partially blunted with high doses of benzodiazepine drugs (e.g., lorazepam) and other prescription agents. Likewise, people who want to quit cigarettes must stop smoking, and their cravings can also be blunted with drugs, but the irritability, nausea, and other withdrawal phenomena cannot be avoided and must be endured to rid their bodies of the effects. The body adjusts to the constant flow of chemicals, whether from alcohol, cigarettes, or grain; remove these chemicals and the body's physiology needs to readjust.

> *"The first day was the most difficult,*
> *recognizing the full-blown addiction. Each*
> *day was easier; by day 3: no desire.*

> *"I had low-grade flulike symptoms*
> *(headache, nausea) for about a week,*
> *diminishing a little each day.*
> *The desire for wheat diminished as*
> *the ability to resist increased."*

> —TERESA, ANNAPOLIS, MD

Just as an alcoholic can stop the tremors, paranoia, and hallucinations of alcohol withdrawal with a calming shot of whiskey or a wannabe non-smoker can quell the out-of-control anxiety and nausea of withdrawal with a few puffs on a cigarette, so you can turn off the process of grain withdrawal by consuming any wheat, rye, barley, or corn product. But you'll also halt your return to health, and you'll have to start the process all over again, suffering all of the same symptoms. The entire process of withdrawal, thankfully, can be partially softened by a number of strategies that we discuss next.

GRAIN WITHDRAWAL: SMOOTH THE TRANSITION

You are facing the prospect of withdrawal, a tumultuous physical and emotional storm. This can be terrifying, especially now that you know that it can involve fatigue, nausea, anxiety, headache, light-headedness, leg cramps, and depression, as well as powerful cravings for the foods you are avoiding. Many people have had a small taste of this syndrome after brief lapses in grain intake, though they probably didn't recognize it as grain withdrawal, often dismissing the anxiety and headache, for instance, as the effects of hunger, impending flu, or marital annoyances. But with the complete removal of grains from your diet, those feelings are going to persist.

Is there an emotional electroshock therapy that might zap you out of this experience, an antidote to this opiate, a laxative that purges the poison, *anything* you can do to smooth the grain withdrawal syndrome?

Yes, there is. Nothing completely ablates the experience, but you can soften the blow. Here are a few strategies.

CHOOSE A NONSTRESSFUL PERIOD TO EXPERIENCE WITHDRAWAL. If you have the luxury of managing your time, choose a period when you don't anticipate high stress. Don't choose, for instance, the week an annoying mother-in-law is planning to visit, the start of a new and challenging project at work, or the week before your dissertation is due. Ideally, choose a long weekend or vacation. And pamper yourself a bit: Watch movies, laugh, enjoy a glass of wine, lie in the sun, get a massage. Like a bad hangover, this will pass.

DON'T EXERCISE. Don't torture yourself by exercising—and don't feel guilty for *not* exercising during this process. At most, do something at a leisurely pace: Go for a walk in the woods or neighborhood, or take a casual bike ride. But it would be counterproductive to force yourself to jog, bike hard, or strength train, as the effort will make you feel worse.

HYDRATE. The precipitous drop in insulin caused by removing grains also reverses the sodium retention of wheat and grain consumption,[2] causing fluid loss (diuresis) and a reduction in inflammation. If you don't compensate by hydrating more than usual over the first few days, you may experience light-headedness, nausea, and leg cramps. (If you're hydrated, your urine should be nearly clear, not a dark, concentrated yellow.) A great habit to start the day right is to drink 16 ounces (2 cups) of water immediately upon awakening, since we awake dehydrated after lying supine and mouth breathing for 8 or so hours.

USE SOME SALT. Specifically, sprinkle sea salt or another mineral-containing salt on your food to compensate for the loss of urinary salt that develops due to the drop in insulin levels. Salt, along with water, addresses the light-headedness and leg cramps that commonly occur during withdrawal. (On page 152, we will discuss why strict sodium restriction is a bad idea for most people, but know that it is especially bad during grain withdrawal, as it can result in extreme light-headedness or even passing out.)

SUPPLEMENT WITH MAGNESIUM. Magnesium deficiency is widespread and is associated with osteoporosis, hypertension, higher blood sugar, muscle cramps, and heart rhythm disorders. Magnesium deficiency is common, especially in people who have consumed grains for a long period of time, and it can magnify some of the symptoms of withdrawal from grains, particularly leg cramps and sleep disruptions. Magnesium supplementation can have dramatic benefits during wheat withdrawal, but unfortunately, most magnesium supplements are better laxatives than they are sources of absorbable magnesium. Among the best absorbed is magnesium malate at a dose of 1,200 milligrams (mg) two or three times per day. (This is the weight of the magnesium plus the malate, not just "elemental" magnesium; this provides 180 mg of elemental magnesium per 1,200-mg tablet or capsule.) Another way to get supplemental magnesium is to make your own magnesium bicarbonate, the most absorbable form. Because it is very hygroscopic (water-absorbent), no manufacturer sells it in dry form, so you have to make it yourself. (See page 341 for directions.)

CONSUME FATS, OILS, AND PROTEINS LIBERALLY. Do what your grandmother did and eat the skin and dark meat on your chicken, and ask for the liver. Don't remove the fat from your steak or pork—eat it, instead, and again, ask for the liver. Save the bones and boil them for soup or stock (see page 333), and don't skim off the fat or gelatin when it cools. Add olive oil and coconut oil to anything and everything you can, even eggs, soup, and vegetables. Have lots of avocados, which are full of fat, and put them in your smoothies. Don't limit your egg consumption; have a three-egg omelet, for instance, with extra-virgin olive oil, pesto, or olive oil–soaked sun-dried tomatoes. Loading up on fats helps eliminate cravings by inducing satiety. Remember: Fat consumption does not make you fat, nor does it cause heart disease. Bury that bit of nonsense with the "healthy whole grain" fiction.

TAKE A PROBIOTIC. Try 30 to 50 billion CFUs (colony forming units, the method used to quantify bacterial numbers) or more per day, and look for a supplement containing mixed species of *Lactobacillus* and *Bifidobacteria*. As you shop, you will recognize that this is a high dose that's provided by only a handful of products; however, this number actually represents a small percentage of the total number of bacteria residing in your gastrointestinal tract. So while fermented sources of healthy bacteria (such as yogurt, kimchi, or kombucha) can be modestly helpful long-term, they are insufficient in the special situation of grain withdrawal, during which rapid repopulation with a broad range of species is desired.

Taking a high-potency probiotic accelerates colonization by healthy bowel flora once the disruptive effects of bowel-toxic grains are absent. This addresses the bloating and constipation that typically accompany grain withdrawal, with relief usually occurring within 24 hours of initiation of the probiotic. You shouldn't need to take probiotics for more than 8 weeks, since the idea is to repopulate your gut with healthy bacterial species after the grains have been removed. (If symptoms such as heartburn or bloating return when probiotics are stopped, this suggests that something else is wrong, such as an issue with the pancreas or with insufficient stomach acid, etc., which may require a formal assessment, or at least a more prolonged course of probiotic supplementation. More on this later.) Among the best probiotic brands are VSL#3, Garden of Life, and Renew Life. A full program for restoration of bowel health through management of bowel flora goes farther than just taking a probiotic supplement and is discussed in Chapter 9.

SUPPLEMENT IODINE. Marginal iodine deficiency is common, particularly in people who avoid using iodized salt.[3] Ironically, the more you avoid processed foods (as we do with grain elimination), the less iodized salt you get. Avid exercisers are also more iodine deficient than average, due to iodine losses via sweat.[4] Iodine deficiency has gotten so bad that I have been finding people with goiters (enlarged thyroid glands due to iodine deficiency) that are reminiscent of the disfiguring protuberant masses that used to plague people in the early 20th century. There was a time when we only saw pictures of these in *National Geographic*, but now they're coming to a mall or school near you.

Even a modest lack of iodine leads to lower output of thyroid hormones, resulting in mild hypothyroidism sufficient to impair weight loss, make fatigue worse, increase LDL cholesterol and triglyceride values, and increase cardiovascular risk. I advise patients to supplement iodine with inexpensive drops, capsules, or kelp tablets (dried seaweed) at a dosage of 500 micrograms (mcg) per day, which is more than the Recommended Daily Allowance (RDA) of 150 mcg per day and, I believe, closer to the ideal intake. Also, see the extended discussion about iodine in Chapter 11.

5-HYDROXYTRYPTOPHAN. Brain serotonin levels drop with weight loss, resulting in food cravings and low mood.[5] Serotonin levels can be increased by supplementing with 5-hydroxytryptophan (5-HTP), a strategy that has proven effective in clinical trials where it has been used to combat depression and even alcohol withdrawal.[6] Some people have experienced reductions in food cravings during grain withdrawal by supplementing with 50 to 100 mg three times per day, while others have taken it when cravings strike, particularly at night, by supplementing with 50 to 300 mg in the evening. Higher doses can be associated with nausea, so it's best to start with a lower dose (around 50 mg) and build up as required for the desired effect.

RHODIOLA. Another nutritional supplement, rhodiola also appears to work by increasing brain serotonin and may thereby address the low mood and cravings associated with grain withdrawal. I'd recommend taking 340 to 680 mg per day, divided into two or three doses.[7] In my experience, effects are modest (generally less than that provided by 5-HTP) but positive, with benefits that can include increased mental acuity.

To simplify your life during the tumultuous withdrawal period, I've included a recipe for what I call the Wheat Whacker Smoothie (see page 336), which includes many of the supplements listed above. Know that, as unpleasant as it may be, withdrawal from grains is a necessary step on the path to regaining total health. And once you survive that process—and you will—you can look forward to the good stuff that follows, which we discuss below.

SKINNY BONES: WEIGHT LOSS

Nothing I have ever come across matches the power of grain elimination to cause weight loss—not counting calories, cutting fat, cutting sugar, or adding extreme exercise. Actually, that's not entirely true: Starvation can match the weight loss effect of grain elimination. But, of course, you are not starving by eliminating grains. Think of excess weight as reflecting a disordered metabolism. When you set your metabolic patterns right, weight is released, and, in this grain-free experience, it is usually released at a surprising pace.

For all the reasons I've discussed—loss of the appetite-stimulating effects of gliadin and related prolamin proteins, unblocking of the leptin hormone, allowing normal appetite signals to operate, freedom from the 2-hour cycle of blood sugar and insulin ups and downs, restoration of the sensation of taste and sensitivity to sweetness, receding inflammation, and loss of water retention—weight typically drops rapidly after grains are eliminated. It is not uncommon for people to be *frightened* at the pace of weight loss, as weight can drop off at the rate of 1 pound per day.

Defenders of the first law of thermodynamics and the conservation of energy say this is impossible: Nobody can lose 3,500 calories of fat per day just by eliminating grains. What they fail to understand is that it is not just fat weight that is lost; there is also edema (retained water) from tissues in the face, arms, legs, and abdomen. Inflammatory phenomena recede quickly and powerfully with the removal of grains, evidenced by such things as the disappearance of facial seborrhea and other skin rashes and reduced joint pain and swelling. Grain elimination typically results in reduced calorie intake by 400 calories per day due to the lack of appetite stimulation. People usually lose 10 pounds during the initial 14 days, though the pace of weight loss slows over time, yielding typical results of 15 to 20 pounds lost the first month and 26 pounds lost the first 6 months.[8]

Once through with the exaggerated cravings experienced during withdrawal, people repeatedly notice that they are *no longer hungry*. Even if you were previously plagued by constant thoughts of food, experienced rumbling hunger that caused you to be on the constant lookout for something to eat, planned your next meal even while chewing the previous one, and were unable to turn away anything placed in front of you, all of that disappears. You will experience a refreshing indifference to foods, even ones you used to find irresistible. Breakfast at 7:00 a.m. may leave you uninterested in lunch or snacks until dinnertime. After-dinner snacking will be long gone. Even hunger itself feels very different: It's no longer a rumbling, rolling, panicky feeling, but instead becomes a soft reminder that at some point it might be nice to eat something.

Notice that nowhere in this book have you read that you should cut calorie intake, count fat grams, reduce portion size, push the plate away, eat many small meals 2 hours apart, or purge your bowels with laxatives—*none* of this is necessary for weight loss once you remove grains and their unnatural effects on appetite and weight. Weight loss will happen naturally.

When substantial weight is lost, especially that concentrated in visceral fat, many of the health conditions associated with excess weight also diminish or disappear: diabetes and prediabetes; high insulin; high blood pressure; distortions of estrogen, testosterone, and prolactin; and body-wide inflammation, along with the long-term risk for cancer, heart disease, and dementia. The reduced load on your joints, along with diminished inflammation, result in further improvements in joint pain, including that in large joints such as the knees, hips, and lower back. The Wheat Belly world is filled with many people who have lost 100, 150, or 180 pounds over a year or more on this grain-free lifestyle, all the while experiencing substantial transformations in health. And provided that you remain free of the effects of grains, the weight does not return.

"Am I Too Skinny?"

This question comes up with some frequency during our social media discussions: People are fearful that they will either lose too much weight or feel they have already lost too much weight with grain elimination. First of all, let's consider the broader perspective of this question: People are worried about losing too much weight—in the midst of the world's worst epidemic of weight gain and obesity. There are literally tens of millions of people who would gladly experience this "problem." Minus grains, the human appetite reverts back to what's required to provide sustenance: You eat what you need, nothing more, nothing less. Weight accordingly returns to your physiological ideal. It is, however, not uncommon for people following this grain-free lifestyle to plateau at a weight that was *lower* than anticipated.

There are indeed issues to consider when the "Am I too skinny?" question arises.

The turning point in my life was Wheat Belly.

I was diabetic and the dietitian told me to eat healthy whole grains in February 2012. But I had read *Wheat Belly*. I was armed with knowledge.

My diabetes was self-inflicted due to poor diet. I went to a diabetes dietitian on the advice of my doctor. The dietitian told me to eat bread and I said no. I was told to eat pasta. I said no. I was told that I was "being uncooperative and I'll have to report that back to your doctor." I asked, "How many people coming through here lose a huge amount of weight and get off the medications related to diabetes?" No answer.

Imagine being told as a type 2 diabetic to eat wheat—my blood sugar would spike, then I was supposed to take metformin or insulin to bring it back down. I said, "Don't eat wheat of any type and don't have the spike in the first place." Dietitians are trained to tell us to eat "healthy whole grains." But it wasn't healthy for me.

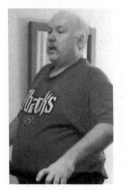
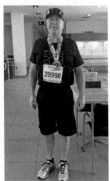

Before   *After*

I was still morbidly fat as I spoke to her, so she had no reason to think I had a clue or would lose even 1 pound. But I was starting to understand my relationship to food and the food industry by this time, and that was life changing.

No wheat. No more fructose. No processed sugar. I would eat vegetables, fruits, chicken, fish, and beef. No more pouring milk over 15 teaspoons of sugar (called cereal) that tasted good, but poisoned me. The first few days of no wheat were very hard. My wheat addiction was very strong. Then it subsided.

I was off insulin by March 2012. I'm off a page full of meds, except for metformin. I hope to be off that soon. I've lost 113 pounds.

In spring 2012 I turned in my old couch potato life for walking, then running. I've done two half-marathons in 2013. I'm training for a full marathon. I was a wheataholic and stopped after reading *Wheat Belly*. I spread the word at every opportunity.

John, Ontario, Canada

Are You *Really* Too Skinny?

Is your weight too low, or are you normal in a world of overweight and obese people and just look skinny by comparison? Watch an old movie or look at old photographs and magazines from the 1950s, for instance, and notice that everyone is "skinny," just like you. They are not too skinny; they are *normal.* More often than not, people who judge themselves to be too skinny are really not—they just feel that way when they're standing next to overweight friends, family, and co-workers.

We Do Not Limit Calories, Fat, or Protein

If you feel that you have lost too much weight, eat *more* avocados and *more* coconut oil. Consume *more* fat from meats or poultry, eat *more* raw nuts, and use grain-free recipes to create muffins, cookies, and pies. Spread or pour *more* organic butter, ghee, or extra-virgin olive oil over your dishes. (The *Wheat Belly Cookbook* and the *Wheat Belly 30-Minute (or Less!) Cookbook* are filled with these sorts of recipes.)

Consider Building Muscle

Weight loss is inevitably accompanied by muscle loss. If you lose, say, 30 pounds total, up to 10 pounds of that lost weight can be muscle. Muscle is easily regained with strength training. That doesn't mean having to spend hours and hours in the gym; just devoting 15 to 20 minutes twice per week and focusing on large muscle groups (such as your upper and lower back, thighs, and pectorals) is sufficient to build back muscle.

The person who teeters on being too thin (this happens very rarely) can increase carbohydrate intake, especially from foods like beans and sweet potatoes, which also stimulate healthy bowel flora. However, be mindful of blood sugar and other metabolic distortions (a rise in triglycerides, the provocation of small LDL particles) that can be triggered if carbohydrate consumption goes too high. In my experience, only rarely can someone safely consume more than 25 to 30 grams net carbohydrates in a single meal without triggering some adverse effect. (More on these issues in Chapter 7.)

THE GRAINLESS BRAIN

Remove grains from your diet and your brain is released from the control of their mind-active components. It is liberating, wonderful, and empowering. Your brain can be restored to its normal alert, energetic, calculating, and creative state. After withdrawal, the benefits that can be experienced include:

IMPROVED MOOD. Once the depression that can accompany withdrawal is past, there is typically a substantial lifting of mood. This develops due to the removal of gliadin and other prolamin protein–derived exorphins, as well as increased levels of brain serotonin. People are happier and more optimistic, and they become better engaged with the people and activities of their lives. Some people experience such dramatic improvements of mood that they are able to free themselves from suicidal thoughts and antidepressant medications.

> *"I was very addicted to bread, it was a very bad problem for me. I ate it a lot: 5 to 12 slices per day, I craved it so much. I skipped meals and I just ate my bread and grains.*
>
> *"I was depressed until I listened to a lecture from Dr. Davis, and then I wondered if my symptoms could be due to the grains. I left the grains after the lecture and 4 days later my depression was so much better. If I eat grains, depression comes back. So I have to be very precise.*
>
> *"I do not have to medicate. I enjoy life more now and smile more often."*
>
> —Susanna-Alessandra, Helsinki, Finland

Dark, suicidal thoughts appear to be among the most easily reprovoked thoughts with any grain reexposure. People who experience this effect, for instance, report being plagued by a week of suicidal thoughts after a single intentional or inadvertent episode of grain exposure. Meticulous avoidance is therefore key. Also, anyone taking an antidepressant medication will need to consult with his or her health-care provider before any effort to reduce or change medication is undertaken, as a trained health-care professional is required to make good decisions in this area.

REDUCED ANXIETY. Many people are plagued by constant low-level anxiety, the sort of pointless and unwarranted unease that makes day-to-day life an unpleasant experience, a layer of worry that is unnecessary, even incapacitating. Typically, such anxieties recede with grain removal. For some, the effect can be dramatic and life changing, sometimes even providing relief from years of phobias such as agoraphobia (the fear of leaving home) or claustrophobia (the fear of closed spaces). For others, it may be a more subtle change, with relief from frequent or pervasive anxieties that darkened your life. Like suicidal thoughts, anxiety is easily reprovoked with any grain exposure, so avoidance is key.

> *"I have both generalized anxiety and social anxiety disorder. I used to get quite big panic attacks a few nights a week resulting in insomnia. Since I gave up wheat last August, I have not had a single panic attack."*
>
> —DANIELLE, CASTLE HILL,
> NEW SOUTH WALES, AUSTRALIA

LIFTING OF MIND FOG. Like the lifting of mood, a lifting of mind fog is also a common grain-free experience. People report that they are better able to concentrate for prolonged periods and are able to think more clearly, make decisions more easily, and speak more effectively. Writers are able to write for longer periods; artists are able to draw, paint, or compose more easily; businesspeople can engage in discussion, perform at meetings, and prepare documents more effectively; and athletes are able to sustain concentration for a longer time and become less reliant on performance crutches such as energy drinks and protein bars. This effect applies to children just as much as adults. Some of the most dramatic stories I've heard have come from parents who report that their children's school performance skyrocketed when they were freed from the fogginess of grain consumption.

ENHANCED LEARNING. Restoration of the capacity for prolonged concentration, clearer thinking, and reduced distractibility add up to an enhanced ability to learn. People listen more effectively, retain more with reading, acquire and synthesize data and concepts with greater ease, and enjoy enhanced recall. They are more focused, more creative, and more effective.

REVERSAL OF SEIZURES. As seizures have been associated with grain consumption, especially consumption of wheat, removal of grains can be associated with relief from seizures if grains were the initiating cause. Most commonly, sufferers of temporal lobe seizures experience a marked reduction or complete relief from these episodes. Although the causal association between grains and grand mal seizures is more tenuous, I am hearing from more and more people who have experienced marked relief from these dangerous events, as well.

REVERSAL OF NEUROLOGICAL IMPAIRMENT. People with cerebellar ataxia (see Chapter 5) usually experience a slow, gradual improvement in coordination, balance, capacity to walk, and bladder control, or at least experience no further deterioration, after grains are eliminated. Likewise, the pain or impaired feelings of peripheral neuropathy (see Chapter 5) recede slowly or stop progressing. Because the nervous system is slow to heal and may do so imperfectly, the process can take months to years, so a long-term commitment is required to gauge improvement. This is very important to recognize, as some people eliminate grains and report 2 weeks later that grain elimination didn't work for them.

Even multiple sclerosis, which results from autoimmune destruction of the myelin covering of nerve tissue, can slowly improve or reverse. It's also critical that you simultaneously correct vitamin D deficiency, as preliminary studies suggest a powerful relationship between vitamin D and this condition. (See the discussion on vitamin D in Chapter 8.)

PREVENTION OF DEMENTIA. High blood sugars that occur day in and day out, many times per day, due to habitual grain consumption are reversed when grains are removed. Clinical trials have demonstrated the powerful association between blood sugars that are around 110 mg/dl— which is *below* the cutoffs for prediabetes and diabetes and considered just above normal—and the development of dementia, with even higher risk presented by the higher blood sugar levels of prediabetes and diabetes. Grain elimination is a powerful means of reversing high fasting and after-meal blood sugars. Some people are also prone to the autoimmune process triggered by the gliadin and prolamin proteins that leads to dementia; it is likewise turned off with elimination of the inciting grains.

Other organs experience different effects when wheat and other grains are removed from the diet. Let's consider these effects.

ACHIEVING 30 FEET OF DIGESTIVE BLISS: THE GRAINLESS GASTROINTESTINAL TRACT

Removing grains and ending the constant beating your poor gastrointestinal tract has endured for many years is the start to a fabulous recovery. In fact, I would argue that ideal gastrointestinal health is *not* possible as long as grains remain a part of your life. This new grain-free path will allow you to start your journey back to gastrointestinal bliss.

> *"After decades of inconsistent fecal combat,*
> *I enjoy a serene, gentle, and tidy regularity."*
>
> —ROBERT R., NEWNAN, GEORGIA

Now that you've found the key to reversing so many of these conditions, just what can you expect? Let's tackle them one by one.

Relief from Acid Reflux and Esophagitis

The majority of people with these conditions, having suffered for years, heave a big sigh of relief with grain elimination. This is among the earliest and most consistent of benefits that develop after ridding your life of the prolamins, lectins, and allergens of grains. It is uncommon for someone with acid reflux to *not* respond to elimination of grains: The effect is consistent and predictable for the majority of people and generally occurs within 5 days of kissing your last bagel, corn chip, and slice of rye toast goodbye. I've even witnessed a growing number of people obtain complete relief from esophageal stricture that had been necessitating periodic balloon dilatation.

For the millions of people prescribed acid-suppressing drugs, grain elimination means having a discussion with the prescribing health-care provider about whether the drug is still necessary as your symptoms improve. Some people will need to wean, rather than abruptly stop, their drugs to avoid a "rebound" increase in stomach acid—a process that may stretch out over weeks or even months.

However, removal of the damaging effects of grains and the need for drugs may unmask an underlying problem: Some people are left with inadequate production of stomach acid (*hypochlorhydria*) that could have been caused by prior grain consumption or infection with the organism *Helicobacter pylori*, which is associated with ulcers. Confusingly, the symptoms of hypochlorhydria mimic those of excessive stomach acid and acid reflux: Consequently, you halt the grains and experience reduced stomach discomfort and heartburn, but you may be left with bloating or a lesser level of discomfort. Inadequate levels of stomach acid not only cause discomfort but also pose health risks because the lack of proper stomach acidification—whether it occurs naturally or due to acid-suppressing drugs—reduces calcium absorption and thereby increases risk for osteoporosis and fractures. Low stomach acid also increases your risk for pneumonia, since the acidic environment of the stomach normally provides a protective barrier against undesirable bacteria. Some people therefore need to address, ironically, *enhancing* stomach acid availability. I discuss this in greater detail in Chapter 9.

Irritable Bowel Syndrome

Irritable bowel syndrome, or IBS, is so common in people who consume prolamin protein–containing grains that it should make us pause and ask whether the humans with IBS are "abnormal" or are just normal people consuming something they should not be consuming. I favor the latter explanation. As with acid reflux, most people experience complete relief from IBS symptoms within 5 days of saying goodbye to grains. People prescribed drugs for IBS symptoms will therefore have to discuss the possibility of discontinuing these drugs with their health-care provider, a very realistic prospect for the majority of sufferers. An occasional person who eliminates grains, however, may be left with residual bloating, constipation, or even diarrhea. In this situation, additional efforts may be necessary, especially efforts to restore healthy bowel flora, as is discussed in Chapter 9.

Gallbladder and Pancreatic Health

Minus grains, the gallbladder and pancreas are permitted to make their important contributions to digestion. Recall that wheat germ agglutinin (WGA) in wheat and the identical lectins of rye, barley, and rice block the glycoprotein receptor for the hormone cholecystokinin (CCK), which stimulates gallbladder contraction to release bile and the pancreas to release digestive enzymes. When you remove grain lectins, sensitivity to CCK is restored and normal gallbladder contraction and pancreatic enzyme release return. This means that the potential for gallstone formation is decreased (as there is less bile stasis) and food is digested more effectively. This effect develops over weeks to months after grain elimination. Interestingly, the heightened responsiveness of the gallbladder to CCK can make some people sensitive to caffeine in coffee, tea, and other sources because it stimulates CCK release and gallbladder contraction.[9] A reduction in caffeine intake may therefore be advisable to reduce loose bowels from gallbladder overstimulation. Occasionally, a person may not experience full restoration of CCK sensitivity. In these cases, typically signaled by reduced but persistent discomfort, bloating, or irregularity despite efforts to address restoration of bowel flora, additional evaluation may be required if digestive health is not restored after several weeks of grain elimination (see Chapter 9).

Inflammatory Bowel Disease

People with inflammatory bowel diseases (generally called IBD, these are ulcerative colitis of the colon and Crohn's disease of the small intestine and colon) have inflammation, pain, and complications that are worsened by WGA, gliadin and other grain prolamins, and grain allergens. These complications are compounded by distortions of bowel flora. Being freed from the worst symptoms or reducing reliance on IBD drugs, minimizing the frequency of flare-ups, or obtaining an outright cure can change the lives of the people who suffer from this condition.

Remove all the bowel-destructive components of grains and IBD symptoms improve in most people: They experience less bloating, diarrhea, and pain.[10] Because IBD involves a more complex collection of phenomena than, say, acid reflux, it generally takes a longer time period to respond. Typically, people with IBD experience less pain and bloating within 1 to 2 weeks of eliminating grains, with gradual reduction in diarrhea over weeks to months. The majority of people experience major improvements in symptoms with grain elimination, but just what proportion of people can experience full relief from their condition requires better quantification in clinical trials. And, of course, going grain-free is an option for people that (1) costs nothing, (2) carries no nasty side effects, and (3) yields benefits outside of intestinal health. There is *nothing* lost in trying.

IBD involves dramatic distortions of bowel flora that discourage the happy coexistence of bacterial species and their human host.[11] Dysbiosis is a major concern in people with IBD, as they have suppressed normal populations and larger populations of undesirable species, such as *E. coli*. All of this adds up to making the disease worse, magnifying the bloating, pain, and diarrhea, as well as increasing intestinal permeability and body-wide inflammation. This can persist even after grains have been eliminated from the diet. Some experts have advocated the use of antibiotics to wipe out abnormal bacterial species, and therefore their negative contributions, in IBD, although this provides little to no reassurance that a more desirable collection of bowel flora will step in to take their place once the antibiotics have run their course.[12] It also risks the emergence of nasty, undesirable species, such as *Clostridium difficile*, which are very destructive. The bulk of studies demonstrate that people with ulcerative colitis and Crohn's disease benefit from supplementation with a high-potency probiotic to repopulate their intestinal tracts with healthy bowel flora.[13] In one study of children with ulcerative colitis, 92.8 percent of participants experienced remission when a high-potency probiotic (VSL#3) was added to standard drug therapies, compared to 36.4 percent responding to drugs alone.[14] Several clinical studies have demonstrated an enhanced likelihood of remission of IBD with specific bacterial species, such as *Bifidobacterium breve*, *Bifidobacterium bifidum*, and the yeast *Saccharomyces boulardii*, as well as the high-potency combination of species in the VSL#3 preparation.[15] And while most people only need to take probiotics for a few weeks to repopulate after the offending agents—grains—have been removed, people with IBD generally benefit from taking probiotics for an extended period, perhaps even years, to facilitate healing. Because of this uncertainty, long-term, even lifelong, attention to bowel flora and use of probiotics may be required. These sorts of complex issues are best managed with the assistance of a knowledgeable health-care provider. If your health-care provider has failed to discuss the benefits of probiotics and normalization of bowel flora with you, then you have been done a grave disservice that needs to be addressed.

An emerging role is being recognized for so-called "prebiotics." These fibers, such as fructooligosaccharides and inulin from sources such as tubers and legumes, are indigestible by humans but digestible by bowel flora, which convert these fibers to short-chain fatty acids such as butyrate. Butyrate is proving to play an essential role in maintaining a healthy intestinal lining, including repair of "tight junctions" between intestinal cells disrupted by grain consumption. This repair restores normal barrier functions against undesirable components from other bacteria and reduces colon cancer risk.[16] Restoration of desirable bowel flora restores the capacity for species such as *Lactobacillus* to generate butyrate.[17] With IBD, more so than with other conditions, prebiotic intake should be built up slowly, or else plenty of gas and discomfort can result. Practical ways to supplement prebiotics are discussed in Chapter 9 (see page 193).

For those with IBD, a search for nutrient deficiencies above and beyond those experienced by the average grain-consuming individual is in order. In particular, people with IBD are prone to deficiencies of vitamin D, calcium, folate, vitamin B_{12}, and zinc. Omega-3 fatty acid supplementation and reduced exposure to omega-6 fatty acid sources (such as vegetable, corn, and safflower oils) may also have outsize benefits in people with IBD.[18]

People with IBD may see an added benefit by avoiding specific foods beyond grains. A systematic elimination diet, in which foods associated with symptom flare-ups are eliminated one by one, has been shown to maintain remission in 62 percent of people over 2 years and 45 percent over 5 years, without medication.[19] Beyond grains, dairy and fructose are also frequent sources of symptom recurrence. Intolerance to dairy can originate with either lactose or an abnormal immune response to various milk proteins.[20] People with Crohn's disease, in particular, are prone to fructose malabsorption, which can worsen symptoms.[21]

Celiac Disease

Many of the issues that apply to inflammatory bowel disease also apply to celiac disease, the autoimmune disease of the small intestine triggered by gliadin and other prolamin proteins (including the zein of corn and perhaps the avenin of oats). Just as in IBD, people with celiac disease typically experience dramatic relief from abdominal pain, cramps, bloating, and diarrhea within days to weeks of strict grain elimination.

Because celiac disease, more so than IBD, is associated with damaging effects beyond the intestinal tract, phenomena outside of intestinal symptoms can also clear up. Sufferers may experience relief from joint pain, rashes (especially dermatitis herpetiformis, seborrhea, eczema, and psoriasis), reversal or improvement in anemia from iron and vitamin B_{12} deficiency, partial reversal of reduced bone density, and gradual reversal of neurological deterioration.

As in IBD, people with celiac disease begin with a high prevalence of dysbiosis, with similar reductions in healthy bacteria and dominance of unhealthy species.[22] Just removing grains is usually not enough to correct the situation. It is therefore not uncommon for people diagnosed with celiac disease to experience only a partial recovery after eliminating grains because of persistent distortions of bowel flora. When assessed, the majority of people with celiac disease following a gluten-free diet are found to have dysbiosis.[23] In other words, "gluten-avoidance" is *not* enough. Probiotics taken over the long term, prebiotic fibers, and fermented foods eaten as a means of obtaining fermenting bacteria are all part of the solution, as are antibiotics in the most difficult situations. (See Chapter 9 for further discussion.)

In many ways, celiac disease can be viewed as the extreme expression of grain intolerance, so it should not be surprising that issues such as hypochlorhydria, inadequate pancreatic enzymes and bile, as well as bile stasis—issues that are experienced by people without celiac disease—are experienced with increased frequency in people with celiac disease. Many of the same nutrient deficiencies experienced by those with IBD are also experienced by people recovering from celiac disease, including deficiencies of vitamin D, calcium, folate, vitamin B_{12}, and zinc. These deficiencies will need to be assessed with the assistance of your health-care provider and corrected to facilitate full restoration of health.[24] Likewise, when those with celiac only partially recover in response to the elimination of grains, correction of dysbiosis, and correction of nutrient deficiencies, they'll need to consider a possible intolerance to other foods, especially dairy (both lactose and dairy proteins).[25]

GRAIN ELIMINATION: A JOINT TASK FORCE

Remove the joint inflammation–provoking components of grains— prolamin proteins that trigger autoimmunity, inflammation-provoking lectins, visceral fat that fans the flames of inflammation, and disrupted bowel flora—and joint inflammation and pain can powerfully recede. This will not make bone or cartilage regrow, but it will allow the inflammatory swelling and pain to subside.

Most typically, people report relief from pain and stiffness in the fingers and wrists within 5 days of grain elimination. Large joint discomfort, such as that in the hips, lower back, and knees, requires a longer period before relief develops, typically several weeks to several months. (This is not to say that *all* large joint pain goes away with grain elimination. Some pain, particularly in those people with "bone-on-bone" arthritis, in which the cartilage has eroded and allows direct contact between bones without cushioning or lubrication, will not.) Even if relief from joint pain and stiffness is not complete, it is often sufficient to reduce or eliminate reliance on anti-inflammatory drugs such as aspirin, naproxen, ibuprofen, rofecoxib, and other common nonsteroidal anti-inflammatory drugs. And, unlike such drugs, grain elimination provides health benefits outside of joint health without the range of side effects common to these drugs.

Grain-free athletes without joint disease but who deal with the rigors of high-intensity training and competition also report marked reduction in joint stiffness and pain after training and faster recovery after the physical demands of competition. Similar observations are made by people who simply exercise or engage in physically demanding work: Without grains, they experience less joint and muscle pain and stiffness and a more rapid recovery.

If joint pain and stiffness are being driven by an autoimmune process, such as that associated with rheumatoid arthritis, psoriatic arthritis, or lupus, then the more complex inflammatory responses that define these conditions will require months or longer to respond. But, more often than not, they *do* respond, providing substantial relief and reduced reliance on medication. For example, people with rheumatoid arthritis who eliminate grains report substantial improvement, sufficient to reduce reliance on drugs.[26]

Long-term elimination of grains allows the glycation of proteins to slow to its natural, low-grade rate, as is reflected in dropping hemoglobin A1c (HbA1c) values. This means that the destruction of your cartilage is slowed to a minimum. Unfortunately, cartilage tissue does not regenerate—it's one of the few tissues in the body that lacks this capacity—but you will slow further deterioration and best preserve what you've got.

BREATHE A SIGH OF RELIEF: THE RESPIRATORY SYSTEM AND ALLERGIES

Grain proteins act as allergens themselves, as well as worsening susceptibility to other allergens, such as pollens, pets, and other foods. For many people, removing grains provides relief from a range of allergies after years of struggling with antihistamines, nasal inhalers, oral asthma inhalers, and even steroids. Elimination of wheat, rye, barley, and corn can provide such dramatic relief to many people with asthma that they can often cut back on or eliminate using inhalers. (This should be accomplished, of course, with the knowledge and assistance of a capable healthcare provider.) It is wise, however, to keep a rescue inhaler handy even if you obtain full relief. There's always the small chance that an episode could occur with grain reexposure or exposure to another allergen.

Likewise, sinus congestion, sinus drainage, and repeated sinus infections are typical grain-related conditions that recede within days of saying goodbye to grains. This can happen even after years of struggles with these problems. If these conditions do *not* respond, it's important to consider the presence of nasal polyps, which are common with a long history of nasal allergies. Polyps require a specific treatment (e.g., a prolonged course of inhaled nasal steroids) before relief can be obtained, even with removal of the offending allergens.

Other nongrain allergies can recede with grain elimination, but the effect is highly variable. It is not uncommon, for instance, to remove grains and discover that the egg allergy you had for many years or the seasonal allergy that would visit you every spring has disappeared. Because the response is variable, each instance needs to be approached individually. Allergies are often determined through step-by-step elimination, allergen skin testing, or a variety of blood tests that identify immune and allergic sensitivities. Naturopaths, some chiropractors, and practitioners of functional medicine who focus on biochemical and nutritional strategies have become the most accessible experts in these situations.

SKIN: GOODBYE REDNESS, PUFFINESS, AND RASHES

Seeing is believing, and you can actually watch it happen: Many rashes recede with the elimination of grains, and we can observe obvious and rapid changes in skin health. Interestingly, the skin and the gastrointestinal tract, organ systems that interact with the outside world, often demonstrate simultaneous relief, so if you can see positive changes on the outside, you can bet that positive changes are happening on the inside, too.

Most commonly, people experience relief from facial seborrhea and dandruff (seborrhea of the scalp) within the first week and from eczema and acne within the first few weeks of going grain-free. These skin developments are typically accompanied, as would be expected, by relief from acid reflux and bowel urgency, as well as enhanced absorption of nutrients and improved digestive function.

"I've had eczema since I was a young child. Many times, it was so bad my skin would crack and bleed. The doctors always just gave me steroids. When I stick to a wheat-free/grain-free diet, though, my skin clears up within days. If I lapse and eat pizza or something else with wheat, I break back out."

—Dana, Shreveport, Louisiana

More immunologically complex skin conditions such as psoriasis or the rash of lupus can require many weeks, or even months, to respond. And again, as expected, many of the people who experience such changes notice relief from gastrointestinal complaints at the same time.

It is very common for women, in particular, to report improvements in appearance. They report that years of facial puffiness (edema) and redness (usually seborrhea) disappear, skin color improves, and they look more vital and vibrant. Such skin changes are, I believe, a big part of the reason many people look younger after grain elimination. (It's also, interestingly, one of the fascinating phenomena responsible for the growing Wheat Belly social media audience, with readers posting "before" and "after" face transformations online that are nothing short of jaw-dropping.)

Of course, not all rashes recede or disappear with grain elimination, but *most* do. As with all other grain-free experiences, however, there is nothing lost in assessing the effect. And if no response is experienced, as in partially responsive gastrointestinal conditions, there may be advantages to be gained by fully addressing bowel flora restoration (see Chapter 9) and identifying other food sensitivities.

A GRAIN-FREE SEX CHANGE

Yes: Grain elimination yields astounding changes in the status of sex hormones. While the changes are not as drastic as, say, surgically changing a man into a woman or vice versa, the shifts in hormones without wheat, rye, barley, and corn can nonetheless be astounding. Given the complex disruptive effects of grain consumption on sex hormones, we would expect much or all of this disruption to right itself with grain elimination. And it does, and is further improved by losing the excess visceral fat gained through grain consumption—provided you don't muck your health up with some other misguided blunder (like taking prescription estrogens sourced from horse urine).

Women with celiac disease experience dramatic changes in sexual and reproductive health with grain elimination, including the restoration of regular menstrual cycles, which bring an end to spontaneous miscarriages and impaired fertility and prevent premature menopause. Some of the most heartbreaking stories of repeated miscarriages originate with celiac disease that went unrecognized for years, but they can be followed by stories of miraculously normal pregnancies and deliveries after the elimination of wheat, rye, and barley. Women without celiac disease who give up all grains experience less dramatic but similar benefits. This plays out most clearly in overweight and obese women, especially in those with excess visceral fat who struggle with disrupted menstrual cycles, reduced fertility, and increased risk of miscarriage, and who are at risk for undesirable effects on the baby in utero. Upon losing weight and visceral fat, these women experience marked improvements in libido, sexual frequency, menstrual regularity, and fertility.[27]

Women with polycystic ovarian syndrome (PCOS) experience all the problems experienced by other women when overweight, but with exaggerated gains in visceral fat and exaggerations of other weight-related phenomena, such as high blood sugar. They also experience masculinizing effects, such as thicker mustache hair. Accordingly, after weight loss and grain elimination, women with PCOS experience even greater improvements than most other women, including increased fertility.[28]

Likewise, men with celiac disease who eliminate grains can expect to experience a boost in testosterone, accompanied by increased energy and heightened mood, improved libido, and gains in muscle strength, along with decreased estrogen levels. Oddly, some men with celiac experience a complex disruption of hormonal status and have higher, rather than lower, testosterone levels with grain consumption, due to heightened pituitary activity. They still experience symptoms of low testosterone, though, due to unresponsiveness to that hormone. This likewise reverses with grain elimination.[29]

Overweight men without celiac disease who go grain-free experience a reduction in abdominal visceral fat and its testosterone-to-estrogen converting action. As a result, testosterone levels increase and estrogen levels decrease, leading to increased libido, improved erections, improved mood, protection from the common midlife "blues" experienced by many men, and increased muscle mass and strength.[30] Correcting the testosterone-estrogen effect, combined with decreased prolactin from the pituitary, leads to shrinkage of breasts.[31]

In the grain-free world, with the distortions introduced by grain consumption removed, men are men and women are women, and they all feel and perform as well as they should.

My endometriosis pain decreased significantly.

When I ditched the grains, I lost 20 pounds and 6 inches off my waist. I have no more headaches, no sinus issues, no mood swings, no digestive issues, and no joint pain. My energy has increased, I sleep like a rock, and—best of all—my endometriosis pain has decreased significantly.

I was taking Vicodin for the pain, which was excruciating. I would be doubled over in agony every month. I could make no plans, as I was pretty much out of commission for a week or so each month. I started following *Wheat Belly* and my first cycle that month was much lighter and less painful. My husband and I thought it was just a fluke, but then it happened again the next month, and the month after that! Well, it wasn't a fluke—it was because I changed my diet!

Wheat Belly works and I am able to enjoy my life again.

Dottie, Center Line, Michigan

DÉJÀ EWWW: WATCH OUT FOR THE REEXPOSURES

As you may have gathered from our discussion so far, no human fully adapts to the range of detrimental effects experienced by consuming grains. People often fail to recognize, for instance, that their hip pain is caused by breakfast toast, their cataracts at age 56 are the result of too many pancakes and tortillas, or their child's type 1 diabetes was caused by animal crackers. Nobody can fully acclimate to the head-to-toe adverse effects of grains, but there does indeed appear to be a *partial* tolerance. This is suggested by the very common phenomena I call grain "reexposure reactions."

Most typically, someone will have been grain-free for several months, experiencing all of the health benefits. Then they have a reexposure, either inadvertently (due to something like a gravy or roux that they failed to recognize as grain-containing) or intentionally (such as by having a small slice of birthday cake at their child's birthday party or a single canapé at the office holiday party). Wham! They're hit with gastrointestinal fireworks: excessive gas, cramps, and diarrhea that typically last 24 hours, much like a bout of food poisoning. The common gastrointestinal complaints of acid reflux and irritable bowel syndrome can return full blast, lasting up to several days. They may experience joint pain, especially in the hands and wrists; recurrent joint pain in larger joints, if they experienced this during previous grain-consuming times; and mental effects including mind fog, impaired concentration, anxiety, headache, depression, and even recurrent suicidal thoughts if they had them previously. And some symptoms, such as joint pain and acid reflux, can strike even if you *didn't* have them during your grain-consuming days, suggesting that you had previously developed a partial tolerance to the components of grains—a tolerance now lost due to their elimination.

Grain-derived opiates go to work again, too, and stimulate appetite, occasionally producing an effect I call the "I ate one cookie and gained 30 pounds" effect: One indulgence unleashes the floodgates of appetite, and you can't stop at just one cookie or one handful of pretzels. You tell yourself, "Just one can't hurt. I'll be extra good tomorrow. I'll exercise an extra 20 minutes." But before you know it, you've eaten the whole bag of Oreos or pretzels and you feel awful, all while you're looking for your next treat. You may recognize your mistake and swear to do better, but the cycle continues and you regain 30 pounds in a month. The key: Recognize that this can happen should you have any grain exposure, and do your absolute best to avoid grains altogether.

People who experienced asthma or sinus congestion previously can have recurrences with reexposure. The asthma can be especially dangerous, as some asthmatics become so confident that their asthma has disappeared with the grains that they fail to keep their inhaler prescriptions up-to-date. For this reason, a rescue inhaler should be maintained, as discussed above, or you should at least talk to your doctor about the situation. If the doctor doesn't understand or doesn't care, find one who does.

People who experienced relief from autoimmune inflammation in their joints, skin, or intestinal tract can have especially bad reexposure reactions, not uncommonly triggering joint swelling and pain, as well as diarrhea, cramps, and bleeding. Recurrent symptoms may be immediate, or they may be delayed for 3 to 4 days and then can last for weeks or even months. People with autoimmune conditions should therefore meticulously avoid problematic grains.

People diagnosed with celiac disease must absolutely avoid wheat, rye, and barley, but they are also well advised to avoid corn and oats, due to the potential structural and immunological overlap of the zein and avenin proteins with gliadin. (This differs from the advice commonly given to

I have polycystic ovarian syndrome (PCOS), and I was experiencing excruciating pain in my abdomen.

My diagnosis came in 2006. I couldn't figure out why I couldn't get pregnant. I wasn't having normal cycles. When I did, it was extremely painful and caused me to be laid up in bed for days at a time. My doctor said I would probably never conceive unless I lost more than 100 pounds. At that time, I weighed 365 pounds, my heaviest weight. He prescribed metformin and told me to eat more veggies and less of everything else.

I wanted a baby more than anything. I tried everything, but I just couldn't stick to it. I felt so deprived. I read *The Atkins Diet* and *The South*

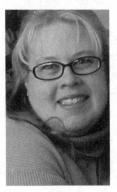 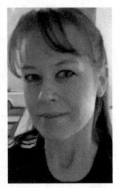

Before   *After*

Beach Diet. I never really followed any one diet, but I just made my own rules that worked for me. I cut all grains, beans, sugars, and starches from my diet and allowed myself to eat as much whole "good" foods—like veggies, berries, and meat—as I wanted. I constantly read what worked for other women with PCOS.

I took bits and pieces of knowledge and applied it. The things that worked, I stuck with: healthy fats, coconut oil, fish, even butter, lots of veggies, and low-glycemic fruit with a high fiber content. I love *Wheat Belly* because it explained the science of why this nutrition plan works for me. The hardest part for me was giving up bread. When I ate bread, I would want more bread. Sometimes I would eat an entire loaf of bread in a day and not even realize it. With cutting it out completely, I don't have the cravings or black-out eating moments.

I have been morbidly obese my entire life, and this process took a very long time: 3 years of consistency. I fell off the wagon a few times and, when I did, it showed immediately: I got puffy and unhappy. So having lost and maintained the loss, I am no longer hungry from the second I wake until I sleep. I have remarried. I feel so much more alive.

PCOS is a hormonal imbalance; it affects insulin and how insulin works with the liver. I had prediabetes that went away completely. I have had completely normal 30-day cycles. I haven't had a burst cyst in years. Now I am pain-free. PCOS causes hair growth and, when I was bigger, I didn't even realize how hairy I was due to all the extra testosterone in my system, but now it's completely manageable. I believe I cured my symptoms by a simple change in my diet.

I have maintained a 160-pound weight loss just by cutting out wheat and sugar. I went from a 67-inch waist to a 36-inch one—31 inches disappeared. I went from a size 32 or 4XL to a size 14 or medium, and I am happy where I am. I am now a personal trainer and motivator. I love who I have become through all of my trials, and I know without a doubt that this would never have happened for me if I had not made the decision to cut the wheat.

Kersten, Sandy, Utah

celiac patients, who are usually told that corn and oats are safe. They are not and should be avoided entirely.) It may also be advisable to minimize rice consumption because of its low quantity of lectin, not to mention its arsenic content. Avoiding gliadin and related prolamins is especially important, as even occasional reexposures escalate the risk for serious complications such as lymphoma of the small intestine, autoimmune conditions, and distortions of bowel flora (such as SIBO).

The key is to recognize what reexposure looks and feels like in your own individual experience. I've actually witnessed people who did not realize, for instance, that their explosive diarrhea or swollen knee was nothing more than a reaction to the bread crumbs on chicken or the crust on a slice of pizza. Because of this, they end up spending many hours (and many thousands of dollars) in the emergency room. It's important to prevent reexposure from happening in the first place, or to at least minimize your experiences, and to recognize what it looks and feels like should it occur.

People often ask if there are ways to reduce some of the phenomena of grain reexposure. Beyond hydration for diarrhea and conventional solutions like acetaminophen for headache, I know of no specific strategies that blunt this experience, except to do your best to keep it from happening in the first place. There are supplements advocated by some to reduce the consequences of gluten exposure; these contain enzymes that digest gluten and gliadin. I urge people *not* to take these supplements in the hopes that they will turn off all the undesirable effects of grain consumption. First, not all the gluten or gliadin is digested, allowing their effects to break through. This is no small matter in people with celiac disease, as it means a dramatically increased intestinal cancer risk and disruption of bowel flora. In people without celiac disease, it can trigger all of the same phenomena experienced with previous grain consumption. Second, supplement manufacturers are guilty of the same sort of overly simplistic thinking practiced by gluten-free food manufacturers who regard wheat, rye, and barley as nothing more than vehicles for gluten. You now know better, as these grains have many other components that are detrimental to your health, and those components are untouched by these supplements. The *only* situation in which the use of these supplements makes sense is for people who are exceptionally gluten or gliadin sensitive who, when desiring to eat at restaurants or in social situations, suffer recurrent symptoms with even the modest exposures of cross-contamination (such as when a frying pan is used to fry something coated with bread crumbs, not cleaned thoroughly, and then is used to sauté their dinner). Reliance on such supplements can reduce or minimize the consequences of inadvertent exposure, but I believe it is foolhardy and wrong to think that such products make grain consumption safe. This is simply not true.

Given the wonderful health benefits of grain elimination and the emotional and physical reactions caused by reexposure, once you're grain-free, you should always be grain-free.

HOMO GRAINLESS: A NEW KIND OF HUMAN

We do not really create a new strain of humans when we eliminate grains. However, we do make such a gigantic leap in every sphere of human health and life that we might as well regard ourselves as having an entirely different experience from that endured by grain-consuming humans these last 300 generations—those who've lived since making the miscalculation of embracing the seeds of grasses as food. With their removal, our perceptions change, our sense of taste changes, our vision changes, our internal dialogues and sleep content change, and our moods and capacity for intellectual accomplishment change. And they all change for the better.

Next we'll discuss the nitty-gritty, day-to-day details of just how to rid your life of the ubiquitous seeds of grasses.

CHAPTER 7

GRAINLESS LIVING DAY-TO-DAY

*What if I'm so broken I can never do something as basic as feed myself? Do
you realize how twisted that is? It amazes me sometimes that humans still exist.
We're just animals, after all. And how can an animal get so removed from
nature that it loses the instinct to keep itself alive?*
—Amy Reed, *Clean*

IF YOU HAVEN'T already done so, this is the place where we make a
raging bonfire of wheat, rye, barley, corn, rice, and other seeds of grasses, and
then we roast some marshmallows. Anything left over, we feed to the cows.

I still recommend that people follow the same approach as outlined in
the original *Wheat Belly* book, but I've also learned a few new tricks in the
years since it was published. I believe these lessons can make this lifestyle
easier, more satisfying, and more effective, plus make the world you live in
a better place.

In this chapter, I discuss just what it means to live with all traces of
grains, the commoditized foods used to control the diet of the world while
extracting maximum profit, removed from your dietary experience. It
does not mean that you can't fill your gas tank with corn-derived ethanol
or use wheat for cat litter. You just don't want the products of the seeds of
grasses in or on your body.

There's really nothing intrinsically wrong with grasses. They're beautiful, swaying in the wind, covering large swaths of the earth. Like other
plants, they process carbon dioxide and produce oxygen. Animals eat
them. The problem is that our species of primate, *Homo sapiens*, simply
lacks the means to digest them as food. When we try, acute and chronic
health pandemonium ensues. When we stop, our health begins to revert
back to its natural state.

WHY ARE GRAINS IN *EVERYTHING?*

As you set out to remove all grains from your life, examining labels for anything that might contain the seeds of grasses, you will quickly throw your hands up in the air and declare, "This is impossible! Grains are in everything!"

Indeed, grains are in salad dressings, seasoning mixes, licorice, frozen dinners, breakfast cereals, canned soups, dried soup mixes, rotisserie chickens, soft drinks, whiskeys, beers, prescription drugs, shampoos, and conditioners. Your observation is correct: Wheat and corn, in particular, are in virtually every processed food on grocery store shelves, as well as in cosmetics and toiletries. Grains such as oats, millet, teff, and sorghum are more obvious and less commonly used in various hidden or modified forms. Wheat or corn, however, can be found in practically everything on store shelves, sometimes clearly listed as wheat flour or cornstarch, other times listed under not-so-obvious names, such as hydrolyzed vegetable protein or maltodextrin. Barley malt and rice flour make frequent appearances, as well.

Why are grains so ubiquitous? There are legitimate and practical reasons for including the products of grains in foods, such as to improve texture, taste, thickening, and consistency. Likewise, in cosmetics and toiletries, grains provide a low-cost way to obtain specific textures or performance characteristics. But there are some other not-so-desirable reasons—at least not for the consumer. Grains are a way to bulk up a product inexpensively, making you think that the deep-dish pizza you purchased for only $8.99 is a bargain. Grains, after all, have been converted into commodities: cheap, high-volume products that provide calories and short-term sustenance, satisfying hunger for a few minutes or hours. They provide the appearance of plenty, but really they're just cheap filler.

A metric *ton* (2,200 pounds) of whole wheat flour can be purchased for $400 to $800 wholesale. That means the huge plate of breads and rolls served before dinner at a nice restaurant costs literally pennies in materials (not counting labor costs), while conveying the appetite-stimulating effects of grain-derived opiates to paying customers. Likewise, the wholesale price of cornstarch is just a few pennies more, and still no more than around 50 cents per pound. High-fructose corn syrup, at prices around $600 per metric ton, or 27 cents per pound, is likewise a great way to bulk up and sweeten cheap, commoditized foods. Feed the masses, cheaply and in a big way, with plates piled high, and their appetites will be satisfied—at least for a few minutes.

But the dirty little secret is that grains, put into every dietary nook and cranny, increase food consumption. The opiates that derive from grains increase appetite and thereby consumption, adding an average of 400 more calories per person, per day, every day. (And it's actually not uncommon for grains to provoke consumption of 1,000 or more additional calories.) Throw in some high-fructose corn syrup derived from corn, with its intense sweetness that comes at a very low cost and is included in every conceivable food, and you increase the expectation of sweetness in the consuming public, further increasing our appetites for other sweet, processed foods.

Of the 60,000 or so processed food products that fill the shelves of the average supermarket, your options will be reduced to more like 1,000—an upheaval, to be sure. The only foods without traces of grains are the foods that are *naturally* grain-free, such as cabbage, eggs, and meats. That observation points us in the direction of a solution: a return to unprocessed, naturally grain-free foods.

BRUSH OFF YOUR LOINCLOTH

Imagine I send you back in time to 100,000 BC, stripped of your smartphone, iPad, car, centrally heated and cooled home, and all other conveniences of modern life, including the nearby supermarket. You wake in your hut, cave, or tree, clothed in only the skins of animals you've killed, hungry for something to eat. There's nothing cellophane-wrapped or microwaveable in this world, just the plants and animals you obtain from your surroundings. Where do you start? Grab your spear, the one you crafted from a sturdy tree branch, sharpened stone lashed to the tip. You'll also need that dried stomach from the ibex you killed, one end tied off to create a bag to collect mushrooms, nuts, and berries, as well as the odd reptile you find. Over time, you become acquainted with the rhythms and patterns of wildlife in your area: where they obtain water, how well they protect their young, how their gait slows when they are aged or weak. You learn their migratory habits, their vulnerabilities. You also come to know which plants are edible and taste good but don't cause diarrhea, hallucinations, or death.

Most people have a tough time imagining such a life—having to gather, hunt, and kill their next meal. But you would get reacquainted with your inner hungry *Homo sapiens* very quickly if you had to go without eating for a week or two. You would likely find that you instinctively know what to do. Armed with the confidence of the desperate, you'd kill, skin, and eat to survive, savoring each bite. Just as there may be no atheists in foxholes, there are no vegetarians among the starving. Killing a turtle, rabbit, deer, gazelle, or wild boar seems like a small price to pay to survive another few days or to keep your family alive, especially if cold weather is on its way. And if you didn't have access to the tools or knowledge to build a fire, you'd quickly become resigned to eating the flesh and organs of your kill without the benefit of cooking it.

In our modern, sanitized world, such thoughts invariably cause revulsion. But humans ate this way until the relatively recent past, and it's been a mere blink of an eye, in anthropological time, since we stopped. But it's this inner wisdom that we hope to tap into, an instinctive knowledge of what and how to eat.

While it is an easy thing to imagine consuming the flesh of an animal or a piece of wild fruit, it is not so easy to imagine how you might come to consume the seeds of grasses. We have to give a little credit to those starving humans who, 10,000 years ago, figured this out, mimicking the eating habits of the aurochs and ibex, ruminants grazing on grasses, without recognizing the Pandora's box of health they were opening.

Most of us won't be tracking and killing our next meal, of course, nor will we gnaw on liver that's been freshly retrieved from the abdominal cavity of a creature we've just speared. But we need to style a way of eating that mimics such instinctive habits, drawing from the inner wisdom that is already deep inside each of us.

THE THREE-STEP PROCESS TO GRAINLESSNESS

Many people find the prospect of grain elimination daunting or even overwhelming, having been inundated for years with the advice to make grains the dominant part of their diet. So when I say it's all utter nonsense, a fundamental misinterpretation of the science, advice crafted for top-down control and commoditization of the world's diet, and the underlying cause for an astounding list of health problems, it's like having the dietary rug pulled out from under your feet. To make the transition to grain-free doable for you, I've broken it down into three bite-size, grain-free pieces.

The three steps to living grainlessly are:

1. Eliminate grains.
2. Eat real, single-ingredient foods.
3. Manage carbohydrates.

It's that simple. Yes, there are additional steps to take to regain body-wide health, and we'll discuss them later in the book. But the effort to convert your diet from that of unwitting, helpless, weight-gaining, disease-causing grain-filled diet to that of health-empowering, performance-enhancing, feel-great-again grain-free diet is just this easy.

Don that loincloth, brush the dirt off your backside, sharpen your figurative spear, and set out to eat the way you were *supposed* to eat by tuning into the internal wisdom gained during 2.5 million years of adapting to life on this planet. As best you can, push aside notions of "healthy" eating inflicted upon you by ignorant or biased agencies. When humans eat foods we are adapted to consume, there are no concerns about saturated fat or fiber, there is nothing carbonated, nothing sugared-up, nobody counts calories, and there are certainly no products made from the seeds of grasses. We return to the foods that allowed our species to survive and thrive, foods that we consumed to provide sustenance, grow, and reproduce.

Step 1: Eliminate Grains

If you are already familiar with the *Wheat Belly* approach, then you have taken steps to eliminate the worst of the worst: foods made with modern semidwarf wheat. To complete the first step as discussed here, you need only extend your elimination efforts to include that of all other grains, something that most wheat-free people find they can do easily.

Yes, grains are everywhere. Living grainlessly means eliminating all foods that are obvious products of grains, such as breads, pastas, bagels, pizzas, pretzels, muffins, cakes, pastries, pancake mixes, corn chips, tacos, taco chips, tortillas, and oatmeal. It is not uncommon for modern people to obtain 50 percent or more of their daily calories from grains. I am now proposing that we yank that big chunk out of our diets. It is, without question, a disruptive prospect. But the health gains are so extraordinary that you will be glad you did. This is, by far, the most important step, as the next two steps naturally follow Step 1 to a substantial degree. It helps to understand Steps 2 and 3, but just getting Step 1 right often automatically helps you get the subsequent steps right. This is because, by eliminating grains, you eliminate the appetite-stimulating effects of prolamin proteins—effects that encourage consumption of junk carbohydrates.

FOODS TO ELIMINATE DURING STEP 1

All wheat-based products: breads, breakfast cereals, noodles, pasta, bagels, muffins, pancakes, waffles, doughnuts, pretzels, cookies, crackers, wheat-brewed beers, wheat-brewed liquors

All bulgur and triticale (both offspring of wheat)

All rye products: rye bread, pumpernickel bread, crackers, rye whiskey, rye vodka

All barley products: barley, barley breads, soups with barley, beers made with barley malt

All corn products: corn, cornstarch, cornmeal products (chips, tacos, tortillas), grits, polenta, sauces or gravies thickened with cornstarch, corn syrup, high-fructose corn syrup

FOODS TO MINIMIZE OR ELIMINATE DURING STEP 1

Rice products—white rice, brown rice, wild rice

Oat products—oatmeal, oat bran, oat cereals

Amaranth

Teff

Millet

Step 2: Eat Real, Single-Ingredient Foods

Eliminate hidden sources of grains by avoiding the processed foods that fill the inner aisles of the grocery store. Almost all of these are thickened, flavored, textured, or otherwise adulterated with the seeds of one or more grasses. Living grainlessly means avoiding many foods that you never thought contained grains, such as taco seasoning, canned soup, dry soup mix, Twizzlers, soy sauce, just about every frozen dinner, and certainly all breakfast cereals, hot and cold. It means being able to recognize the common labels for grains, such as wheat flour, cornstarch, and barley malt, but also the many grain aliases, such as hydrolyzed vegetable protein, seitan, panko, maltodextrin, and modified food starch. (See Appendix B for a more complete listing of such stealth labels.) Examine all labels and avoid any food that contains grains in any shape or form. This does *not* mean that you will never have a salad with dressing again, or a delicious soup; you can make your own versions with no unhealthy grains to booby-trap them, or you can identify the few brands that have no grains added. (Yes, there are a few!)

It's also not a bad idea to avoid foods with labels, which makes label reading easy. Cucumbers, spinach, and pork chops, for example, don't come with labels (except perhaps to show weight). Avoiding labels means you'll be buying foods in their basic, "minimally changed by misguided human intervention" forms.

Avoiding grains means choosing foods carefully. It means not consuming about 59,000 of the 60,000 foods offered by your local supermarket. It does *not* mean a lack of variety or choice, though, as the 98 percent of foods now considered off-limits are (1) virtually all comprised of the same few ingredients—wheat flour, cornstarch, high-fructose corn syrup, sucrose, and salt; and (2) almost always able to be re-created using no products derived from the seeds of grasses.

Focusing on real, single-ingredient foods means enjoying unlimited quantities of many foods.

VEGETABLES. Eat all the fresh or frozen veggies you want, except for potatoes (see "Step 3: Manage Carbohydrates," below—unless you're consuming them raw, as is discussed in Chapter 9). Minimize consumption of canned foods due to bisphenol A in the lining. Explore the full range of choices: spinach, chard, kale, broccoli, broccolini, collard greens, lettuces, peppers, onions, mushrooms, Brussels sprouts, zucchini, squash, and so on. (Though I criticize agribusiness for its grain tactics, one benefit of a worldwide agricultural system is year-round availability of many vegetables.)

RAW NUTS AND SEEDS. Raw almonds, walnuts, pecans, hazelnuts, pistachios, Brazil nuts, cashews, macadamias, pumpkin seeds, sunflower seeds, sesame seeds, flaxseed, and chia seeds are all good choices, as are dry-roasted peanuts (but not those roasted in oil). Choosing raw nuts and seeds whenever possible means you avoid the hydrogenated cottonseed or hydrogenated soybean oil used to roast nuts, as well as the wheat flour, cornstarch, and maltodextrin used to coat them.

MEATS. This includes red meats, pork, fish, chicken, turkey, buffalo, ostrich, and eggs. Consider pasture-fed, free-range, grass-fed, and organic sources whenever possible. And try to overcome the modern aversion to organ meats, the most nutritious components of all, especially liver and heart. Save your bones in the freezer to make soups and stocks.

FATS AND OILS. Choose coconut, extra-virgin olive, extra-light olive, macadamia, and walnut oils, as well as butter, ghee, and avocado. Minimize polyunsaturated oils (corn, safflower, mixed vegetable, and sunflower). Avoid hydrogenated or partially hydrogenated oils.

BEVERAGES. Enjoy tea, coffee, water, unsweetened almond milk, unsweetened coconut milk, coconut water, and hemp milk.

CHEESES. Eat real cultured cheeses only (not Velveeta or single-slice processed cheese). Read labels carefully before eating blue cheese, Gorgonzola, and Roquefort, which are occasionally sources of wheat.

MISCELLANEOUS. Go for guacamole, hummus, unsweetened condiments (e.g., mayonnaise, mustard, oil-based salad dressings), ketchup without high-fructose corn syrup, pesto, tapenades, and olives.

Step 3: Manage Carbohydrates

The third step is to manage carbohydrates to squeeze even further benefits from the power of your nutritional program.

Nothing matches the power of grain elimination if you're looking to recover health, reduce appetite, and drop weight. But carbohydrate management still plays a role, as eating no grains but drinking four cans of sugary soda every day means you can still trip up your health. Four cans of soda per day provide more than 40 teaspoons of sugar, more than enough to mimic the blood sugar effects of grains in your diet and thereby negate at least some of the health benefits of grain elimination. Given the extraordinary ubiquity of diabetes and weight gain over the past few years, it's necessary to manage foods that contribute to these modern epidemics, even after grains have been eliminated. Diabetes and obesity were not health struggles primitive humans had to contend with, and so we must factor carbohydrate management into our thinking. Grain elimination does not therefore give you carte blanche to do everything else wrong with your diet.

Carb management is easier than it sounds, even in people who have a sweet tooth. Ridding your life of grain-derived opiates and lectins results in both reduced appetite and a reawakened sense of taste, including a heightened sensitivity to sweetness. It means that goodies you formerly thought were tasty will now taste sickeningly sweet. It also means that your desire for sweets will almost certainly diminish or disappear. As wacky as it sounds, people will often say things like, "Avocados and carrots taste so good now that I don't need sugary snacks anymore," which is just as it should be.

Managing carbohydrates means restricting carbohydrate intake to a level that keeps blood sugars at or below 100 mg/dl at all times, including after meals. This is low enough to avoid generating big spikes in blood sugar, which means insulin is minimally triggered, insulin resistance backs down, and excess glycation does not result.

(continued on page 146)

The Dietitian's Folly: Glycemic Index (GI)

Glycemic index, or GI, describes how high blood sugar climbs over 90 minutes after consuming a food compared to glucose.

The GI of a chicken drumstick? Zero: No impact on blood sugar. How about three fried eggs? Also zero. This is true for all other meats, oils, and fats and most nuts, seeds, mushrooms, and nonstarchy vegetables. You eat any of these foods, and blood sugar doesn't budge. No glycation phenomena follow, no glucotoxicity, no lipotoxicity.

There is nothing intrinsically wrong with the concept of the GI index or the related concept, glycemic load (GL), a measure that also factors in the quantity of food. The problem is how the values for GI and GL are *interpreted.* For instance, categories of GI are arbitrarily broken down into high glycemic index (70 or greater), moderate glycemic index (56 to 69), and low glycemic index (55 or less).

This is like being a little bit more or less pregnant. By this scheme, cornflakes, puffed rice, and pretzels have high GIs (above 70), while whole grain bread, oatmeal, and rice have low GIs. A typical nondiabetic person consuming a typical serving of cornflakes (1 cup of cereal in ½ cup of milk) will thereby experience a blood sugar in the neighborhood of 180 mg/dl. This level is very high, and it's more than sufficient to set the process of glycation and glucotoxicity on fire and add to adrenal disruption, cataract formation, destruction of cartilage, hypertension, heart disease, and neurological deterioration or dementia.

How about a low GI food, such as 1 cup of cooked oatmeal in ½ cup of milk? A typical response would be blood sugar of 170 mg/dl—lower, yes, but still quite awful, triggering all the same undesirable phenomena as the high-glycemic cornflakes. This is why I believe "low" GI would be more accurately labeled "less high" GI. Alternatively, we could just recognize that any GI above single digits should be regarded as high because it's not until you get to single digits or zero that blood sugars no longer rise to destructive levels.

The concept of glycemic load tries to take this into account by factoring in portion size. Under this system, the GL of cornflakes is 23, the GL of oatmeal is 13, and the GL of whole wheat bread is 10. GL is usually broken down as high glycemic load (20 or greater), moderate glycemic load (11 to 19), and low glycemic load (10 or less).

Once again, this lulls you into thinking that foods like oatmeal and whole wheat bread don't raise blood sugar—but they do. They don't have low glycemic loads; they have *less high* glycemic loads.

The value that truly appears to count and predict whether or not we will have a blood sugar rise? Grams of carbohydrates. Specifically, net grams of carbohydrates as calculated by subtracting fiber:

$$\text{Net carbohydrates} = \text{total carbohydrates} - \text{fiber}$$

The concept of net carbohydrates was popularized by the late Dr. Robert Atkins, who recognized that fiber has no impact on blood sugar despite being lumped together with other carbohydrates. (Fiber is technically a carbohydrate, or polysaccharide, but humans lack the enzymes to digest most fibers into sugars.)

If you were to test blood sugars with a common finger-stick glucose meter (as many of us, diabetic and nondiabetic, often do to gauge the effects of different foods) 30 to 60 minutes after consuming a food, you would see that it takes most of us 14 to 15 grams (g) of net carbohydrates before we begin to see our blood sugar rise. However, the peak can actually occur before or after this 30- to 60-minute time frame, depending on the mix of protein, fat, and fiber; the amount of water or other liquids; the pH and temperature of the food, and other factors. By testing during this time frame, you can perform a single finger stick, rather than sticking yourself every few minutes. What we *don't* do is check blood sugar 2 hours after eating, as is advised by most physicians interested in blood sugar control while on diabetes medications. Doing this seems obvious, but it is a point of disagreement when discussed with doctors who view blood sugar rises as either of no consequence or as signaling a "need" for blood sugar medication.

Ideally, *little to no rise* in blood sugar is allowed after eating any food. This turns off any excess levels of glycation and glucotoxicity, undoes the effects of high insulin and insulin resistance, and allows fasting blood sugars to drift downward over time.

There is a common fiction—or perhaps *half-truth* might be a better term—offered by the dietary community that tells us that if a high-glycemic index food is consumed along with proteins, fats, or fiber (foods with low or nonexistent glycemic indexes), the *net* glycemic effect will be much improved. For this reason, dietitians often advise people to consume, say, bread with peanut butter, theorizing that the high blood sugar potential of the bread is blunted by the low-glycemic protein, fat, and fiber in the peanut butter. As often occurs in the flawed logic of nutrition, this is another example of something being less bad, but not necessarily good. For instance, a typical blood sugar in a middle-age, mildly overweight male after consuming two slices of multigrain bread made with whole wheat flour, oats, and millet on an empty stomach might be 170 mg/dl—high enough to provoke insulin, cortisol, insulin resistance, visceral fat accumulation, inflammation, glycation, and glucotoxicity, and to add to his dementia risk. But if the same man again starts with an empty stomach and consumes two slices of multigrain bread with several slices of turkey (mostly protein), mayonnaise (mostly fat), and lettuce (mostly fiber and water), his blood sugar will be around 160 mg/dl. Better, yes, but still pretty awful and more than sufficient to generate all the negative effects of a blood sugar of 170 mg/dl, including brain atrophy. *Less bad is not necessarily good.* Feel free to count your carbs, but ignore the misleading concepts of glycemic index and glycemic load. Use any tables of glycemic index that you might have to line your box of cat litter, but don't use them to construct a healthy diet.

The ideal way to tailor carbohydrate intake to your unique level of metabolic tolerance, even as it changes over time, is to perform finger-stick blood sugar tests *30 to 60 minutes* after starting a meal to capture the blood sugar peak (see "Blood Sugar: Tool at Your Fingertips"). Ideally, your blood sugar 30 to 60 minutes after a meal should be no higher than your blood sugar prior to eating. This simple insight provides extraordinary control over metabolism, helps rapidly reverse diabetes and prediabetes, and can even accelerate weight loss.

Blood Sugar: Tool at Your Fingertips

A blood sugar meter used pre- and post-meal can be a very powerful tool for weight loss and the reversal of metabolic distortions like high blood sugar. But you have to know how to apply the information.

Many people are frightened at the prospect of getting their blood checked for anything, and they are particularly frightened by the prospect of checking it themselves. They're frightened that it could be painful or expensive, or that it would make them feel like they have diabetes. As diabetics and anyone else comfortable with checking blood sugars will attest, the process is easy. It is not painful, as the devices used to prick the finger are spring-loaded and cause minimal discomfort. And costs are modest, especially if you obtain a device and test strips from your physician, who will often just give them to you. (The device manufacturers give them away to physicians, since their money is made on the repeat sales of test strips.) If worse comes to worst, you might have to shell out the equivalent of the cost of a nice dinner at a restaurant to purchase a glucose meter and test strips for glucose and ketones (if desired; we discuss this below).

There are a number of devices that can test your blood sugar. I've had good experiences with the OneTouch Ultra, Accu-Chek Aviva, Bayer Contour, and ReliOn brands. The Precision Xtra tests for both glucose and ketones, using different test strips for each. Instructions are provided with each device, and it will take about 15 minutes to get any of these up and running. Once you get comfortable with the process, it requires just 1 to 2 minutes to obtain a blood sugar or ketone value.

Here are some tips to help you get reliable readings.

- Try using the soft pads of your fingers first, though you can test just about anywhere on your body, including the sides of your fingers or even the back of your hand.

- Swab with an alcohol wipe first to ensure that the surface you choose is clean and free of hand creams, lotions, etc.

- Don't "milk" your finger to get an adequate drop of blood. If the blood that results from your finger stick is too small, repeat using a deeper setting on your finger-stick device and/or use firmer pressure on the device. You can also bend over and lower your hand toward the floor for 30 seconds before performing the finger stick, as this will encourage blood to pool in your hands.

- Rotate finger-stick sites to avoid making one site sore.

Remember: The goal here is not to control blood sugar with medication or insulin but to identify problem foods that provoke blood sugar and insulin, thereby impairing weight-loss efforts. To do this, we check blood sugar immediately prior to a meal and then 30 to 60 minutes after the start of the meal.

Aim for no change in blood sugar when you take these two readings. If the after-meal value jumps up to, say, 138 mg/dl, look at that meal and identify the carbohydrate source that was too much for you, and then either slash your portion size or eliminate that food. (In the meantime, go for a walk, ride a stationary bike for 20 minutes, or engage in some other light activity to drop your blood sugar back to its starting level.)

If you don't like the idea of checking finger-stick blood sugars, consider having your doctor measure a value called hemoglobin A1c (HbA1c). This value reflects blood sugar fluctuations experienced over the previous 90 days. The typical primary care doctor will say something like, "Your HbA1c is less than 6.5 percent, so you're okay," meaning that you don't have diabetes and don't need diabetes medication. What he or she is not saying is that your HbA1c is ideal and does not have implications for health, because that's just not the case. In fact, people with HbA1c values in the "normal" range—say, 5.6 percent—are still at an increased risk for heart disease, cancer, hypertension, and dementia. An HbA1c value of 5.0 percent or less represents the ideal level; it approximates the level enjoyed by a primitive human hunting and foraging for food and spared the health problems that come from uncontrolled high blood sugars. If your doctor won't test you, you can buy at-home test kits for HbA1c from the pharmacy. After you test yourself, make sure you find a new doctor.

Another way to manage carbohydrate content is to count carbs. This method is the least precise and least individualized, as it does not take into account whether you are a slender 23-year-old woman who runs marathons or a 297-pound, sedentary 63-year-old accountant with lots of pretax stress. Nonetheless, most people do well by keeping net carbohydrate exposure to 15 g per meal or less, particularly while trying to achieve substantial weight loss. You will need a resource for looking up the composition of various foods, such as an inexpensive book with tables of the nutritional content of foods. Smartphone apps are also useful on the go. (Search for "nutritional analysis" in your application source.) There are also many Web sites that list nutritional analyses of foods.

There are a few additional tips that are useful when managing carbohydrate intake.

WATCH YOUR FRUIT. Limit yourself to no more than 15 g of net carbohydrates per meal within a 4- to 6-hour period. Choose your fruit wisely by referring to this list, which ranks each type from best to worst: berries of all varieties, citrus, apples, nectarines, peaches, and melons. Minimize (ripe) bananas, pineapples, mangoes, and grapes, and when you eat them, do so only in small quantities, since their sugar content is similar to that of candy. An exception to the fruit guidelines is avocado, which is high in fats, rich in potassium, wonderfully filling, and low in net carbs (3 g per avocado), so eat as much of it as you like.

AVOID FRUIT JUICES. If you must drink fruit juice (such as pomegranate juice for its health benefits), drink only real, 100 percent juices (not fruit "drinks" made with high-fructose corn syrup and a little added juice) and only in minimal quantities (no more than 2 to 4 ounces per 4- to 6-hour digestive period, i.e., the period of time required by most people to clear the effects of a meal), as the sugar content of juice is very high.

One 8-ounce glass of orange juice, for example, contains the equivalent of 6 teaspoons of sugar.

LIMIT DAIRY PRODUCTS. Have no more than 1 serving per day of milk, cottage cheese, or unsweetened yogurt (preferably full fat). Remember: Fat is not the problem. We limit dairy due to both the lactose sugar content and the peculiar ability of the whey protein to provoke insulin, which can impair weight loss and encourage insulin resistance. Cheese is the least problematic form of dairy, as the culturing process reduces lactose and much of the whey is skimmed off during production.

MEASURE YOUR LEGUMES, BEANS, PEAS, SWEET POTATOES, AND YAMS. This is where carbohydrate counting and blood sugar finger-stick testing are useful. In general, however, you should eat no more than ¼ cup of any of these in any 4- to 6-hour digestive period, as larger quantities tend to start blood sugar fireworks. I do believe that such foods *should* be consumed, however, as they provide important benefits to bowel flora. (See Chapter 9 for information on how to restore important prebiotic fibers for bowel flora and bowel health without messing with blood sugars.)

INDULGE IN SOME DARK CHOCOLATE. Choose chocolate that's no less than 70 to 85 percent cocoa, and eat no more than 40 g (approximately 2 inches square) per day to limit sugar.

STAY AWAY FROM SUGAR-FREE FOODS. Avoid foods sweetened with sorbitol, mannitol, lactitol, or maltitol, as they act much like sugar and cause plenty of diarrhea and bloating, too. (See the discussion below about safe sweeteners used in *Wheat Belly* recipes.)

Managing carbohydrates to improve control over metabolism and health goes hand in hand with not consuming gluten-free foods made with junk carbohydrates (cornstarch, rice flour, tapioca starch, and potato flour). Cornstarch and rice flour are ground from the seeds of grasses, so they should be off your list anyway. If you need another reason to avoid them, remember that all four popular wheat- and gluten-free replacements are guilty of provoking blood sugars higher than *all* other foods: higher than wheat flour, higher than sucrose, higher than candy bars. Nothing raises blood sugar higher than the gluten-free junk carbohydrates in, say, gluten-free multigrain bread or gluten-free pasta. Blood sugar that results from eating two slices of whole grain gluten-free bread made with potato flour, rice flour, and millet can easily top 180 mg/dl over the first hour after consumption, regardless of what was contained within the sandwich. Unfortunately, this has not stopped the gluten-free industry from selling awful, unhealthy products made with these junk carbohydrate ingredients.

You will notice that there are no restrictions on oil or fat intake here, which means eating the way you may remember your grandparents did: Eat the fat on your beef, pork, lamb, poultry, and fish. Save the fats in a container and refrigerate them to use as cooking oil. Save the bones (or buy them from a butcher) to make soup or stock. Don't buy lean meats. Eat dark poultry meat as well as white. Consider eating bone marrow. Use oils generously, especially coconut oil, extra-virgin or extra-light (when you don't want the vegetal flavor of extra-virgin) olive oil, organic butter or ghee, avocado oil, macadamia oil, flaxseed oil, and walnut oil. (There are occasional genetic exceptions to the notion of unrestricted fat intake, generally suggested by very high total and LDL cholesterols. See the additional discussion about this issue in Chapter 10.)

I also encourage people to consider consuming organ meats, such as liver, heart, tongue, and thymus, as they are among the most nutrient dense of all foods. Liver, for instance, is packed with vitamin C, vitamin B_{12}, iron, vitamin A, vitamin D, coenzyme Q10, and fats. By consuming organ meats, we mimic the eating habits of humans going back to our adaptive beginnings. How did primitive humans who lacked access to fish or shellfish obtain omega-3 fatty acids, without which you perish? They ate the brains of land animals. How did these humans obtain iodine, since iodine is present only in the ocean, fish, shellfish, seaweed, and foods grown along the coasts? By eating the thyroid gland of animals. In other words, humans require nutrients that, in many settings, could only be obtained by consuming the organs of animals. Get over it: Have some liver.

If you're just getting started with eating organ meats and related dishes, the easiest and most convenient way to do this is to purchase uncured liver sausage and chicken livers (since they are easy to handle). You can also make soup or stock from bones (see the recipe on page 334). Choose organs, as well as meats, from organic, pasture-fed animals to minimize your exposure to contaminants. Just as in humans, if an animal was raised in a contaminated area, the meat and organs will be contaminated. Because of their roles in detoxification, organs can concentrate heavy metals, such as mercury and lead. There have been reports that kidneys, in particular, can have higher levels of heavy metals.[1]

There are also foods outside of grains that cause enough of an undesirable health effect that they essentially should never be a part of your diet. Of course, if you find yourself stranded on a deserted island with nothing else to eat, go ahead and have the loaf of stale bread, fried onions, and fat-free cookies. But if you are not stranded and have choices, you should never consume the foods listed here.

Gluten-free foods made with rice flour, cornstarch, tapioca starch, or potato flour	Cured meats (hot dogs, sausages, bacon, bologna, pepperoni fixed with sodium nitrite)
Fried foods	Fat-free or low-fat salad dressings and other low-fat or nonfat processed foods
Fast foods	
Hydrogenated trans fats	

ADDITIONAL STEPS FOR TRULY HEALTHY EATING

In our modern age of mass-produced commercial foods, we have to be aware of several other important issues to maximize health. None of these achieve the outsize benefits of grain removal, but just as quitting cigarettes yields terrific health benefits that you could partly sabotage by drinking too much bourbon, we don't want to botch up the wonderful grain-free start we obtain by making unhealthy choices outside of grains.

MEATS SHOULD BE UNCURED AND UNPROCESSED AND SHOULD NOT CONTAIN SODIUM NITRITE. Sausage, pepperoni, bacon, salami, and other processed meats often contain the color-fixing chemical sodium nitrite. Upon cooking, sodium nitrite reacts with amino acids in meat, yielding nitrosamines that have been linked to gastrointestinal cancers.[2] This is a confusing issue, and the science has been misinterpreted by many. The related compounds called nitrates (NO_3), for instance, occur in green vegetables and are converted into nitrites (NO_2) that are further converted in the body to nitric oxide, which is beneficial, reducing blood pressure and yielding other health benefits. This has caused some to dismiss the issue of nitrates and nitrites. However, they overlook the fact that nitrites in cured meats react with the meat itself, especially when the nitrites are heated, yielding high levels of nitrosamines which, in every animal experimental model, have caused gastrointestinal cancers and, in several human epidemiological studies, have been associated with greater cancer incidence.[3] Instead of meats cured with sodium nitrite, look for meats that are processed naturally and do not contain sodium nitrite. (They often contain nitrates that do not react to form nitrosamines in meat.) Of course, also make sure they contain no wheat, cornstarch, or other hidden grains.

CHOOSE ORGANIC DAIRY PRODUCTS. Because many commercial, high-volume dairies milk pregnant cows throughout pregnancy (rather than the more limited milking period practiced by organic farmers), products made from this milk contain more estrogen. Avoid this problem by choosing milk, sour cream, cheese, yogurt, and butter from organic producers.[4] By choosing organic products, you'll also avoid consuming bovine growth hormone.

CONSIDER FERMENTED FOODS. Coconut or dairy yogurt, kefir, fermented radishes, fermented cucumbers, and fermented onions are among the many delicious and healthy ways you can add some exotic spice to your vegetables while obtaining healthy quantities of bacteria that benefit bowel health. The process of fermentation is different from that of pickling; fermentation yields probiotic-like healthy bacteria to repopulate bowel flora, while pickling yields no special health benefits. (Fermented foods are wonderfully easy to make yourself: See page 328 for some guidelines.) Yogurts and kefirs provide delicious breakfasts, desserts, and snacks. Fermented foods can be eaten as is, added to salads, or dipped into hummus or salsa.

DON'T LIMIT SALT. At this point, it should be no surprise that "official" advice may not just be ineffective, but may actually *cause* health problems. And so it goes also with the advice to severely restrict salt use. That advice has been retracted in view of clinical studies demonstrating increased cardiovascular death with salt restriction to levels below 1,500 milligrams (mg) per day.[5] Average salt intake in the United States is 3,400 mg, which may be a perfectly fine level, although the Institute of Medicine stands by its advice to limit salt to no more than 2,300 mg per day. There can be problems, however, with unlimited salt use, as salt intakes in or above the 6,000 to 10,000 mg range per day can indeed be associated with adverse cardiovascular effects. Also, a minority of people, such as people with kidney disease, do have sensitivities to salt and should not engage in unrestricted salt intake. If you have such a condition, a sodium prescription should come from your doctor. For the vast majority of us engaging in a grain-free lifestyle, however, light to moderate use of (preferably) mineral-rich forms of salt, such as sea salt, is actually healthier than severely restricting salt, particularly when that salt is combined with healthy foods rich in potassium (such as vegetables, avocados, or coconut).

USE SAFE SWEETENERS. Those of you already familiar with the Wheat Belly lifestyle know that we can re-create cookies, muffins, cakes, and other goodies using safe sweeteners with little to no downside. The *Wheat Belly Cookbook*, the *Wheat Belly 30-Minute (or Less!) Cookbook*, and the *Wheat Belly* blog, www.wheatbellyblog.com, are all sources of grain-free recipes that put such sweeteners to work when needed. Among the safe sweeteners are pure liquid or powdered stevia; stevia with inulin, but not maltodextrin; monk fruit (also known as Lo Han Guo); erythritol, and xylitol. (Be careful with xylitol around dogs, as it is toxic to them.) An occasional person will experience triggering of their sweet tooth with these sweeteners, leading to cravings for other sweet foods, but it is uncommon.

AVOID FRUCTOSE-CONTAINING SWEETENERS. Beyond avoiding grain-sourced high-fructose corn syrup as a source of fructose, it is also important to avoid other sources of fructose. Sucrose (table sugar) is 50 percent fructose, which is not too different from high-fructose corn syrup. And some of the new "healthy" sweeteners, such as agave nectar (90 percent fructose—the worst of all) and coconut sugar, are really nothing more than sources of sucrose or fructose. Some people choose to use honey and maple syrup, as they are natural sources, but both are high in fructose and should be used sparingly.

CHOOSE ORGANIC VEGETABLES AND FRUITS. Whenever they're available and your budget permits, make organic your first choice. This is most important when the exterior of the food is consumed, as with blueberries and broccoli, for example. If the exterior is not consumed, as with bananas and avocados, it is not as important, though pesticides and herbicides can still penetrate to the interior. If you cannot choose organic, at the very least rinse fruits and veggies thoroughly in warm water to minimize residues of pesticides and herbicides such as perchlorates, which can block thyroid function.

MINIMIZE EXPOSURE TO BISPHENOL A (BPA). This compound is found in polycarbonate plastics (clear hard plastics with recycling code #7) and the resin lining of cans and is suspected to exert endocrine disruptive effects leading to congestive heart failure, diabetes, thyroid dysfunction, and weight gain.[6] Canned coconut milk is therefore a potential source of exposure, though Native Forest and Natural Value are among the first brands to declare that they use BPA-free cans. As the controversy over BPA heats up, more manufacturers are converting to BPA-free linings.

AVOID SOFT DRINKS AND CARBONATED BEVERAGES. The acid effects of carbonation erode bone health, as carbonic acid is neutralized by extracting calcium salts from bones. Instead, drink water (squeeze in some lemon or lime or keep a filled water pitcher in the refrigerator with a few slices of cucumber, kiwi, mint leaves, or orange), teas (black, green, or white), infusions (teas brewed from other leaves, herbs, flowers, and fruits), unsweetened almond milk, unsweetened coconut milk (carton variety from the dairy refrigerator, or other BPA-free type), coconut water, hemp milk, and coffee.

AVOID HYDROGENATED FATS. The hydrogenated fats, or trans fats, that fill processed foods contribute to heart disease, hypertension, and diabetes.[7] Margarine is the worst culprit, made with vegetable oils hydrogenated to yield a solid stick or tub form. Many processed foods, from cookies to sandwich spreads, contain hydrogenated oils and should be avoided for their trans fat content as well as their grains and sugars.

MINIMIZE EXPOSURE TO HIGH-TEMPERATURE COOKING. Any method of cooking that involves temperatures that exceed 450°F will provoke reactions called glycation or lipoxidation, reactions between carbohydrates or proteins with the fats in foods. These contribute to hypertension, formation of cataracts, arthritis, heart disease, and cancer.[8] These reactions develop with deep frying (not sautéing, a relatively low-temperature process), broiling, and any form of cooking that involves charring the food's surface.

Bottom line: Stick with real foods that require no labels and are least processed by manufacturers. You can be confident that these foods are safe to serve to your family and don't contain obvious or hidden seeds of grasses.

Belly Up to the Grain-Free Bar

Having a glass or two of wine, brandy, or a cocktail is perfectly in line with the grain-free lifestyle, but you will have to be selective. The price of a poor choice can be reigniting an autoimmune condition, provoking high blood sugar, triggering an inappropriate emotional outburst that ruins your evening, or regaining 15 pounds. The reward for choosing wisely can be a wonderful time spent with friends without such problems. Also, recognize that *any* amount of wine, cocktails, or beer can stall weight loss.

Wine is as close to a perfect wheat- and gluten-free beverage as it gets, regardless of varietal or vintage. Combined with the probable health effects that derive from light wine drinking (no more than two 4-ounce glasses per day) due to the combination of alcohol, anthocyanins (which provide the red-purple color of red wine), and perhaps resveratrol, wine drinking is proving to be both pleasurable and healthy.

Rarely, gluten is used as a clarifying agent. Bovine spongiform encephalopathy ("mad cow disease") raised doubts about the safety of gelatin, and gluten emerged as an alternative, though very few winemakers use it. Even less commonly, a wheat flour–containing paste is used to seal the barrels used to age wines. The presence of gluten in wine is therefore uncommon. Even if gluten were used as the clarifying agent, it is unlikely to pose sufficient exposure to generate an immune response.[9] Note that **wine coolers** typically contain barley malt, not to mention higher carbohydrate and sugar levels, and should be avoided.

Virtually all **ales, beers, malt liquors, and lagers** are brewed from grains and are therefore off the list, as there are measurable grain protein residues present—generally 1 to 2 g per 12 ounces. This is not a lot, but it's enough to stimulate appetite, provoke inflammation, and initiate autoimmunity. People with celiac disease or the most extreme forms of gluten sensitivity should avoid beers altogether, except those designated gluten-free. (Though I have my doubts about even the gluten-free products, since all are brewed from the seeds of grasses.) If a beer is designated gluten-free, no gliadin or gluten should be present (the official cutoff is fewer than 20 parts per million), but there is still potential for uncertain reactions from other grain proteins. Those who do not have celiac disease or gluten sensitivity seem to do okay with beers brewed from sorghum and rice but which also include barley malt, though you may have to experiment and see how your body reacts to these beers before you decide whether or not to consume them regularly. Of all alcoholic beverages, beer is the most hazardous, so be careful. If you must drink it, here are a few of the least problematic brews.

Bard's gluten-free beers. Brewed from sorghum without barley, this beer is truly gluten-free. As with many gluten-free beers, however, it's high in carbs, and therefore you should not drink more than one per day (14.2 g carbohydrates per 12-ounce bottle).

Bud Light and Michelob Ultra. Bud Light, made by Anheuser-Busch, is brewed from rice but also contains barley malt. The most severely gluten-sensitive people should therefore *not* indulge in this beer because of the gluten content. But most of us who are just avoiding wheat but who aren't gluten-sensitive can safely consume this brand without exposing ourselves to the undesirable effects of grains. One 12-ounce bottle contains 6.6 g of carbohydrates. Michelob Ultra is likewise brewed from rice with barley malt. It is also low in carbohydrates, with 2.6 g per 12-ounce serving.

Redbridge. Redbridge is brewed from sorghum and is not brewed with wheat or barley. It is therefore confidently gluten-free, though it's still brewed from the seed of a grass. The carbohydrate content is a bit high at 16.4 g per bottle; have more than one beer and the carbohydrates begin to stack up.

Green's gluten-free beers. UK brewer Green's provides several gluten-free choices made from sorghum, millet, buckwheat, brown rice, and "deglutenised" barley malt. They are not grain-free and have low quantities of grain proteins. So tread carefully here, and make judgments based on your individual experience. The carbohydrate content of these beers is slightly less than most others, ranging from 10 to 14 g per 330-ml bottle.

In addition to these choices, I have seen some microbreweries starting to jump on the gluten-free bandwagon. Look for beers brewed from chicory and other ingredients.

Avoid **vodkas** brewed from grains if you have an extreme gluten sensitivity or celiac disease. Wheat-sourced vodkas include Absolut, Grey Goose, Ketel One, SKYY, and Stolichnaya. Nonwheat but grain-sourced vodkas include Belvedere (rye), Finlandia (barley), Van Gogh (wheat, barley, and corn), and Smirnoff (corn). For the rest of us, the low grain protein content in these beverages (they contain gluten and other prolamins at less than 20 parts per million) means they are likely safe to consume. The safest vodkas, however, are free of any grain proteins; this includes Chopin (potatoes) and Cîroc (grapes). Beware of the flavored varieties, as they tend to be loaded with sugar or high-fructose corn syrup. In general, simple unflavored vodkas are safest.

Most **whiskeys** are not safe for those highly sensitive to grain proteins, since they are distilled from rye, barley, wheat, and corn. Whiskeys nearly always test below 20 parts per million for gluten, which is the limit the FDA considers safe for people with celiac disease and gluten sensitivity. Nonetheless, some people still seem to react to whiskeys distilled from grains. This means that by consuming many popular whiskeys, such as Jack Daniels (barley, rye, and corn), Jameson (barley), and Bushmills (barley), you are risking a gluten (gliadin) reaction. People without extreme sensitivities are likely to be just fine, given the very low quantity of grain proteins.

Brandies and cognacs are generally safe, since they are distilled from wine. Safe brands include Grand Marnier, Courvoisier, and Rémy Martin. There are occasional exceptions (such as Martell) that add caramel coloring, which is a potential grain exposure.

Rum is distilled from sugar cane and does not contain any residues of grain proteins. Be careful of any flavored or spiced rums, though, which may contain a grain-based ingredient, excessive sugar, or high-fructose corn syrup.

Safe **liqueurs** include Kahlúa (contains dairy), fruit liqueurs like triple sec and Cherry Kijafa, amaretto, and Bailey's Irish Cream (contains dairy). The most gluten-sensitive may have to avoid those blended with whiskey, as the source of whiskey is often not specified. Also, note that liqueurs tend to be high in sugar.

WHAT TO EXPECT WHEN LIVING GRAINLESSLY: A TIMELINE

In Chapter 6, I discussed what happens to members of our species when we cease consumption of the seeds of grasses: At first, it isn't pretty. But I'd like to cover this topic again, this time with a timeline of what to expect when you banish all grains from your diet. Note that timelines are approximate, depending on, for instance, the quantity of grains consumed previously, status of bowel flora, thyroid status, age, sex, form and intensity of inflammatory or autoimmune response, and other factors. Nonetheless, a rough timeline can be constructed to help you anticipate how and in what sequence your grain-free experience may play out.

WEEK 1: This is, for about 40 percent of us, the worst part of the experience. This is the period plagued by withdrawal from the opiates of grains, resulting in fatigue, nausea, headache, and depression—all the features of opiate withdrawal syndrome—and cravings for foods made of grains. Recognize that this does not represent a "need" for some component of grains, but just withdrawal from the opiates in gliadin and related proteins. Light-headedness and muscle cramps can develop, so be sure to hydrate, use mineral-rich salt, and take magnesium supplements.

Despite the rigors of withdrawal, weight loss can nonetheless proceed, often rapidly. Many, though not all, people experience weight loss at the rate of 1 pound per day for the first week, losing a combination of visceral fat and water. It is also at the end of Week 1 that sleep begins to improve: It becomes deeper and more restful, with fewer restless leg tendencies.

WEEKS 2 THROUGH 4: For most people, Week 2 marks a big turnaround in emotions, energy, joint health, and skin health. Typical observations during this period include relief from acid reflux and heartburn; relief from the bowel urgency of irritable bowel syndrome; relief from joint pain in fingers and wrists; relief from depression; relief from appetite stimulation, including the 24-hour-a-day food obsessions experienced by people with bulimia and binge eating disorder; and relief from common skin conditions such as eczema, acne, and seborrhea.

For the majority of people, weight loss continues, though it may slow from the rapid pace of the first week. Most people feel a surge in energy at this time, and many people who experience chronic migraine headaches experience partial or total relief. Women with painful and turbulent premenstrual syndrome symptoms may begin to feel them recede at Week 2 or just beyond, depending on when in their cycle they began the grain-elimination process.

WEEK 5: The early period of opiate withdrawal should have passed by now, and those people who developed metabolic reliance on carbohydrates during their former grain-consuming lives should begin to acquire higher levels of energy. Depriving the body of carbohydrates, especially grain amylopectins, results in a drop in energy until the body adapts by ramping up the process of fat mobilization. Once that occurs, energy increases and mood improves.

If you chose to exercise during the first few weeks of grain elimination, you probably noticed that running, swimming, biking, and other activities were difficult, with reduced energy, slower times, and overall poor performance. Once you reach Week 5, though, performance for most athletes *surpasses* levels achieved prior to grain elimination. Carb-loading is no longer necessary and carbohydrate supplementation needs are much reduced during prolonged efforts. Less-serious exercise efforts, such as jogging 5 miles, biking 20 miles, or doing aerobics for an hour, do not require carb-loading, energy drinks, energy bars, or other supplementation, as your body is more efficient at drawing energy from its fat stores.

People with chronic fatigue syndrome or fibromyalgia typically respond at about this time, partially or completely, with surges in energy and mood and relief from muscle pain, joint pain, and stiffness. Hormonal issues, such as tumultuous menstrual periods in women and enlarged breasts in men, typically require this long to improve. The hormonal distortions that cause these issues, such as inappropriately high estrogen levels and inflammatory phenomena, recede with visceral fat, which should, by this time, have shrunken dramatically.

WEEK 6 AND ONWARD: Six or more—sometimes many more—weeks are usually required for more complex conditions that involve autoimmunity and inflammation to recede or reverse. Autoimmune conditions such as rheumatoid arthritis, lupus, multiple sclerosis, Hashimoto's thyroiditis, polymyositis, polymyalgia rheumatica, psoriasis, and others typically start to respond at about this time, with continuing improvement over the next several months. (See Chapter 13 for how to improve the likelihood of full response by autoimmune conditions.) Inflammatory conditions, such as osteoarthritis of the hips and knees, also respond more slowly, providing relief over the following few months. The degree of response is highly variable, depending upon the extent of bony damage, which does not reverse with grain elimination.

Neurological conditions also require more time to respond, given the slow and limited potential for nervous system tissue to undergo repair. Multiple sclerosis, the impaired coordination of cerebellar ataxia, and the tingling and pain of peripheral neuropathy can require months to years to respond or, at least, stop progressing further. Neurological impairment from grain consumption should be treated in the same way as autoimmune conditions, and the strategies discussed in Chapter 13 should be considered in order to maximize the long-term likelihood of recovery.

Wheat Belly *did not change my life—it saved my life.*

My trainer and nutritionist both told me, "You *must* read *Wheat Belly!*" I did. And so started a journey in which I lost 200 pounds in less than 2 years.

Before reading and acting on the advice of *Wheat Belly*, I was morbidly obese (more than 400 pounds) and sick all the time. I had chronic migraines and chronic heartburn and indigestion. I had zero energy, was severely depressed, and was addicted to food.

I was about 17 years old the first time I had a horrible migraine. I remember trying to drive to the local drugstore to get medicine, but it was so painful that I could hardly drive. Over the course of the next 2 decades, I continued to struggle with headaches. I had MRIs, tried different drugs, went to occupational therapy, worked with a headache "specialist"—nothing helped. In addition to the chronic migraines, I developed acid reflux 10 years ago. I had it so bad that I went to the emergency room because I thought I was having a heart attack.

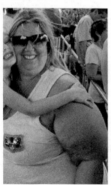
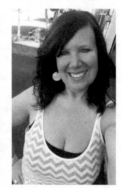

Before   *After*

I had EKGs, stress tests, and numerous other tests. They diagnosed me with acid reflux and started me on acid blockers. I was taking up to four different pills per day to try to help control the heartburn.

I knew I needed to lose weight. A cardiologist told me, "The only way you will ever lose weight is with gastric bypass surgery." I talked with a nutritionist and doctor. They both told me to cut out the "whites": white sugars, white rice, white flour, and so on. Stick to whole wheat. I switched to whole wheat bread, whole grain cereals, whole wheat pasta. I did that for a bit more than a year. I was miserable. I gained 2 pounds that year. All I thought about was food! I would eat a sandwich and an hour later I would not be able to stop thinking about another sandwich. I was irritable all the time, and my skin looked awful. I always had a bit of acne, but, over the course of that year, it got much worse. I cried a lot. I was not sleeping properly. The life I was living was awful. It was unfair to my daughters, my husband, my family, and myself.

I turned to a local gym in February 2012 and sought the advice of both a trainer and a nutritionist. The one thing they both told me in my first meeting with them was "You must read *Wheat Belly!*"

Two weeks later, I went back to step on the scale. I had lost 29 pounds. Chronic migraines: gone. Chronic severe heartburn: gone. I quit taking all the drugs I was on for both migraines and heartburn. To this day, nearly 2 years later, I have not had a single migraine nor have I battled heartburn. I have gone on to lose 200 pounds! I feel amazing.

I had an enlarged heart. My recent follow-up indicated my heart was normal. My resting heart rate is under 60—it used to be 90. I am no longer depressed, I can focus, and I sleep great. My energy is through the roof! I absolutely feel like a different person. Yes, I worked out. Yes, I made some other dietary changes. But the change that impacted my life and my health the most was following the advice of *Wheat Belly* and going wheat- and gluten-free.

I am so grateful to *Wheat Belly* for giving me a life I never dreamt possible without any sort of radical stomach surgery.

Amy, Chaska, Minnesota

REDUCING THE COSTS OF A GRAIN-FREE LIFESTYLE

Some people balk at the prospect of following this lifestyle because they're concerned that the increased reliance on pasture-fed and organic vegetables and meats will end up costing them an arm and a leg. They worry that this shift in diet will blow the lid off their grocery budget, and they worry about a life without quick, inexpensive convenience foods.

These concerns are entirely unwarranted. Sure, you will be purchasing more costly foods, but the net cost is typically unchanged or less. Many people who budget their monthly grocery bill actually report a modest cost savings with this lifestyle. Do the math: Banished from your life are the foods that stimulate appetite, and so you no longer have to purchase 400 additional calories per person, per day. In a family of five, that's 2,000 or more calories per day that you no longer have to buy—60,000 calories over the course of a month. It is not uncommon to witness family-wide reductions of 3,000 to 4,000 calories *every day* with grain elimination: no more corn chips, rye crackers, frozen dinners, breakfast cereals, endless snacking and bingeing. It's like no longer having to feed an extra invisible person with a large appetite. Over a month's time, that's about 90 meals you no longer have to purchase or prepare.

Nonetheless, there are a number of strategies that you can use to keep a lid on costs as you make your new food choices. Not everybody can or wants to follow each and every strategy, but incorporating just a few of these can further trim costs. Remember: We evolved in a world in which the foods we consumed were without cost because we gathered and hunted them from our surroundings. Bearing that in mind, the more we revert to such practices, the closer we get to consuming foods that are not only free, but also healthier.

Consider these cost-saving strategies.

GROW YOUR OWN. Grow your own green beans, tomatoes, cucumbers, and fruit every spring. You don't need a big, fancy garden (though that would be wonderful), just a simple 5- by 5-foot or similar plot, fertilized with coffee grounds and composted organic materials. If you have never gardened before, choose the vegetables that are easiest to grow, such as cucumbers, zucchini, and squash, and save your seeds for the next year. (Not all seeds will germinate, such as those from hybrids. Ideally, start with an heirloom plant or seed, then simply propagate year after year by saving the seeds for next season.)

PRESERVE YOUR HARVEST. If you grow your own, you may be left with more than you can consume. Freeze, can, or ferment the excess whenever you have more than you and your family require. (See Appendix A for instructions on fermenting your own foods.)

CULTIVATE HERBS. Grow your own fresh basil, oregano, mint, and other herbs in a windowsill planter indoors. You will no longer have to pay $3.99 for a few fresh leaves of basil, but will simply pull a few off your own plant, which will regrow in just a few days.

GROW BERRIES. Berry vines, such as raspberries, are wonderfully easy to grow and allow you to pick your own delicious fruit year after year. Plants typically cost just a few dollars, or you can obtain cuttings from someone else eager to cut back their endlessly propagating berry vines. Within a year or two of planting, you will be fighting your vines as they try to overtake your entire backyard. Grapes are another prolific fruit to grow.

PLANT FRUIT TREES. Nothing beats picking your own apples, pears, and cherries. Obviously, this is a long-term strategy, as these trees require a few years to mature. But once they do, you will have more than you will ever need. Those of us living a grain-free lifestyle limit fruit consumption because of the sugar content of most modern strains, so a little will go a long way.

PICK EXCESS FRUIT IN YOUR NEIGHBORHOOD. It is shocking to see the number of apples, pears, and cherries in colder climates, and oranges, lemons, and grapefruit in warmer climates, that just fall to the ground or rot on the tree. If local laws or neighbors allow, why not gather them? And, if you are so inclined, join the growing number of people foraging. Just be sure to learn from a knowledgeable expert which leaves, flowers, and mushrooms are safely edible before you take this path.

EAT FATTY OR LESS COSTLY CUTS OF MEAT. We embrace fat: It is essential for life and is good for health. It is also satiating. Buy fatty cuts of meat, such as chuck, rib eye, tongue, and fatty ground meat. Or just eyeball the cuts with the fat left on—and don't cut it off before eating. Round, brisket, and shank, while not rich in fat, tend to be less costly cuts. If the cuts you choose are tough, pound them with a meat mallet before cooking or use a slow cooker.

SAVE FATS FROM MEATS. Save fats in a nonplastic container (such as a clean jar), and set them aside to cool. Use the saved fats as your cooking oil, which is healthier and cheaper than buying bottles of polyunsaturated oils.

SAVE BONES. Or purchase them from the butcher or meat section at the grocery store. (Sometimes they will just give them to you without charge.) Boil them for soup with added inexpensive cuts of meat. Three pounds of bones and a pound of inexpensive meat (with chopped onions, carrots, celery, etc., and some tomato paste) will yield a rich and delicious soup that lasts for days. If you use the bones to make stock, add it to vegetables and other dishes to enhance their flavor at virtually no cost.

EAT MORE EGGS. Eggs, combined with vegetables, oils, olives, herbs, and other ingredients, make wonderful frittatas or quiches (with nut meal crusts; there are recipes for these in the *Wheat Belly* cookbooks) that can be used for exceptionally low-cost breakfasts, or even dinners. Buy large quantities of eggs from family farms and they will also be healthier, with delicious orange- or red-colored yolks, if the chickens were allowed to range and forage freely.

DEHYDRATE FOODS. This is one of my favorite strategies, as it allows you to dehydrate leftover meats, vegetables, and fruits to convert them into delicious snacks. Spice them up with turmeric, ground red pepper, sea salt, and other spices prior to dehydrating. A dehydrating device can be purchased for as little $30 to $40 and will pay for itself after just a few uses.

SHOP AS CLOSE TO THE SOURCE AS POSSIBLE. By eliminating the middleman and avoiding high-end stores, you shave off substantial added costs. Purchase vegetables from a farm or farmers' market. Subscribe to a community supported agriculture (CSA) group (though you may want to split the subscription with another family, given the high volume typically provided) for vegetables, eggs, and meats. Increasingly, a market style of CSA is emerging in which you pick and choose each week what you desire, rather than receiving a predetermined variety or quantity.

PRACTICE INTERMITTENT FASTING. While I don't view the practice of intermittent fasting as a money-saving maneuver, it is so easy in this grain-free lifestyle and it packs so many benefits that it can indeed result in diminished food costs. If, for instance, you fast for 36 hours every 10 days, that means you do not have to shop, cook, or eat for 4½ days per month—all while feeling terrific, reducing blood pressure, restoring insulin responses, and reducing risk for heart disease. Plus, you'll have a greater appreciation for the flavors and textures of foods when you resume eating. Fasting means eating no food but maintaining vigorous hydration, or else light-headedness and nausea can result. (More on this in Chapter 14.)

The ultimate way to save money would be, of course, to have a full-size garden and scavenge for edible leaves, tubers, and mushrooms while hunting wild game, fishing, and gathering shellfish. Wild turkey and deer are plentiful, and just a few hunting excursions can yield a freezer full of meat. Unfortunately, most people simply have neither the time nor the inclination to return to their scavenging, hunting, and gathering origins to this degree. But I believe that human health is enhanced by always remembering that you and your family are really just a small clan of hungry primates making your way through the world.

Beyond the money saved by choosing just one or more of the above cost-saving methods, you and your family will need fewer (or no) antacids, prescription drugs for acid reflux, antihypertensive drugs, cholesterol drugs, pain medications, and antidepressants. You'll also make fewer visits to the doctor, emergency room, or hospital. So does grain elimination cost you money? Heck, no. In many, if not most, instances, the net effect of grain elimination is that it saves or makes you money.

A GRAINLESS PRESCRIPTION

If grain elimination were a prescription dispensed by your doctor, it would be unlike any other: There is no need to run to the pharmacy to get it filled, shell out full cost or a co-pay, get it refilled every month, and then endure side effects while experiencing only partial benefit.

The "prescription" of grain elimination is something you can conduct by yourself, in the comfort of your own home, with no pharmacy hassles involved. This prescription costs nothing and often yields cost savings. The only side effects experienced are that your body will revert to its normal state, which is not a side effect in the usual sense. Aside from personal fears of the withdrawal process and concerns about convenience, I can conceive of no reason why you should not fill this prescription to release yourself from the appetite traps set by grains and allow your body to declare its grain-free health.

PART III

BE A GRAINLESS OVERACHIEVER

The Next Steps to Reclaiming Grain-Free Total Health

CHAPTER 8

CORRECT NUTRITIONAL DEFICIENCIES CAUSED BY GRAINS

Populations that depend on grains and legumes as staple foods consume diets rich in phytic acid... This compound binds tightly to important mineral nutrients such as iron and zinc, forming salts that are largely excreted. This phenomenon can contribute to mineral depletion and deficiency.

—Victor Raboy, US Department of Agriculture

YOU'VE BEEN LOST at sea for 5 days, clinging to a piece of driftwood. Sunburned, dehydrated, starving, sores all over your body from getting nipped by curious fish, you miraculously get saved. But you're not physically better yet. You've got some eating, drinking, and healing to do, along with a promise to yourself that you will never go sailing again. And so it goes after you've been rescued from a life of "healthy whole grains": It's time to heal the wounds and address the deficiencies.

Yes, you've experienced nutritional deficiencies—calorie surpluses, but nutritional deficiencies. The idea that grains cause nutritional deficiencies is, of course, contrary to conventional advice. Conventionally minded dietitians and nutritionists insist that grains are absolutely necessary for good nutrition and that without them you will suffer nutritional deficiencies, succumb to numerous diseases, be thrown off your softball league, and be barred from setting foot in church again. They even advise us to eat more grains to solve existing nutrient deficiencies. Such advice is again guilty of flawed logic. Yes, it is true that replacing white flour products with whole grain products gives you the benefit of B vitamins and fiber, because replacing something bad with something less bad does indeed yield incremental health benefits. But it most definitely does not mean that consuming plenty of whole grains is better than consuming no grains at all. The absurdity of conventional advice becomes clear when we view the catalog of problems presented by grains and various nutrients (see Chapter 4). This is the reason that all grain products are sold fortified: to partially overcome their nutrition-impairing effects.

The combination of digestion-impairing components in the seeds of grasses exposes you to a collection of poorly digested, toxic, allergic, and disruptive agents—no surprise, since we are not suited to consuming anything from the grasses of the earth. A cow or goat can obtain all of its nutrition from the seeds of grasses, but you cannot, and fortification doesn't change that.

In Chapter 4, I detailed many of the ways in which grains impair nutritional status. I touched on the use of nutritional supplements in Chapter 5 as specifically applied to the process of withdrawal from grains. Here I discuss the nutrients that are typically deficient and require correction after grain withdrawal has run its course. You are in the process of healing after being rescued, but it's going to take more than just being tossed a life preserver.

PUMP SOME IRON

After blood loss, grain consumption is a common cause of iron deficiency. Not eggplant, turnips, Brazil nuts, or pork loin—only grains, and more specifically wheat, rye, and barley. As discussed in Chapter 4, this explains why cultures heavily reliant on grains experience high levels of iron deficiency anemia, seen especially in growing children. Iron deficiency, despite grain availability and even iron fortification, remains a worldwide problem, affecting as many as two billion people.[1] As discussed on page 60, anthropologists have concluded that the genetic condition hemochromatosis represents a mutation that compensates for impaired iron absorption. Recall that as little as 50 milligrams (mg) of phytates in a typical serving of grains can slash iron absorption by 80 to 90 percent, and absorption is worsened if any form of intestinal inflammation enters the picture.

Iron deficiency is signaled by symptoms such as low energy, light-headedness, inappropriate feelings of coldness (also caused by hypothyroidism), breathlessness, and difficulty maintaining concentration. Removal of grains permits normal iron absorption to resume, and supplemental iron intake is only necessary if low levels of the iron storage protein, ferritin, or iron deficiency anemia are identified. In these situations, several months of either over-the-counter or prescribed iron supplements may be necessary and can accelerate correction over just the increased iron absorption of grain elimination.

Animal products are rich in the heme form of iron, meaning the iron in hemoglobin (from red blood cells) or myoglobin (from muscle), while plant sources provide nonheme iron. Approximately 30 percent of heme iron is absorbed, while approximately half as much nonheme iron is absorbed.[2] This means that the best sources of iron are eggs, meats, and organs, such as beef, pork, poultry, liver, and shellfish. The richest non-grain sources of nonheme iron are spinach, chard, kale, molasses, pumpkin seeds, lima beans, and kidney beans. The Recommended Daily Allowance (RDA) for iron is 8 mg per day for adult men, 8 mg per day for nonmenstruating women, 18 mg per day for menstruating women, and 27 mg per day for pregnant women. (All quantities refer to elemental iron, i.e., weight of the iron alone.) Growing teenagers have 50 to 100 percent greater iron needs than nonmenstruating adults. Vegans and vegetarians may need to double their RDA of iron, as they only get iron from nonheme iron sources.

Iron supplements come in the ferrous form: ferrous fumarate, ferrous sulfate, and ferrous gluconate. Of these, ferrous fumarate is the best absorbed (33 percent absorption) and gluconate is the least (12 percent).[3] The various supplements should be dosed by the quantity of elemental iron, not the total weight of ferrous fumarate, for example. (There are also ferric forms that are poorly absorbed and are not recommended.) Because of limited absorption, even of the ferrous forms, typical dosing regimens of prescription forms of iron provide 50 to 60 mg of elemental iron per day, divided in two or three doses to maximize absorption. They're generally taken for only 1 to 2 months, and doses this high should not be taken unless prescribed by a doctor. Heme iron forms are also available, such as Bifera and Proferrin, and they may be absorbed better and cause less gastrointestinal upset. Iron supplements should not be taken without a diagnosed iron deficiency, ongoing blood loss (such as through menses or pregnancy), and careful monitoring, as iron overload can occur and can be toxic, especially when excess visceral fat is present. Note that cooking in iron cookware and even stainless steel can increase the iron content in food, especially if acidic foods are cooked, such as tomato sauce, citrus, or vinegar-containing dishes. Typically 1 to 6 mg of iron are added to a serving, especially when cast-iron pots and pans are new, when prolonged cooking times are used, and when lots of stirring is involved.[4]

Due to inflammation of the small intestine, people diagnosed with celiac disease and Crohn's disease may require iron supplementation for longer than usual to compensate for reduced absorption. Iron deficiency, especially mild degrees as represented by low levels of ferritin but without anemia, are a common performance-impairing issue in competitive athletes. Athletes should consider an evaluation that includes a ferritin level and CBC to document iron status; female and vegetarian athletes, in particular, should consider a low-dose supplement to correct any abnormalities or to prevent deficiency. (This should be performed under the supervision of someone knowledgeable about athletes and sports performance and who will continue monitoring ferritin levels.) People with hypochlorhydria, low stomach acid that can result from years of grain consumption, may also require more prolonged iron supplementation to correct iron deficiency and may benefit from efforts to increase stomach acid (see page 203 for more information).

ZINC: THE MISSING LINK

The phytates that impair iron absorption also impair zinc absorption, resulting in widespread deficiencies among grain-consuming people. Zinc deficiency accounts for a variety of symptoms, including skin rashes, distortions of taste, unexplained diarrhea and other gastrointestinal distress, impaired growth and development in grain-dependent children, increased susceptibility to infection, poor wound healing, impaired learning, and other chronic health problems. Grains are also low in zinc, compared to meat, poultry, shellfish, and organ meats.[5] Grain-consuming vegans and vegetarians, in particular, can develop severe zinc deficiencies.

Twenty-five percent of the world's population experience zinc deficiency due to limited availability of meat and other animal products and reliance on grains for calories.[6] Zinc availability is therefore becoming a hot topic for worldwide health.

As the human body needs 15 mg of zinc per day to permit all zinc-dependent immune, neurological, reparative, and other functions to proceed, supplemental intake can be important. It is especially important during your first few grain-free months, as your gastrointestinal health recovers from the destruction previously wrought by grains. The RDA of zinc for adults is 11 mg per day for men, 8 mg per day for women, 11 mg for pregnant women, and 12 mg per day for lactating women. Much of your daily zinc needs can be obtained through food. For example, 6 ounces of beef chuck roast provides 6 mg of zinc; 2 slices of pork loin provide 5.8 mg; 4 ounces of chicken breast provides 1.0 mg; 3 ounces of Alaskan king crab provides 6.5 mg. More modest quantities are obtained from vegetables, nuts, cheese, other dairy products, and other seafood—generally less than 1 mg per serving.

Nutritional supplements such as zinc gluconate, zinc sulfate, and zinc acetate can supplement dietary intake; look for the quantity of *elemental* zinc in the preparation, not total weight. Because zinc supplements are indeed meant to supplement dietary intake, a modest additional intake of 10 to 15 mg of elemental zinc per day is reasonable. Because vegans and vegetarians don't eat zinc-rich animal products and commonly rely on legumes that also contain phytates that block zinc absorption, they typically require larger supplemental doses, such as 15 to 25 mg per day. (It is wise not to exceed 35 to 40 mg total—dietary and supplemental—intake per day, since zinc can also be toxic in excessive quantities.) Soaking legumes for several hours reduces their phytate content—a useful strategy for people with marginal zinc intakes. People who begin their grain-free journey with inflammatory bowel diseases, have other malabsorptive conditions, or take thiazide diuretics (such as hydrochlorothiazide, chlorthalidone, or metolazone) may already have a severe zinc deficiency, so higher levels of supplementation may be required. Blood zinc levels are of limited usefulness, as they can often underestimate tissue levels. Nonetheless, if a blood level is obtained and is below the quoted reference range or is at the lower end of that range, zinc deficiency is likely. Zinc supplementation of 10 to 15 mg per day in this situation is safe and effective.

MILKED OF MAGNESIUM

Magnesium deficiency is alarmingly common, given our reliance on filtered water that has had all magnesium removed, the reduced content of magnesium in modern crops, and the widespread use of proton pump inhibitors—drugs for acid reflux and ulcers that reduce magnesium absorption.[7] To make matters worse, phytates reduce magnesium absorption by 60 percent, even with a single bagel or sandwich.[8] The more grain is consumed, the more magnesium is blocked. Add it all up, and magnesium deficiency is the rule, rather than the exception. A diet rich in "healthy whole grains" virtually assures deficiency.

The RDA of elemental magnesium is 320 mg per day for adult women and 420 mg per day for adult men. Most people obtain about 245 mg per day—well below the RDA—while not even factoring in the impaired absorption caused by grains or drugs. I view the intake set by the RDA as just enough and not necessarily the ideal intake, so most of us fall way below an ideal intake of magnesium. Magnesium deficiency has real health implications. Because magnesium provides structural integrity to bone tissue, a lack of magnesium contributes to osteoporosis.[9] Magnesium deficiency is also associated with hypertension, higher blood sugars, muscle cramps, low birth weight in infants, migraine headaches, and heart rhythm disorders such as premature atrial and ventricular contractions, atrial fibrillation, and sudden cardiac death.[10] (Anyone who has worked in a hospital cardiac unit recognizes the power of magnesium replacement to miraculously subdue life-threatening heart rhythms.) Magnesium deficiency can show itself to an exaggerated degree during withdrawal from grain-derived opiates. It is typically experienced as leg cramps and disruption of sleep during those first few days.

Magnesium repletion provides substantial benefits. Women supplementing magnesium demonstrated a 1.8 percent increase in bone density over 1 year, compared to a reduction in bone density in women not taking magnesium.[11] In a study of combination nutrients, 25 mg of elemental magnesium as part of a panel of nutrients improved bone density by 4 percent over 1 year, which was more than that achieved by the prescription drug alendronate (Fosamax).[12] Magnesium repletion also reduces blood pressure: Supplementing with 410 mg of elemental magnesium per day reduces systolic pressure by 3 to 4 mmHg and diastolic pressure by 2 to 3 mmHg.[13]

Increasing your consumption of magnesium-rich foods helps correct the situation: Almonds and other nuts have 80 mg per ounce; peanuts have 50 mg per dry-roasted ounce; peanut butter has 50 mg per 2 tablespoons; and spinach has 156 mg per cooked cup. The real magnesium superstars are seeds, though: Pumpkin seeds have 191 mg per ¼ cup; sesame seeds have 126 mg per ¼ cup; and sunflower seeds have 114 mg per ¼ cup. Spinach and seeds are therefore the richest magnesium sources. For additional information on magnesium supplements, see page 109.

RUN NAKED IN THE TROPICAL SUN... OR JUST SUPPLEMENT VITAMIN D

Humans were meant to roam the savanna with plenty of skin exposed to the bright sun (activating vitamin D) while also consuming the organs of animals (also rich in vitamin D). When humans migrated north and south out of the savanna to colder climates, we learned how to wear clothes that covered, by necessity, much of our exposed hairless surface area, we developed lighter skin to increase our capacity to activate D, and we continued to consume the organs of animals. But even these adaptations have proven inadequate, given modern habits such as living and working indoors, wearing clothes that cover skin surface area, aversion to the consumption of organ meats (just since the mid-20th century), and, of course, the disruptive effects of grains. Factor in that we lose the ability to activate vitamin D in our skin with sunlight exposure after age 40, and it all adds up to a widespread and common deficiency with substantial implications for health.[14] In fact, I believe that restoration of vitamin D is second only to grain elimination as among the most powerful of health strategies.

Vitamin D deficiency allows a number of abnormal health phenomena to occur.[15]

- Greater inflammation, as is reflected in higher C-reactive protein levels, tumor necrosis factor, and others

- Higher blood sugar and resistance to insulin (the conditions that lead to diabetes)

- Injury to pancreatic beta cells that produce insulin
- Weight gain
- Greater risk for osteoporosis and fractures
- Periodontal disease
- Higher risk for cancer, especially breast, prostate, colon, ovarian, and melanoma
- Higher risk for heart attack, heart failure, and cardiovascular mortality
- Preeclampsia and eclampsia during pregnancy
- Depression and seasonal affective disorder
- Autoimmune conditions

For many of these, the association between lower levels of vitamin D and the disease is powerful. For example, vitamin D deficiency provides as much as a 50 percent increased potential for diabetes.[16] Accordingly, all of the above phenomena are improved or reversed with the restoration of vitamin D to healthy levels, including the facilitation of weight loss.[17] However, note that achieving an ideal level of vitamin D is key—not too low, but also not too high. What level of vitamin D, measured as 25-hydroxy vitamin D, is ideal remains open to debate; however, applying epidemiological observations to the above diseases, combined with studies that demonstrate vitamin D's relationship to minimizing unhealthy levels of parathyroid hormone that can impair bone health, suggest that 60 to 70 ng/ml is the ideal range.[18] Too much vitamin D is also not a good idea. Besides provoking abnormal calcium deposition in tissues, vitamin D levels that exceed 100 mg/dl are associated with increased potential for the abnormal heart rhythm called atrial fibrillation.[19] The majority of people require vitamin D doses of 4,000 to 8,000 international units (IU) taken in an oil-based gelcap form to achieve the target value of 60 to 70 ng/ml. Vitamin D should be taken as D_3, or cholecalciferol, the form that occurs in the human body and is widely available as a nutritional supplement, not the form found in mushrooms (D_2 or ergocalciferol), which is also the form in prescription vitamin D. This is an instance in which the nutritional supplement form is superior to the prescription form. Ideally, your vitamin D level should be reassessed every 6 to 12 months to maintain desired levels, as needs can change over time.

People with a history of Crohn's disease, malabsorption, or celiac disease may have difficulty absorbing vitamin D. They usually start with more severe degrees of deficiency and may not respond to the usual doses, particularly at the beginning of a grain-free journey, before intestinal healing has occurred.[20] Higher doses may therefore be required, adjusted by a health-care provider monitoring 25-hydroxy vitamin D blood levels. (It really helps to have a health-care practitioner who is confident with the use of vitamin D, as very high doses are occasionally required to overcome poor absorption.) Rarely, absorption is so poor that injectable vitamin D has to be used until intestinal healing has occurred.

THERE'S NOTHING FISHY ABOUT OMEGA-3S

Relatively infrequent consumption of seafood, avoidance of consuming the brain tissue of land animals, and overreliance on processed omega-6 oils in modern foods have led to deficient levels of omega-3 fatty acids in modern people. Of course, the seeds of grasses, with all their absorption-blocking and inflammatory effects, add to the problem. Once grains are removed, omega-3 fatty acid absorption may improve, but intake may still remain low.

There are plenty of reasons to supplement omega-3 fatty acids. We have, for instance, an abundance of clinical studies that demonstrate that omega-3 fatty acids, as eicosapentaenoic acid (EPA) and docosahexaenoic acid (DHA) obtained from fish, yield reductions in sudden cardiac death, heart attack, heart rhythm disorders (such as atrial fibrillation), autoimmune inflammatory conditions (such as rheumatoid arthritis and lupus), and a variety of cancers.[21] These potential benefits apply only to the EPA and DHA of fish oil, not to the linolenic acid of flaxseed, chia seeds, walnuts, and other sources. While linolenic acid is biochemically an omega-3 fatty acid and is, for other reasons, a truly healthy oil, it does not yield the same collection of benefits provided by EPA and DHA. There have been some naysayers lately who've claimed an increase in prostate cancer risk with omega-3 fatty acids (an assertion based on a flawed analysis of the data) or lack of cardiovascular benefit, but the overwhelming bulk of data suggest otherwise. Omega-3s are essential fatty acids with a clear-cut deficiency syndrome when they are lacking. Our need for omega-3 oils makes sense from an evolutionary standpoint, too, as we require them for brain development, cellular signal transduction, and a multitude of other bodily functions.

Omega-3 fatty acids have special relevance to the grain-free experience. Once grains are removed from the diet, weight loss proceeds at a rapid clip for most people, a process that involves mobilization of fatty acids into the bloodstream. This natural part of the weight-loss process is the reason why cholesterol panels and other laboratory assessments are best avoided during weight loss and for 4 weeks after weight loss has plateaued. Blood drawn during active weight loss can show increased triglycerides, reduced HDL cholesterol, and even higher blood sugar, all of which are transient and correct themselves when the flood of fatty acids subsides, accelerated by omega-3 fatty acids' ability to activate the enzyme lipoprotein lipase. These ill-timed test results are often misinterpreted by physicians who, unaccustomed to witnessing the effects of weight loss, declare, "See, I told you that *Wheat Belly* stuff was killing you!"

Fish oil is the only reliable and sufficiently potent source of EPA and DHA. Krill oil, while interesting for its astaxanthin content (a carotenoid similar to beta-carotene), provides only a trivial amount of EPA and DHA. Krill oil is often marketed as having a more highly absorbed phospholipid form of omega-3s, which is true, but it contains so little that you'd have to consume an entire bottle every day to yield a sufficient quantity of EPA and DHA. I advocate an intake of 3,000 to 3,600 mg per day (the dose of combined omega-3 fatty acids, EPA and DHA, not of fish oil), divided into two doses taken before breakfast and before dinner. This quantity yields a level of omega-3 fatty acids in the bloodstream of 10 percent or more, meaning that 10 percent of all fatty acids in red blood cells are comprised of EPA and DHA, the level that provides maximal protection from cardiovascular disease and a variety of anti-inflammatory benefits. The best fish oils come in the liquid triglyceride form, as the triglyceride form is better absorbed (particularly the DHA) and re-creates the form of omega-3s as it occurs in fish. Excellent brands include Ascenta NutraSea and Nordic Naturals. Liquid fish oil is not fishy in odor, but it must be stored tightly sealed in the refrigerator. Most fish oil in capsule form is the less-well-absorbed ethyl ester form. You can still do just fine with capsules; absorption just won't be as complete as with the triglyceride form.

Recently, concerns have been raised that the widespread use of statin drugs for cholesterol reduction may impair the potential for omega-3 fatty acids to yield benefits, since statins preferentially divert fatty acid metabolism to yield higher levels of omega-6 fatty acids.[22] While omega-6 fatty acids, such as linoleic (not to be confused with linolenic) acid, are among the essential fatty acids, most modern people are overexposed to omega-6s due to our widespread reliance on corn, mixed vegetable, safflower, cottonseed, and other oils—a situation that amplifies the potential for inflammatory phenomena. My choice, whenever possible, is to avoid the use of statin drugs while preserving the natural health benefits of omega-3 fatty acids.

IODINE: "KEEP YOUR FAMILY GOITER FREE" AND OTHER LESSONS RELEARNED

While we cannot blame grains for disrupting iodine status, iodine deficiency is such a common stumbling block in people who eliminate grains that it is worth knowing how and when to correct deficiency to remove this impediment to total health. Most people have forgotten that, until the first half of the 20th century, disfiguring goiters occurred in 20 percent of the population: large bulging thyroid glands on the front of the neck caused by a lack of iodine. This was a serious problem in inland areas away from ocean sources of iodine (and in people who failed to consume the thyroid glands of land animals, which are rich in iodine). The connection between goiter and iodine deficiency was recognized around 1920 and led to the introduction of iodized salt in 1924. The FDA then urged the public to use more salt. (The Morton iodized salt slogan in the early 20th century was, "Help keep your family goiter free!") It worked: Goiters essentially disappeared as enthusiastic use of iodized salt became the rule. Even today, iodized salt is considered a great public health success story, and most people younger than 50 years old have never even seen a goiter. Unfortunately, excessive salt consumption caused health issues in some susceptible individuals, prompting new advice: Reduce salt and sodium exposure. Now, in the 21st century, health-conscious people proudly declare their avoidance of iodized table salt. Others have turned to alternative sources, such as sea salt (very little iodine content), kosher salt (no iodine), and potassium chloride–based salt substitutes (no iodine). As a result, iodine deficiency and goiters are staging a comeback.

Iodine is an essential trace mineral for health. Just as deficiency in vitamin C will lead to the loose teeth, open sores, and inflamed joints of scurvy, so does iodine deficiency lead to serious health problems. Simply meeting the RDA of 150 mcg per day will prevent a goiter from developing and maintain a normal level of thyroid hormone production for most people. If iodine is unavailable to the thyroid gland, production of thyroid hormones T3 and T4 (the 3 and 4 refer to the number of iodine atoms per molecule of these hormones) begins to flag and hypothyroidism (underactive thyroid) ensues. Iodine deficiency over time leads to a thyroid gland that enlarges—a goiter. However, it is not necessary to have a goiter for thyroid dysfunction to be present.

Iodine deficiency slows metabolic rate and is therefore a common reason someone may be unable to lose weight. Athletes and people engaged in frequent heavy physical effort are at a higher risk for iodine deficiency because of iodine loss through perspiration.[23] Vegetarians who avoid seafood and iodized salt also have a greater likelihood of iodine deficiency than omnivores do.[24] Iodine is also proving to be important for breast health, as deficiency has been associated with fibrocystic breast disease, a potential precursor to breast cancer. (Luckily, iodine replacement is associated with reversal of this disease.[25]) The salivary glands also concentrate iodine, providing protection against undesirable microorganisms in the mouth. What is not clear is just how much iodine we need for optimal health. Does alleviating goiter also mean that thyroid function is optimized? To further complicate the situation, what quantity of iodine is required in the presence of ubiquitous environmental blockers of thyroid function and iodine? Many industrial chemicals have been shown to block thyroid hormone production; having sufficient iodine helps prevent these chemicals from entering thyroid tissue,[26] but how does this factor into our decisions when choosing a dose of iodine?

There are no confident answers yet. Simply adhering to the RDA of 150 mcg or thereabouts per day for adults is likely just enough for most people to avoid a goiter. Many multivitamins and multiminerals contain the RDA for iodine. Relying on iodized salt is a flawed method of obtaining iodine because salt increases blood pressure in a minority of susceptible people, causes fluid retention, and can accelerate osteoporosis. It's also tough to know precisely how much iodine you are obtaining simply by shaking your salt shaker over food. Iodine in salt is also inconsistent and volatile, evaporating from the container within 4 weeks of opening it.[27] (The canister of iodized salt that's been sitting in your cupboard for 6 months therefore contains little to no iodine.) If there is any indication of hypothyroidism, such as inappropriately cold hands and feet, low energy, constipation, or thinning hair, and certainly if an enlarged thyroid is present, an increase in iodine to the 500 to 1,000 mcg per day range may increase thyroid hormone output *if* lack of iodine is the limiting factor. Iodine is readily obtained from supplements such as potassium iodide drops, capsules, or kelp tablets (a dried seaweed form that approximates the natural, ocean-derived source).

Thyroid testing can suggest iodine deficiency with the pattern of a free T4 at the lower end or below the reference range, along with a slightly higher than optimal TSH of 1.5 mIU/L or greater. This is usually corrected after 3 to 6 months of iodine replacement if iodine deficiency is the cause, especially if any thyroid enlargement is present. Rarely, someone with hypothyroidism or goiter will develop an abnormal hyperthyroid response to iodine. This occurs because the iodine deficiency present before correction distorts thyroid function; adding iodine can worsen the situation temporarily by activating hyperthyroidism with palpitations, sleeplessness, and anxiety. Iodine replacement may therefore be best undertaken alongside monitoring of thyroid function, as well as other assessments of thyroid status (such as some form of thyroid imaging), by your health-care provider. Once cleared of trouble spots (such as abnormal thyroid nodules), some people succeed by increasing their dose of iodine gradually, starting at the RDA of 150 mcg per day and gradually building up by 50 to 100 mcg increments over 6 months until the desired dose (500 mcg per day) is achieved.

Note that in addition to iodine deficiency, grain consumption over a period of years can also activate autoimmune thyroid gland inflammation, Hashimoto's thyroiditis, or Graves' disease. This can result in a damaged thyroid that underproduces thyroid hormone (hypothyroidism), a situation that does not respond to iodine supplementation. Anyone with a history of Hashimoto's thyroiditis, Graves' disease, thyroid cancer, or thyroid nodules should supplement iodine under the supervision of a knowledgeable health-care provider.

Additional information about thyroid health and the details behind thyroid hormone replacement can be found in Chapter 11.

VITAMIN B$_{12}$: SIDESTEP DEFICIENCY

I view vitamin B$_{12}$ absorption as something like a complicated salsa or rumba series of dance steps: Great if you get it right, but there's plenty of opportunity to misstep and botch up the dance. Because several steps are required for absorption, B$_{12}$ is easily interrupted, resulting in a deficiency that may persist for months or even a lifetime after grains are removed, especially if hypochlorhydria (low stomach acid) is present.

Most cases of mild to moderate B$_{12}$ deficiency are unaccompanied by symptoms but present as macrocytic anemia, as the red blood cells, while fewer, are larger than normal. (Note that anemia is not something you want to diagnose yourself, as a blood test is required and a cause needs to be identified to distinguish it from conditions such as iron deficiency from colon cancer.)

Lesser degrees of B$_{12}$ deficiency that precede the development of anemia can be identified by assessing a vitamin B$_{12}$ blood level (cobalamin or holocobalamin), with the ideal level being toward the upper half of the reference range, since the symptoms of B$_{12}$ deficiency (peripheral neuropathy, impaired balance, and memory impairment) can occur at the lower end of the normal range.[28] B$_{12}$ assessment is best combined with measurement of methylmalonic acid, which is superior to B$_{12}$ levels alone in detecting earlier or subtle degrees of B$_{12}$ deficiency.[29]

The average diet that includes animal products provides around 4 to 10 mcg of vitamin B_{12} per day, of which approximately 50 percent is normally absorbed—an intake that does not ensure full maintenance of normal B_{12} levels.[30] Low-dose supplementation of B_{12} (or enthusiastic consumption of organ meats and clams) is therefore a good practice. Supplementation of 50 mcg per day can assure most people of long-term adequate intake. Note that there is no B_{12} toxicity and that some people simply choose to supplement B_{12} chronically, a benign and inexpensive practice.

If absorption is not normal, as in pernicious anemia, inflammatory bowel disorders, or hypochlorhydria, then B_{12} may be poorly absorbed from food and long-term B_{12} supplementation is necessary. Sometimes the injectable, rather than the oral, form will be administered to circumvent impaired absorption. B_{12} absorption can be impaired early in the grain-free experience, especially in people 65 years old and older. An easy workaround is to take higher doses to ensure absorption. Doses of 500 to 1,000 mcg are effective in most people.[31] Such higher doses should be taken with occasional monitoring of B_{12} or methylmalonic acid blood levels to ensure that deficiency has been corrected. While there is likely no advantage in oral versus sublingual preparations,[32] there is an advantage in choosing the naturally occurring (though more expensive) methylcobalamin form over the more common synthetic cyanocobalamin form.[33] The methyl form of B_{12} may also be safer, as the cyanide molecule in the cyanocobalamin form can theoretically accumulate in smokers or if kidney function is impaired. (I say theoretically because cyanide toxicity has never been documented with cyanocobalamin supplementation.)

Foods rich in vitamin B_{12} include chicken liver, with 17 mcg per 3½-ounce serving; veal liver, with 85 mcg per 3½-ounce serving; lamb liver, with 130 mcg per 6 ounces; various cuts of beef, with 6 to 10 mcg per 8-ounce serving; Alaskan king crab, with 15 mcg per leg; cooked herring, with 14 mcg per 5-ounce filet; salted mackerel, with 16 mcg per cooked cup; canned sardines (with bones), with 13 mcg per cup; and bluefin tuna, with 18 mcg in 6 ounces. In general, organ meats (such as liver, kidney, pancreas, heart, and brain) contain much greater quantities of vitamin B_{12} than the muscle cuts do. Clams are also a rich source, though they vary in B_{12} content with variety, but generally supply more than finned fish, ounce for ounce.[34] Vegetables, nuts, seeds, flaxseed, chia seed, coconut, and mushrooms contain no B_{12}, explaining why B_{12} deficiency is such a common concern for vegans and vegetarians. In short, eat no grains but include liver, meats, and seafood in your diet to choreograph your way back to repleting vitamin B_{12}.

FIGURE OUT YOUR FOLATE NEEDS

Folate deficiency is much less common nowadays, as folic acid has been added to grain products in the United States and Canada. While the incidence of spina bifida has decreased as a result of this, there may be undesirable consequences, as well, including increased cancer risk. With grain elimination, of course, we are removing the fortification as well as the additional risks it carries.

Folate status is readily assessed by measuring the quantity of folate in red blood cells (called RBC folate), a better measure of tissue levels than blood levels of folate.[35] The RDA for folate is 400 mcg per day for adult men and women, 600 mcg per day for pregnant women, and 500 mcg per day for lactating women.[36] Most of us eating a grain-free diet can readily obtain sufficient quantities of folate simply by eating healthy, folate-rich foods. Rich sources of natural folate include beef liver, with 430 mcg in 6 ounces; spinach, with 262 mcg per cooked cup; asparagus, with 178 mcg in eight spears; Brussels sprouts, with 156 mcg per cooked cup; romaine lettuce, with 64 mcg per cup; and eggs, with 66 mcg in three.[37] In general, green vegetables (*folium* is Latin for leaf), nuts, seeds, meats, fish, legumes, and eggs add to a healthy intake of folate. Most people who do not have celiac disease, gluten sensitivity, or inflammatory bowel disease can obtain healthy levels of folate just by eating real, single-ingredient foods. People who do have these conditions, as well as women of childbearing age or who are pregnant, should consider supplementation.

Folate is exceptionally easy and inexpensive to supplement in its synthetic form, folic acid. The US Public Health Service, the Centers for Disease Control and Prevention, and the Food and Nutrition Board of the Institute of Medicine all advise women of childbearing age to supplement with 400 mcg of folic acid per day to reduce the risk of congenital defects.

However, it is important not to overdo it, as folic acid is an example of something that's unhealthy whether you take too little or too much—especially when it's consumed as synthetic folic acid. Several studies have suggested that doses of folic acid of 800 mcg or more per day may increase cancer risk, and while folic acid supplementation in grain products has indeed reduced the incidence of neural tube defects in newborns, higher folic acid intake may be associated with increased colon and prostate cancer risk.[38]

For these reasons and because there are differences in how foodborne folates and synthetic folic acid are metabolized, it is preferable to supplement with the 5-methylfolate form because it does not result in abnormally high levels of unmetabolized folic acid in the bloodstream.[39] The 5-methylfolate form is also proving to be more effective in situations such as treatment of depression, with several clinical trials demonstrating dramatic responses with or without conventional antidepressant therapy.[40] However, we should be careful even with the 5-methylfolate form, as it remains unclear whether high doses of this form have potential for increasing cancer risk. Anyone concerned about folate intake and their grain-free lifestyle would likely do fine by supplementing with 400 mcg per day in the 5-methylfolate form. This is enough to address deficient intake from diet but not enough to invite concerns about cancer.

FIBER: QUIT YOUR PUSHING

Getting more fiber is a common justification for encouraging us to consume more grains, since greater fiber intake has been associated with reduced heart disease, diabetes, weight gain, and colon cancer. And grains are indeed rich in fiber, much of it indigestible, just like the many other components of the seeds of grasses. Conventional wisdom holds that greater fiber intake is good for bowel health and encourages regularity. We are advised to consume whole grains—the seeds of grasses—as breads and breakfast cereals, even if they taste like cardboard with a bit of sugar added.

Primitive humans, who generally enjoyed much higher total fiber and prebiotic fiber (discussed further in Chapter 9) intake than modern humans do, obtained fiber from legumes, tubers, vegetables, fruits, nuts, and seeds—not grains. The belief that grains must be among our sources of fiber is a recent notion, and it's one that is at odds with human nutrition over the past 2.5 million years. Total fiber, as well as prebiotic or resistant fibers, can be reliably obtained in adequate quantities without grains.

Much of the fibers provided by grains are of the indigestible cellulose form—the same polysaccharide structure found in wood. Cellulose and related fibers are indigestible by humans and indigestible by bowel flora, and therefore they pass through, yielding "bulk" that has been associated with bowel health. Minus grains, plentiful cellulose-type fibers can be obtained from nuts and seeds to reach the 30 grams (g) or so per day advised by most health agencies. For example, almonds provide 6 g per ½ cup; Brazil nuts provide 5 g per ½ cup; peanuts provide 6 g per ½ cup; pecans provide 5 g per ½ cup; sesame seeds provide 13 g per ½ cup; sunflower seeds provide 6 g per ½ cup; and walnuts provide 3 g per ½ cup. (Peanuts are listed here despite being a legume, since they are consumed much like nuts.)[41] Don't worry: Without grains, you can still get plenty of wood in your diet.

Vegetables, mushrooms, and fruits are other important sources of fiber, a mixture of digestible and indigestible forms. One cup of spinach, cooked, for instance, provides 4 g total fiber; two stalks of broccoli provide 12 g; 10 spears of asparagus provide 3 g; ¼ cup of coconut flour provides 9 g; one avocado provides 9 g; and five large strawberries provide 5 g. If ideal daily intake of fiber is estimated to be 25 to 40 g or more per day, obtaining this value is no problem if you include some nuts and seeds in your diet, some sources of prebiotic fibers (ideally 10 g or more per day; see Chapter 9), and some vegetables and fruits. Adding some ground golden flaxseed or chia seed can boost fiber intake considerably: ½ cup of flaxseed adds 23 g of total fiber; ¼ cup of chia seed adds 15 g fiber.

Provided your diet is not rich in foods like candy bars, chewing gum, and soft drinks, but rather is rich in nuts, seeds, vegetables, mushrooms, and fruits, as well as sources of prebiotic fibers, obtaining healthy quantities of all forms of fiber is virtually effortless, no pushing required.

THE GRAIN DEFICIENCY SYNDROME

One thing you do *not* have to do is correct deficiencies that develop as a consequence of eliminating grains. There is no such deficiency (putting aside the folate deficiency that can develop during pregnancy in any woman, grain-consuming or not). There is no deficiency of riboflavin, niacin, or thiamin; no deficiency of vitamins A, C, or E; no deficiency of protein, fat, or fiber. In fact, the opposite is often true: Nutrient status *improves* without the nutrient-blocking effects provided by the indigestible seeds of grasses.

If you replace the lost calories of grains with chips, soda pop, and French fries, then many deficiencies can indeed appear. But if you replace them with healthy foods, such as vegetables, meats, fish, and nuts, you will obtain nutrients and fiber in the same way that humans did for the first 99.6 percent of our time on earth. It's okay to skip the nutritional mistakes made during the grassy detour that has consumed the last 0.4 percent of our time here.

CHAPTER 9

FULL RECOVERY FROM POST-TRAUMATIC GRAIN GUT SYNDROME

*I don't stop eating when I'm full. The meal isn't over when I'm full.
The meal is over when I hate myself.*
—Louis C. K.

IF THERE'S ONE problem area in the world of grain-free living, it's the gastrointestinal tract. We've previously discussed how grains do their dirty work in disrupting gastrointestinal health and how grain elimination unravels these effects. Now we'll discuss how to restore ideal gastrointestinal health in the aftermath of grain removal.

It's truly a uniquely human experience to have gastrointestinal function, adapted to the wide food variety of omnivory, go so wrong. Surely a wolf, consuming a diet almost exclusively carnivorous with virtually no plant fiber, does not have to struggle with hard, dry stools, constipation, and hemorrhoids. I believe we would have to search long and hard to find a goose who struggles with explosive and inconvenient loose stools or who has to take a surprise break from his flock while flying in formation. Yet humans are *plagued* by an astounding variety of gastrointestinal difficulties, from annoying to life threatening.

Why? Is it because humans are so poorly adapted to consuming the food on this earth and converting it to the essential components of our bodies that one in three of us experiences an abnormal gastrointestinal condition at any given time—conditions that sometimes last years, decades, or even an entire lifetime? Are we so evolutionarily challenged that we need to take drugs for decades to reduce stomach acid, or remove an entire colon and replace it with an artificial orifice for our stool to emerge, just to allow painless digestion? Or could there be a thing or things we are exposed to that have altered our ability to adapt, distorted our relationship with foods, and upset the usual subconscious and painless process of converting nutrients into human tissue?

The answer, of course, is that turning to the seeds of grasses and regarding them as food was an error of monumental proportions. The food of ruminants served us well in times of desperation, but they were never meant to be consumed in times of plenty, and they were certainly never meant to dominate the human diet. Humans simply cannot digest the components of grasses, including that of their seeds. Such indigestible or poorly digestible seed components include wheat germ agglutinin (WGA), which emerges totally unscathed after its mouth-to-anus journey, and gliadin, which increases intestinal permeability and initiates autoimmunity. Likewise, the various forms of grain proteins are incompletely digested by our bodies. Grains contain a virtual Who's Who of gastrointestinal destruction.

Toss in all the other varied disruptions of gastrointestinal function wrought by the components of grains, and your esophagus, stomach, and small and large intestines look like a nuclear testing site in the Nevada desert. Remove the disruptive components of grains after the blast has done its damage and it is indeed followed by "fallout." Not the sort that involves radiation injury, of course, but the type that leaves a digestive landscape of destruction, disrupted nutrition, distortions of hormonal signaling, disordered digestive control, and a bacterial population that's confused by this new world.

This is why it's common for someone to remove grains and experience rapid relief from acid reflux, heartburn, and bowel urgency but be left with bloating and constipation that don't respond to the usual maneuvers, such as fiber supplementation. Because we also make efforts to undo the insulin resistance of prediabetes and diabetes that affects so many people, we limit carbohydrates, a strategy that can have undesirable effects on bowel flora and that needs to be addressed with specific fiber strategies—though certainly not the fibers from grains. Additional efforts and insights can therefore be important to fully recover and rebuild a normal, healthy gastrointestinal system that works in an orderly, predictable fashion and is replete with healthy bowel flora.

So how do you rebuild full gastrointestinal health on the scorched and damaged scene that remains after you've removed grains?

REPOPULATE WITH FRIENDLY FLORA

Years of grain consumption disrupt the composition of bowel flora in your intestinal tract. Remove the disruptive effects of grains, and your bowel flora begin to shift back to a more healthy profile—but not immediately. This shift can require months, and your flora do not always return fully, as your body cannot create bacterial species it lacks, just as a dirty pile of rags cannot spontaneously generate rats or a pile of dust generate fleas. Residual abnormalities, such as hypochlorhydria (reduced stomach acid), can also prevent normal bowel flora from getting reestablished. It's also important to reduce the overgrowth of bacteria that typically ascends up from the colon into the normally thinly populated ileum and jejunum. Under normal conditions, the colon is heavily populated with trillions of bacteria, there are fewer bacteria higher up, and there are fewer than 1,000 bacteria per milliliter up in the duodenum and stomach.[1] When gastrointestinal health is disrupted, undesirable species increase in numbers, not uncommonly working their way up the 20-some feet of small intestine, duodenum, and even stomach. These marauding bacteria are potentially responsible for continued gastrointestinal symptoms despite the removal of grains.

Up to 35 percent of people with no other gastrointestinal disease and no symptoms have bacterial overgrowth (dysbiosis) or other distortions of bowel flora composition. Even though many doctors regard irritable bowel syndrome (IBS) as a benign condition, 30 to 85 percent of people with IBS have varying degrees of dysbiosis at the time of their diagnosis— it is not benign.[2] Overgrowth of unhealthy bacteria is common in people who have low stomach acid due to acid-blocking drugs (such as Prilosec, Prevacid, Protonix, and Pepcid) or reduced stomach acid provoked by prior grain consumption; people who have taken antibiotics repeatedly or chronically; people with diabetes; people who take narcotics that slow bowel function; people with chronic constipation, which also slows bowel function; and people with fibromyalgia, Crohn's disease, ulcerative colitis, celiac disease, and autoimmune diseases. Even rosacea and restless leg syndrome have been associated with dysbiosis.[3] In short, if you have lived a modern life, you probably have some degree of dysbiosis.

There is debate over how to diagnose such distortions of bowel flora. While sampling the contents of the upper small intestine with an endoscope yields the most confident assessment, it is invasive and costly. Other methods include breath tests that look for the altered products of metabolism provoked by abnormal bacteria and tests that examine stool samples using a number of different methods. Thankfully, only an occasional person needs to undergo such evaluations, since the methods discussed here restore normal, healthy bowel flora in the majority of people.

It's therefore time to repopulate the gastrointestinal tract with healthy species such as *Lactobacillus* and *Bifidobacterium*. Some of this is accomplished simply by an increase in their numbers, while some healthy species also produce bacteriocins—small proteins that act as natural antibiotics on unhealthy bacteria.[4] The most effective species to employ in probiotics may be those that are best at producing effective bacteriocins. A wonderful thing happens when the disruptive effects of grains are removed and healthy bacterial species reenter the picture in large numbers: They outcompete the undesirables for nutrients, reducing their number, while the number of desirable species increases as they feed and reproduce. Bowel health and multiple other facets of health improve as a result.

Probiotics: Call In the Reinforcements

While your bowels are likely to repopulate with healthier bacterial strains over months or years as you get exposed to bacteria from other humans, contaminants in food, doorknobs, and other sources, the judicious use of a probiotic preparation simply abbreviates the timeline. It also increases the odds of acquiring a wider range of desirable species, as there is a healthy synergy that derives from inoculating your bowels with a wide variety of bacterial species. You can accelerate the conversion to healthier bowel flora by supplementing with a high-potency probiotic that provides a broad collection of bacterial species believed to be part of healthy bowel flora. (Nobody knows just what precisely constitutes the full range of healthy species that may have prevailed in the age prior to grain consumption, despite the useful insights provided by coprolite analysis discussed on page 27. The composition of probiotic preparations therefore constitutes our best guess at what may be necessary for restoration of bowel health.) Probiotics supply a range of healthy bacteria that deprive undesirable species of nutrients, produce bacteriocins, restore the normal mucous barrier of the intestine, provide greater quantities of butyrate, and facilitate normal immune responses.[5]

Among the best probiotics are VSL#3, Garden of Life, and ReNew Life brands, all of which offer high-potency products in the multibillion CFU range, which work better than lower-potency preparations that run in the millions or tens of millions. While 30 billion or more bacteria sounds like an awful lot, that quantity represents only a fraction of the trillions of bacteria inhabiting the gut. Typically, probiotics contain a range of bacteria from *Lactobacillus* and *Bifidobacterium* species, the two broad groups generally agreed to have health benefits. Species include *L. plantarum, L. brevis, L. acidophilus, L. casei, L. paracasei, L. rhamnosus, L. salivarius; B. bifidum, B. lactis, B. subtilis, B. breve, and B. longum.* The key with probiotics is therefore to supply sufficient numbers and a broad range of species—typically a dozen or more. Some probiotic preparations contain a yeast, *Saccharomyces boulardii*, either as part of a panel of bacterial species or by itself (as in the product Florastor), because clinical studies have demonstrated effects such as protection from *Clostridium difficile* infection, which can develop after antibiotic use.[6]

Rarely, the dysbiosis or small intestinal bacterial overgrowth (SIBO) at the start of a grain-free journey is so bad and intestinal health is so disrupted that a probiotic is inadequate and a course of antibiotics is required along with the probiotic. This can accelerate the elimination of truly pathogenic species, such as *Escherichia coli, Klebsiella pneumoniae, Enterococcal* species, and some clostridia that may have become dominant. This is more common in people with diagnoses such as Crohn's disease, ulcerative colitis, celiac disease, and malabsorptive syndromes, as well as in people who have been subjected to multiple courses of antibiotics for other infections. This two-pronged approach is something that should only be undertaken under the supervision of someone well acquainted with the issues of small intestinal bacterial overgrowth. Unfortunately, this is usually not the province of a gastroenterologist, a specialty that typically concerns itself with what can be viewed via an endoscope, but is best managed by practitioners of functional medicine, naturopaths, or other more naturally minded practitioners.

Living Off the Leftovers: Prebiotics

Recall that the human intestinal tract is populated by trillions of bacteria—a couple pounds of teeming life hungry to survive and living off the things you put in your mouth and swallow. We are meant to live in a happy, mutually beneficial coexistence. But bacteria have had to accept a second-class life: They only get your leftovers. You eat breakfast, which gets chewed into fragments, broken down, and absorbed by your own digestive process into amino acids, fatty acids, and glucose. By the time digestive remains make it to the colon, where the majority of bacteria reside, there's not a lot left. Some of what remains are indigestible fibers, so bacterial species able to scavenge undigested fibers found their niche and flourished—provided we continue to consume such indigestible polysaccharide fibers. In return, bacteria metabolize the polysaccharides into fatty acids acetoacetate, propionate, and butyrate, which nourish intestinal cells. Butyrate is particularly interesting, as it is also a primary source of energy for the intestinal lining and is necessary for its health. Because such indigestible fibers cause healthy bowel flora to proliferate and thrive, they are often called *prebiotics*, also known as *resistant starches*, because they are resistant to human digestion. Prebiotics are important: They can make or break an effort to restore bowel health and healthy bowel flora. In particular, the lactose-fermenting families of *Lactobacillus* and *Bifidobacteria* that humans have harbored in their bowels for millions of years thrive on prebiotic fibers.

Prebiotics are often called "fibers," though they do not look nor act like what we usually associate with fibers, such as those in wheat bran. They are indeed fibers in the sense that they are polymeric (multiunit) polysaccharides. In the past, they were often called *viscous* or *soluble* fibers, as they were gooey and soluble in water solutions, though such distinctions have blurred as we've identified a wider variety of fibers. Prebiotic fibers are, however, distinct from the cellulose fibers of grains and grasses. Humans have almost no capacity to digest cellulose. Ruminant mammals likewise lack the enzymes to digest cellulose, but they harbor bacteria that has this capacity in their four-compartment stomachs and spiral colons.

Because prebiotic fibers are a preferred energy source for lactose-fermenting bacteria, enriching the diet with prebiotic fibers encourages growth of *Lactobacillus* and *Bifidobacteria* species that yield greater quantities of butyrate for intestinal health. Accordingly, it is becoming clearer in clinical studies that prebiotics are associated with reduced potential for colon cancer.[7] Prebiotics are also proving to be useful for reducing blood sugar and improving sensitivity to insulin, reducing blood pressure, and achieving other improvements in metabolic markers. In addition, supplying plentiful prebiotic fibers to your bowel flora reduces intestinal reabsorption of bile acids, an effect that reduces cholesterol production in the liver and leads to reductions in LDL and total cholesterol.[8]

Primitive humans used sticks, bone fragments, and stones as tools to dig up the energy storage organs of plants—roots and tubers—which are rich in indigestible polysaccharide fibers. This practice is documented in the anthropological record as far back as pre-*Homo* Australopithecines and is thereby deeply rooted in human dietary adaptation.[9] We would likely find most such roots and tubers inedible, as they were dense, tough, fibrous, and not very tasty. Unfortunately, our modern roots and tubers, such as white potatoes and sweet potatoes, tend to be hybridized forms chosen for their high starch content. And because they are eaten cooked, rather than raw, their fibrous starches are converted from an indigestible polysaccharide form to a highly digestible sugar form that results in high blood sugars, as evidenced by the exceptional glycemic index of a baked white potato (70 to 111).

While grains contain prebiotic fibers—one of their few redeeming features—they simply come with too much unhealthy baggage. Non-grain foods that contain such prebiotic fibers include vegetables (especially Brussels sprouts, cabbage, garlic, and onions), fruits, and nuts. But the superstar sources of such fibers are starchy legumes and tubers, such as beans and potatoes. Legumes (such as kidney beans, black beans, pinto beans, other starchy beans, and lentils), when consumed in modest quantities (¼ to ½ cup per serving, or no more than 15 grams (g) net carbohydrates), can be used as a source of prebiotic fibers. Potatoes consumed *raw* can provide another source, as do green, unripe bananas; because the fibers remain in the indigestible form, the high glycemic potential is not expressed. Inulin fibers from chicory root or Jerusalem artichoke are other sources.

The foods with the greatest prebiotic fiber return are:[10]

Raw white potato (peeled): 10 to 12 g fiber per ½ medium

Hummus or roasted chickpeas: 15 g fiber per ¼ cup (10 g net carbohydrates in ¼ cup)

Lentils: 2.5 g fiber in ½ cup (11 g net carbohydrates)

Beans: 3.7 g fiber in ½ cup (22 g net carbohydrates)

Green bananas and plantains: 27 to 30 g fiber in one banana

Inulin: 5 g fiber per teaspoon

As with probiotics, a mixture of prebiotic fiber sources is ideal. I like to slice or chop raw potatoes to include in salads, blend a chopped raw potato or green banana into a smoothie, and dip vegetables or grain-free crackers into hummus. (See recipes in Appendix A.) Inulin can be purchased as a powder, and it's in the erythritol sweetener mix Swerve (see Appendix D). Powdered inulin can be used to add a sweetening effect to foods, as well as provide better mouthfeel in ice creams and iced coconut milk. It is also available as a powder or supplement that you can add to foods, such as fermented coconut yogurt or kefir. Note that such fibers should be consumed *unheated* for their prebiotic benefits, since heating tends to break them down into sugars.

While the average person obtains around 5 g of prebiotic fibers per day from his or her diet, we can fall below even this average intake when we eliminate grains. It is not known what the ideal daily intake of prebiotic fiber is; measurable increases in butyrate production get under way with intakes of 8 to 9 g per day, but 10 to 20 g or more per day is likely ideal, judging by the many observations of short-chain fatty acid production and metabolic consequences, such as reductions in blood sugar. (Interestingly, intake of prebiotic fibers may have been as high as 135 g per day in primitive lifestyles.)[11]

If symptoms such as bloating or intermittent loose stools are present due to inadequate intake of prebiotic fibers, several weeks of supplementation are required before you'll feel relief. This is likely due to the slow healing of low-grade colitis, a process that develops over several weeks of "feeding" bacteria the fibers they prefer. Note that substantial intestinal gas can be a problem at the start, but this effect wears off over several weeks. Many people find it easier to start with a low dose, such as 5 g per day, and slowly increase to the desired intake over time. And because healthy bowels, just like a healthy, thriving garden, require constant care and feeding, ideal bowel health develops by following prebiotic strategies for a lifetime.

Fermentation Nation

Fermented foods represent another long-term strategy worth incorporating into your diet to maintain healthy bowel flora and bowel health. Fermentation is as old as humans, as the natural process of decay—rotting—occurs whenever any food sits exposed to the air for more than a few hours. Humans discovered that the food beneath the rot—not exposed to air, but in an anaerobic environment—was not only safe to consume, but was also tasty. We now know that it is also healthy.

Prior to the age of refrigeration, fermentation was used to preserve foods. If lactate-fermenting bacteria are among the bacteria that contaminate the leaves you've gathered or the meat of the wild boar you've speared, lactic acid will be among the by-products produced through the process of fermentation if the food is not exposed to air. The lactic acid reduces pH and kills dangerous organisms. (Alcoholic fermentation to produce beer and wine proceeds by a different set of reactions.)

Fermented foods are therefore a source for lactate-fermenting organisms such as *Lactobacillus* and *Bifidobacterium*. The number of bacteria contained within the fermented food varies widely depending on what food it is, how long fermentation was allowed to proceed, the ambient temperature, the availability of other nutrients such as amino acids and fatty acids, and other factors. The number can range from trivial, as in most commercial yogurts and kefirs, to substantial, as in naturally fermented dairy products, kimchi (fermented Korean cabbage), sauerkraut (uncanned and unheated, not the stuff sold in grocery stores that is pickled in vinegar rather than fermented), and other fermented vegetables. Cheese and cottage cheese do *not* provide substantial probiotic bacteria, as the whey fraction that is removed after fermentation contains much of the bacterial content. Just about any fruit or vegetable can be subjected to fermentation. Some other sources include kombucha (a fermented tea); takuan (Japanese fermented daikon radish); natto (fermented soybeans that are exceptionally rich in vitamin K_2); and garum (fermented fish sauce). Bacterial content can also be modified by adding probiotic bacteria to a fermented product after the fermenting process has finished. Some commercial yogurts contain greater numbers of bacteria for this reason.

Interestingly, there is a wonderful intersection between lactic acid fermentation and human health, as the bacteria contained in fermented foods are also among the species that have been found to exert the greatest health benefits in humans, such as reductions in LDL cholesterol, improved intestinal health, and weight control.[12] The downside to these foods is that the majority of them have just one or two, and rarely more than four, dominant *Lactobacillus* or *Bifidobacteria* species. (Contrast this with probiotic supplements, which stack the odds in your favor by containing multiple species.) While bacterial counts in these foods can occasionally range into the billions, they more commonly number in the millions of CFUs per serving.[13] Commercial yogurts and kefirs are also typically made with excessive sugar, high-fructose corn syrup, and other undesirable ingredients. You can make your own healthier versions of yogurt and kefir, and you can ferment your own cabbage, cucumbers, and other vegetables, as well (see Appendix A).

The relatively low CFU counts and limited range of species in fermented foods can be useful to *maintain* healthy bowel flora, but these foods may not be the best way to rapidly regain bowel health early in your grain-free journey, after taking an antibiotic, or when you're recovering from celiac disease, Crohn's disease, or ulcerative colitis. In these situations, there is a clearly documented benefit to taking large quantities of a wide variety of probiotic bacterial species, not the limited species and numbers provided by fermented foods.

If you aren't up for making your own fermented foods, which is exceptionally easy and satisfying, look for fermented foods in the refrigerated section of health food stores or supermarkets. The label will usually say "contains live cultures" or something similar. Avoid canned or bottled fermented foods, as the canning or bottling process kills the bacteria.

Additional dietary strategies to encourage healthy changes in bowel flora include eliminating sugary foods and lactose-containing dairy foods. (Milk, cottage cheese, and yogurt are the biggest risks; butter, ghee, and cultured cheese are less offensive from this standpoint.)

INCREASE YOUR ODDS OF RECOVERY FROM CROHN'S DISEASE, ULCERATIVE COLITIS, AND CELIAC DISEASE

The intestinal devastation experienced by people with these chronic intestinal inflammatory processes can affect many facets of digestive health. Removing grains is a huge step toward recovery, but it's often *insufficient*, even with celiac disease, which is often viewed as nothing more than a form of intolerance to gluten. Additional steps are nearly always necessary to correct persistent disturbances.

This situation is similar to the experience of many people without celiac disease or inflammatory bowel diseases who fail to regain full health despite the removal of grains. Partial or failed recovery represents many of the same issues seen in nonceliac people, just to a greater degree. For instance, deficiencies of iron, zinc, and vitamin B_{12} can develop even more commonly. Severe disruption of bowel flora, or dysbiosis, also occurs, but worse. It is therefore of equal or greater importance that you remove all grains, gluten-containing and otherwise: Remove all prolamin protein grains (wheat, rye, barley, triticale, bulgur, and corn); remove all wheat germ agglutinin–containing grains (the same grains, plus rice); and remove all phytate-containing grains. In short, remove all grains. Teff and amaranth exert these effects the least of all grains, but they still pose blood sugar and unhealthy bowel flora implications, so either go very lightly or exclude them entirely.

The steps back to total gastrointestinal health may include some or all of the following:

- **Restore bowel flora.** At the start, taking a high-potency, broad-spectrum probiotic is ideal. Because inflammation can be substantial and healing requires a prolonged period of time, you should take probiotics for an extended period, perhaps even years, to allow full healing. Having the assistance of a health-care practitioner skilled at the processes involved in healing these conditions can be crucial. One issue your health-care provider may want to consider is whether dysbiosis is severe enough to justify a course of antibiotics taken along with a high-potency probiotic, which should be continued for an extended period of time after the course of antibiotics is over. This essentially lets your bowel flora start from scratch. Also, avoid all sugars and minimize lactose exposure from dairy to further allow normal, healthy bacterial species to proliferate.

- **Maintain healthy bowel flora and reduce inflammation with prebiotic fibers.** Dramatic additional benefits, including unique anti-inflammatory and healing effects, can be obtained through the use of nongrain prebiotic fibers (see above).

- **Correct nutrient deficiencies.** Iron, zinc, and vitamin B_{12} are commonly deficient due to intestinal inflammation and nutrient-blocking phytates in grains. Blood tests for each of these are easy to obtain and widely available (see Appendix D).

- **Correct vitamin D deficiency.** Restoration of vitamin D is especially powerful for people with inflammatory bowel diseases.[14] In fact, the data are so compelling that, in my view, it is malpractice to *not* address vitamin D when inflammatory bowel diseases are present. Vitamin D deficiency is worse when the bowels are inflamed due to impaired absorption from the modest quantities in foods; restoration of vitamin D levels contributes to reversal of autoimmune and inflammatory injury. I advocate aiming for a 25-hydroxy vitamin D level of 60 to 70 ng/ml. Doses required to achieve that level may be higher if you have Crohn's or celiac disease, due to impaired absorption in the small intestine. While most people require 6,000 international units (IU) per day, people with inflammatory bowel diseases and celiac disease often require more. See page 175 for more information on correcting this deficiency and monitoring your blood levels.

- **Get your fats right.** Excessive quantities of omega-6 fatty acids, along with inadequate consumption of omega-3s, heighten intestinal inflammation. Correcting these imbalances reduces inflammation.[15] This means minimizing use of omega-6 oils, such as corn, mixed vegetable, safflower, sunflower, and grapeseed oils, and supplementing with 3,000 to 3,600 milligrams (mg) of EPA and DHA per day, divided into two doses. For enhanced absorption, liquid forms of fish oil are superior. Note that omega-6s, specifically linoleic acid, should not be completely eliminated, as it is an essential fatty acid, but most people obtain sufficient quantities just by consuming meats, nuts, and seeds.

- **Consider an assessment for residual digestive dysfunction.** Pancreatic dysfunction with resultant incomplete digestion of fats and proteins can prevent full healing, even inviting dysbiosis. This is an important area to investigate should symptoms persist despite grain elimination and a full probiotic and prebiotic strategy.

- **Supplement the amino acid glutamine.** While it is not considered an essential amino acid for body metabolism, the cells lining the intestine (enterocytes) preferentially use glutamine when it's available. Glutamine has been demonstrated to both help prevent injury to enterocytes and, in doses of 25 to 50 g per day, to modestly accelerate healing when injury has occurred.[16]

- **Avoid factors that increase intestinal inflammation or affect intestinal permeability.** Smoking tops the list, followed by use of nonsteroidal anti-inflammatory drugs, such as naproxen, ibuprofen, and aspirin. Additionally, you should minimize use of antibiotics and take them only when truly necessary and avoid using oral contraceptives for women, as risk for bowel inflammation increases with their use.[17] Stress also plays a factor, and though specific strategies have not yet emerged that reduce this association, it is wise to recognize it and minimize stressful experiences whenever possible.

- **Don't sweat the fiber.** The last thing someone with celiac disease, Crohn's, or ulcerative colitis needs is more cellulose fiber of the sort that occurs in grains; insoluble cellulose fibers are *not* protective and may even increase intestinal irritation. Obtain fibers from vegetables and fruits, which nourish the gut flora and have been associated with reduced inflammation, as well as the prebiotic fibers discussed above, which yield anti-inflammatory factors.[18]

- **Consider anti-inflammatory supplementation.** A 100 ml dose of aloe vera gel, twice per day, has been shown to relieve symptoms and improve tissue damage.[19] Curcumin, a component of the common spice turmeric, may exert additional health effects in people with inflammatory bowel disease, especially ulcerative colitis. One gram (1,000 mg) of curcumin, twice per day, reduces relapses of inflammatory bowel conditions.[20] Likewise, taking 900 mg of boswellia (a component of the spice frankincense) three times per day has been associated with increased likelihood of remission of both ulcerative colitis and Crohn's disease.[21]

- **Consider other dietary intolerances.** Dairy intolerances are common and, if present, can sustain inflammation and encourage dysbiosis. Fructose intolerance and allergies to other foods may also play a role. Elimination of suspect foods and testing for intolerances are best conducted under the watchful eye of a health-care practitioner with experience with this issue.

Too many people with celiac disease are told to "just avoid gluten," with no further effort made to achieve a full recovery of intestinal health. Likewise, I have seen countless people with Crohn's disease or ulcerative colitis subjected to drugs and surgery, experiencing an incomplete response with continuing pain, diarrhea, malabsorption, and risk for cancer and autoimmune diseases, but with no effort made to address any of the above issues. It's really not that tough: Stack the odds for full recovery in your favor by completing these important steps following the elimination of nasty grains.

TROUBLE IN PARADISE: PERSISTENT SYMPTOMS AFTER GRAIN ELIMINATION

The gastrointestinal rubble that remains after the nuclear explosion of grain consumption doesn't always allow full recovery without additional efforts. Some people show initial improvement in gastrointestinal distress but experience residual abnormal symptoms, so they're better, but not perfect. The nature of persistent symptoms suggests the underlying residual problem, as well as the solution, as we'll discuss here.

Acid Reflux, Indigestion, and Heartburn

Remove grains, and you remove a disrupter of stomach acid production, gallbladder bile release, and pancreatic function. Combine this with a full probiotic and prebiotic strategy (see above), and the majority of people enjoy wonderful, effortless bowel health. But what if you do *not*, and instead experience persistent acid reflux symptoms, indigestion, nausea, or heartburn? That's when it's worth considering whether grains have done such a complete job of gastrointestinal disruption that you still have not recovered fully. Imagine, for instance, that you had one leg shorter than the other, causing you to spend years compensating with your walking style and resulting in distortions of spinal alignment, as well as inflammation and arthritis. Now imagine that the shorter leg is corrected, but your spine remains inflamed and arthritic. The cause is gone, but consequences remain, and they require specific interventions. So it goes in this world of grain elimination. If acid reflux, indigestion, or heartburn persist after you've gone grain-free, consider whether any of the following issues are present.

- **Persistent dysbiosis.** If this is an issue, a formal assessment (either breath testing or examination of stool composition) may point you in the direction of a solution. A course of antibiotics may be required to eradicate unhealthy organisms before you repopulate with healthy species. Regardless, a prolonged course of probiotics, along with a lifetime of prebiotics and fermented foods, are in your future.

- **Hypochlorhydria.** Long-term grain consumption disrupts digestive function in the stomach and impairs the release of stomach acid to start the breakdown of foods. Unfortunately, even after removing grains, normal stomach acid production may not resume, which results in hypochlorhydria, or inadequate stomach acid production. People who have taken nonsteroidal anti-inflammatory drugs are also prone to this condition. Recall that *low* stomach acid mimics the same symptoms as *high* stomach acid. Some people in this situation attempt a trial of acid-increasing nutritional supplements, such as a teaspoon or two of apple cider vinegar or one or more 500 mg tablets of betaine hydrochloride supplements taken just prior to meals to supply acid.[22] Others choose to undergo a formal evaluation (a safer route) to document hypochlorhydria and determine just how much additional acid may be required to normalize digestive function. Taking such acids inappropriately, such as in the presence of excessive stomach acid, can worsen the situation.

- **Delayed recovery of cholecystokinin (CCK) signaling.** Because the lectins of grains are such effective disrupters of glycoprotein hormone receptors, such as the CCK receptor of the pancreas and gallbladder, recovery of pancreatic or gallbladder function may not occur immediately. It may take months or years. In the meantime, you can supplement with pancreatic enzymes to assist food digestion, supplement with bile acids to emulsify fats, or supplement with curcumin (a component of the spice turmeric) to stimulate the release of bile from the gallbladder.[23] Ideally, such decisions are made under the guidance of a health-care practitioner skilled in such determinations.

- **Consider getting assessed for food intolerances, particularly dairy, fructose, egg, nuts, and soy.** A variety of testing methods can be performed to identify whether a food or foods are allowing inflammation or disruptions of bowel flora to persist.

- **Avoid factors that increase intestinal inflammation or affect intestinal permeability.** This list includes smoking; taking non-steroidal anti-inflammatory drugs, such as naproxen, ibuprofen, and aspirin; and taking oral contraceptives. Stress can also perpetuate a number of abnormal bowel phenomena. Recognize this association and take action to minimize stressful experiences, if possible.

Constipation

Constipation can result from a number of phenomena that occur singly or in various combinations. It's not about "lazy bowels" any more than health problems experienced by grain-consuming people are due to gluttony and sloth. Irregular or infrequent stools are a signal that something is wrong with the normal passage of undigested remains. And the problem certainly is not remedied with laxatives, which should only be regarded as last resorts.

Poor hydration is among the most common causes of constipation, as it causes water absorption *out* of the colon, resulting in dry, hard, and difficult-to-pass stools. The solution: purposeful and consistent hydration. Hydrate with water, not with silly and destructive juices, drinks, or flavored waters. Use simple, real water—the stuff that has sustained humans from the start. Poor mucous production with resultant impaired bowel lubrication can also result in dry, hard stools. Diminished mucous production is most commonly the result of disrupted bowel flora composition. A course of probiotics, along with prebiotic fibers and fermented foods (see pages 193–198), will usually take care of the problem.

Constipation is yet another reason to supplement with magnesium. If you're taking magnesium just to correct or prevent deficiency, then highly absorbable forms, such as malate or glycinate, are preferred. However, if you want to encourage bowel regularity, take 400 mg of magnesium citrate two or three times per day. When constipation gets out of control, you can take 800 to 1,200 mg of the citrate all at once, or 250 to 500 mg of magnesium oxide; both act as osmotic agents, simply pulling water into the colon to expel its contents. (This is distinct from irritative laxatives, such as phenolphthalein and senna, which can result in habituation with repetitive use.)

Fiber supplementation is rarely necessary with the improved bowel function unique to grain-free people. However, if you need more fiber than you're getting from vegetables, fruits, nuts, and seeds, try psyllium seed, ground flaxseed, or chia seeds, all of which can be helpful. Be sure to hydrate well, though, or else constipation can worsen, rather than improve.

Abdominal Discomfort

If low-grade discomfort persists after grain elimination, consider the list of factors discussed above for acid reflux, indigestion, and heartburn. However, bear in mind that it is also possible to develop an abdominal issue that's unrelated to your grain elimination experience and that requires formal attention. Gallstone attacks, appendicitis, stomach ulcers, pancreatic cysts, and diverticulitis are just a few of the conditions generally suggested by abdominal pain that worsens or persists.

Diarrhea

Should diarrhea persist or develop in the midst of your wheat-free experience, it most commonly suggests that dysbiosis persists. There is little to lose by trying a course of probiotics, along with a vigorous effort at prebiotic supplementation, to accelerate repopulation of the colon with healthy bacteria. Should this succeed, hallelujah: Continue probiotic supplementation for at least several more weeks, if not months to years, to allow full recovery of normal bowel health, and continue prebiotic and fermented food strategies for, oh, another 50 or 60 years.

If loose stools do not respond to your own efforts to restore and maintain bowel flora, a formal evaluation is in order to identify the problem and the solution, since there are causes that simply cannot be identified without medical assistance and may require assessment of stool composition to look for undigested fragments, oils and fats, or parasites. Intestinal infections such as *Clostridium difficile* can arise and *must* be treated with conventional medical treatments.

POOP IS PARAMOUNT

All right, go ahead and pooh-pooh the notion that gastrointestinal health, organ function, and bacterial populations can impact digestive, as well as overall, health. But the experience of thousands of people who've found relief from chronic and bothersome—and sometimes incapacitating—bowel problems with a simple shift in diet is nothing short of amazing.

The human gastrointestinal system developed over millions of years, crafting this astounding collection of organs that maximally derive nutrition and are meant to run like clockwork. We screw the whole thing up by introducing this collection of "foods" (seeds of grasses) that were never appropriate for the human diet in the first place and have been made worse by the ambitions of agribusiness. It creates the perfect storm of disrupted gastrointestinal health. Recognize this essential truth and you are empowered to regain total, ideal gastrointestinal health.

CHAPTER 10

GRAINLESS METABOLIC MASTERY: REGAIN CONTROL OVER BLOOD SUGAR, CHOLESTEROL, BONE HEALTH, AND INFLAMMATION

I don't deserve this award, but I have arthritis
and I don't deserve that either.
—Jack Benny

INJECT SOMETHING INTO the human experience that doesn't belong there, such as *Yersinia pestis*, the organism that causes bubonic plague to be passed to humans from infected rats, or LSD, with its frenzied delusions, hallucinations, and flashbacks, and you can quickly discern whether or not such things belong in our lives.

Introduce the seeds of grasses into the human diet and all manner of peculiar health problems crop up. They might involve mental effects, such as impulsive or irrational behavior. They might cause stimulation of appetite, provoking abnormal or incessant eating that makes no physiologic sense. They could cause an odd and annoying rash that won't go away, or unpredictable and explosive diarrhea. They might initiate the process of autoimmunity. Grains are, in a word, an unnatural component in the human dietary experience. Just as no law-abiding member of the workforce can adhere to a daily routine while high on LSD, no member of the species *Homo sapiens* can achieve and maintain optimal health while under the disruptive influence of the seeds of grasses.

After surviving the chronic health disruptions of grains, you removed them. But will all aspects of your metabolism normalize with their removal?

Possibly, but they may not. As powerful as grain elimination can be, it may not allow all the unhealthy metabolic phenomena caused by grains to fully unwind, much as abstinence from alcohol will not correct the nutritional deficiencies and cirrhosis an alcoholic incurs while drinking. For example, if you have diabetes and previously required insulin and oral drugs to control your blood sugar, removing the grains will cause your blood sugar to drop precipitously, along with your need for insulin and drugs—but not always all the way to normal. Are there steps to take that safeguard you from negative effects, such as low blood sugars? Are there additional steps that will maximize your chances of becoming confidently and assuredly nondiabetic, enjoying normal blood sugars and HbA1c without the assistance of drugs? Or if you have hypertension and take three different antihypertensive drugs, going grain-free may drop your blood pressure along with your visceral fat. How do you safely reduce your medications, and what can you do to stack the odds in your favor such that you won't require *any* drugs?

This chapter will address these questions of metabolic health and others that will arise during both your early grain-free period and the rest of your grainless life.

PLAYING WITH FIRE

The concept of metabolism covers a lot of territory. Metabolism refers to all of the chemical processes by which your body uses food, nutrients, and water to grow, heal, and produce energy. It is the bonfire of body energy: It needs kindling and wood to build heat and convert energy from one form to another.

The myriad processes of metabolic activity can be tracked by measuring parameters that show whether it is proceeding in a healthy fashion or has veered off course and is heading toward metabolic disasters such as diabetes, dementia, osteoporosis, heart disease, cancer, or obesity. Many, if not most, common, chronic health conditions involve disruptions of metabolism in some form or to some degree.

I begin this discussion assuming that you have already undertaken your own personal grain-elimination voyage to begin the process of undoing all the metabolic disruption caused by grains. You may have already endured and completed the withdrawal process. You may be starting or be in the midst of transformations that lead to weight loss, reduced inflammation, increased energy, shutting off autoimmunity, and other beneficial metabolic processes. This discussion will help you understand whether, minus grains, the features of your metabolism have normalized or whether additional efforts will be required to achieve total metabolic health. The discussion is limited to the most common forms of residual metabolic disturbances: diabetes and blood sugar, hypertension, abnormalities of cholesterol, and osteoporosis. As you read, you will see that there are substantial commonalities among these conditions that explain why, for instance, someone with diabetes also develops hypertension, heart disease, osteoporosis, and dementia over time. The basic principles discussed here, applied to the most common forms of metabolic disruption, therefore apply to many other forms that are not specifically discussed. Even if you feel you've reached a perfect state of metabolic health, it's worth reading on and acquiring a deeper understanding of how to attain and maintain ideal metabolic status.

BLOOD SUGAR, HBA1C, DIABETES, AND HYPERTENSION: WHAT GOES UP MUST COME DOWN

Though many view diabetes as the price of civilization, we should throw off this yoke of dietary subservience and declare our freedom.

High blood sugar is a defining marker for grain consumption. This makes perfect sense when you realize that grains are largely indigestible except for their amylopectin A content, the carbohydrate that raises blood sugar even higher than table sugar does. This is true for every grain, even the more benign, such as millet, teff, and amaranth. All grains are rich in amylopectin A, and all grains raise blood sugar to high levels. The more grains you eat, the more frequently you eat them, the more you experience high blood sugars (as high or higher than those resulting from eating candy or drinking soft drinks) that oblige high insulin responses. This is the process that sets *resistance to insulin* in motion—higher blood sugars lead to higher insulin, which leads to higher blood sugars, and around and around. Eventually the pancreas (which produces insulin) loses its capacity to keep up; that's when blood sugars climb even higher, sufficient to qualify for the diagnosis of diabetes. Along with diabetes comes increased risk for heart disease, cancer, dementia, hypertension, cataracts, kidney failure, neuropathy, bone fractures, and loss of limb.

Now that we understand the diabetes-causing potential of grains, we can remove them, their blood sugar–raising properties, and their insulin-boosting effects. It's time to unravel the entire process of insulin resistance and high blood sugars.

Diabetes: The Price of Civilization and Modern Health Advice

Diabetes is the inevitable result of converting from a traditional diet to a modern one, as observed in Pima Indians, the Aboriginal people of Australia, and the tribes of the Amazon rain forest. All of these populations experienced virtually no obesity or diabetes on their traditional diet but displayed epidemic levels of obesity and diabetes within just a few years of being introduced to modern foods.

Agencies such as the American Diabetes Association (ADA) advocate a modern diet, too—one reduced in total and saturated fat and containing as much as 300 grams (g) of carbohydrates per day, acquired mostly from grains. I've witnessed it firsthand hundreds of times: People are advised to follow the ADA diet that's rich in grains and low in fat, and blood sugars climb, HbA1c goes up, insulin and oral diabetic drug needs escalate, and weight goes up 10, 20, 30 pounds. The situation worsens when someone transitions to injectable insulin (similar to the insulin your pancreas produces, the hormone of fat storage), increasing visceral fat stores and worsening inflammation and resistance to insulin.

More grains, more amylopectin A, more diabetes. Reject this advice—eat *more* fat and eat *no* "healthy whole grains"—and diabetes powerfully recedes: Fasting blood sugars drop, insulin levels drop and insulin resistance reverses, HbA1c plummets, body weight and waist size shrink, appetite shrinks, inflammation recedes, and the need for insulin and oral drugs to control blood sugar is reduced or eliminated.[1]

Compound these metabolic benefits with several additional strategies, such as correcting vitamin D and magnesium deficiencies and managing bowel flora (discussed below), and you have a powerful means of restoring normal metabolic control and minimizing, if not entirely reversing, the expression of diabetes.

How did agencies like the ADA get it so wrong? Ignorance, cowardice, greed? Let's ignore the rich revenues obtained from the food and drug industries that support such advice. (Cadbury Schweppes, the world's largest candy manufacturer, was a major supporter of the ADA for years, as are diabetes drug manufacturers Novo Nordisk, Sanofi-Aventis, Merck, and Eli Lilly, all contributing millions of dollars to the ADA each year.) You've heard the argument that if whole grains replace white flour products, the likelihood of diabetes is reduced. That is indeed (a little bit) true, and the ADA went for it hook, line, and sinker. The next step—elimination of all grains and their exceptional glycemic potential—is not talked about. But that is when the real power of diet shows itself. It would now take a major act of courage for an organization to reverse this message, complete with plenty of legal repercussions, so don't hold your breath waiting.

It is *not* just a matter of reducing carbohydrates; it is the combined effect of eliminating *all* the factors in grains. Removing the prolamin proteins, which degrade to opiates that stimulate appetite, is a major factor. Removing lectins, which activate inflammation and block leptin, the hormone of satiety, is another. Because grains have come to dominate diet and modern forms have such exceptional glycemic potential, removing grains achieves larger-than-expected reductions in glucose, insulin, and inflammation.

This is such an important issue that it bears repeating: High blood sugars and diabetes recede with grain elimination not just because we remove the high glycemic potential of grains; it is the combination of effects that packs such astounding diabetes-reversing power.

Over time, improvements are compounded by weight loss and the shrinkage of visceral fat, which drives inflammation. That's when most prediabetics experience a return to normal sugars and many, if not most, diabetics become nondiabetic, or at least experience marked improvements in blood sugar with reduced reliance on insulin and other medications. Not all diabetics will be able, unfortunately, to achieve full nondiabetic status. Persistence of diabetes may occur if the years of pre-diabetes and diabetes caused damage to pancreatic beta cells that produce insulin. If, for instance, you ended up on insulin and two oral diabetes medications to keep blood sugar under control and you have lost 50 percent of beta cell function in the process of becoming diabetic, you may be left with inadequate blood sugar control even after removing grains and losing weight. However, you will still enjoy better control over blood sugars and HbA1c, a reduced need for medication, and reduced potential for diabetic complications.

Also, some people (less than 10 percent) diagnosed with type 2 diabetes as adults, as well as a growing number of children and teenagers, have experienced autoimmune damage to pancreatic beta cells similar to that experienced by type 1 diabetics. (Some call this *latent autoimmune diabetes of adulthood*, or LADA.) These people likewise can enjoy better blood sugar and HbA1c control, weight loss, a reduced need for medication, and reduced potential for diabetic complications with grain elimination. They will, however, still need insulin, as their pancreatic beta cells provide insufficient quantities of insulin (unlike the high insulin levels of the typical type 2 diabetic) and they risk developing diabetic ketoacidosis, a potentially dangerous state caused by a lack of insulin. If you have such a condition, the grain-free approach is best pursued under the supervision of a knowledgeable health-care practitioner. A red flag for pancreatic beta cell damage is an inability to reduce blood sugars despite having eliminated grains, curtailing other carbohydrates, and having lost weight, all of which suggest that insulin production is inadequate.

For most people, benefits snowball over time. In the early weeks to months, excess weight and visceral fat shrink as fatty acids and triglycerides are mobilized into the bloodstream, a natural and expected phenomenon in weight loss. (On a cholesterol or lipid panel, this can be seen as a transient rise in triglycerides and a drop in HDL.) This flood of fatty acids and triglycerides blocks the action of insulin, sometimes enough to raise blood sugar and HbA1c during the early stages of grain elimination, or to fail to yield the desired blood sugar drops. But as weight loss continues and eventually plateaus, blood sugars and HbA1c plummet. So time is also a factor, with the full diabetes-reversing effects generally requiring several months to totally evolve. The vigor of this insulin-blocking effect of weight loss is also dependent on how much weight there is to lose: Someone who only needs to lose 30 pounds to achieve her ideal weight may run through this process in just 4 to 6 weeks, while someone with 150 pounds to lose may have to endure this process for a year or longer. It took years of being pummeled by grains to turn you into a diabetic; it should come as no surprise that the whole process cannot be undone in moments.

One critical issue to address: If you start the process with diabetes and are taking either insulin or oral diabetes drugs, there is the potential for dangerous hypoglycemia (low blood sugars) when you eliminate grains. In other words, as your appetite drops and you consume fewer foods that raise blood sugar, responsiveness to your own body's insulin is restored and you lose visceral fat, reduce inflammation, and become less diabetic. The dosages of your medications will no longer be right for your body, and you may experience low blood sugars, much as a nondiabetic person taking diabetes medication might. For this reason, you must take several precautions because *hypoglycemia must be absolutely avoided* (see "Caution: Zero Tolerance for Hypoglycemia").

Caution: Zero Tolerance for Hypoglycemia

For all the hooting and hollering by the American Diabetes Association (ADA) about wanting to cure diabetes, you will not find a single piece of advice in their literature, from their "experts," on their Web site, or anywhere else telling people just how to cure type 2 diabetes. We cannot turn to the ADA, nor to endocrinologists (who are largely responsible for drafting the absurd dietary advice given by the ADA), nor to most practicing physicians to learn just how to safely manage making the journey from diabetic to nondiabetic. So let's reason this through ourselves.

Eat foods that increase blood sugar, and the need for diabetes medications increases. Reduce or eliminate foods that increase blood sugar, and the need for diabetes medications decreases. The equation is really that simple.

But precautions are necessary if you are diabetic and are taking certain diabetes drugs. The potential danger is *hypoglycemia* (blood sugars lower than 70 mg/dl) and, less commonly, diabetic ketoacidosis if you have a form of diabetes in which pancreatic insulin production is inadequate.

You should be aware that many doctors will voice uninformed objections to the idea of reducing your medications, as they have come to believe that diabetes is incurable, irreversible, and a diagnosis for life.

Anyone taking insulin injections in any form will need to reduce her dosage in order to follow a grain-free diet without experiencing hypoglycemia. An immediate reduction in insulin *by half* is typical. Ideally, this is undertaken with a health-care provider with experience in helping patients become less diabetic or nondiabetic. This almost always means identifying a *new* practitioner, as the one who prescribed the insulin in the first place is likely a member of the "diabetes is incurable and irreversible" school. But I cannot stress enough that hypoglycemia must be avoided, even if some higher blood sugars result (though ideally they should be kept below 200 mg/dl throughout this process). Other medications, especially certain oral agents, can cause dangerous hypoglycemia if taken while eliminating grains. For this reason, many people eliminate these oral drugs or reduce doses, even if it means a temporary increase in blood sugars.

Whatever medications you are taking, frequent monitoring of blood sugars is essential on this journey. I tell my patients that high blood sugars (though below 200 mg/dl) are preferable to low blood sugars (below 100 mg/dl) during this transition period. As blood sugars trend downward, you'll need to further reduce your medications. If, for instance, you have fasting blood sugars of 100 mg/dl or less, it is time to reduce or eliminate a medication, such as one taken at bedtime.

For people with type 1 diabetes, latent autoimmune diabetes of adulthood, or markedly reduced pancreatic beta cell function, the need for insulin is lifelong. Their insulin dose and need for oral diabetes medications, as well as drugs for hypertension, inflammation, and other phenomena, can all be reduced dramatically, but they will always be dependent on insulin. The reduced need for drugs and insulin still greatly reduces risk of long-term diabetic complications. Changes in diet, along with reducing insulin and other drugs, should only be attempted under the supervision of a knowledgeable and willing health-care practitioner.

CREATE A WINNING HAND AGAINST DIABETES

Go to Vegas and bet against the house, and chances are you will lose. Become diabetic or prediabetic and gamble by engaging in a diet of "healthy whole grains," and you might as well fold your hand and get a martini: You will definitely lose.

After grain elimination, there are a number of strategies that work with your improved diet and take you closer to minimizing or eliminating your diabetes. These are important and can sometimes make the difference between success and failure, much like holding a couple of wild cards in your poker hand.

Among the most important are:

SUPPLEMENT VITAMIN D. Correction of vitamin D deficiency reduces blood sugar by restoring the body's response to insulin. Vitamin D restoration may even maintain or partially restore the function of pancreatic beta cells that produce insulin—almost nothing else can do this.[2] Vitamin D also exerts an anti-inflammatory effect, better allowing insulin to do its job. (See page 175 for the ideal level of vitamin D to shoot for.)

SUPPLEMENT MAGNESIUM. Magnesium deficiency is especially common among people with diabetes and contributes to higher or erratic blood sugars.[3] Aiming for values in the upper half of the reference range has proven helpful in alleviating the symptoms of deficiency, such as erratic blood sugars, high blood pressure, muscle cramps in fingers and calves, and abnormal heart rhythms. (See page 109 for information on choosing the right type and dose of magnesium for you.)

OBTAIN ADEQUATE POTASSIUM. The easiest, most natural way to obtain abundant potassium is to include green vegetables, coconut, avocado, fish, and unripe bananas in your daily routine. These foods have been shown to exert many health benefits, including reducing blood pressure. Many people also choose to supplement with an alkaline form of potassium, such as potassium citrate or bicarbonate. To ensure adequate potassium intake to reduce blood pressure over time, take three or four 99-milligram (mg) capsules (the form typically sold) per day. Potassium citrate has been shown to reduce systolic blood pressure by 7.9 mmHg and diastolic by 6.4 mmHg after 3 months.[4]

MAKE YOUR BOWEL FLORA HAPPY. An emerging and exciting strategy for reducing blood sugar and improving insulin responses is coming from insights into the use of prebiotic fibers, which are not digestible by human enzymes but are digestible by bowel flora.[5] This should be viewed as a long-term strategy, not the sort of thing you do for a day and see improvements, since changes in bowel flora and metabolic by-products of bowel flora, changes in the health of the intestinal cells, and shifting responses in gut-derived hormones that affect blood sugar and insulin are

The whole reason I chose this path was my health.

I first started my journey because I wanted to get pregnant. After several miscarriages, failed in vitro fertilizations, polycystic ovarian syndrome (PCOS), type 2 diabetes, high blood pressure, and high cholesterol, I decided to do something. I did enough to conceive my beautiful daughter, but failed badly after she was born.

Almost 3 years ago, I jumped on board again for my health. I started at 290 pounds. I have lost 184 pounds to date, and I am not on a single prescription medicine. Eating and living this lifestyle has cured me of diabetes, high blood pressure, and high cholesterol, and my PCOS has not acted up in ages (no pain or crazy cycles). I was not expecting it to cure my irritable

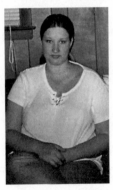
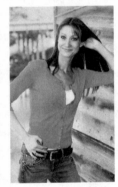

Before *After*

bowel syndrome or touch my thyroid, but my levels are normal now! Oddly, I always had swollen lymph nodes and was always having biopsies. Six months after I went wheat-free, they are gone. All my pains are gone, and I haven't had one migraine in more than 2 years. I used to sleep 10 to 11 hours a night; now I sleep 6 to 7 and feel great. This is life as I imagined it. Without my health issues, I don't think I would have started this journey. My only regret is that I didn't do it sooner!

I'm still scared to talk to people, but now I can walk with my head up and not look at the ground because I'm not scared of what people think of me. I am proud of myself and who I am now.

When I say *Wheat Belly* saved me, I honestly know in my heart that it has. I was ready to give up, but I didn't. I literally owe your wonderful work and research my life. Thank you!

Melissa Ann, Louisburg, North Carolina

required to allow the phenomena of diabetes to recede. Long-term consistency is therefore key: Eat them every day. We can obtain prebiotic starches from nongrain sources, such as legumes and tubers, as well as other vegetables. (See page 195 for a more complete list.)

There are a number of other nutritional supplements purported to reduce blood sugars, including chromium, American ginseng, and pycnogenol. In my experience, such strategies are rarely required, nor are they of much help, as their effects are either too small to make a real difference (as with chromium) or they have consequences that may not be entirely beneficial (for example, American ginseng may stimulate pancreatic insulin release, potentially worsening the demands on an already overworked pancreas). One exception may be cinnamon, since it is already a common component of our diet. Ceylon cinnamon is the variety demonstrated to have a blood sugar–reducing effect, but don't expect too much; it has generally been disappointing in reducing blood sugars, despite reports suggesting a positive effect.[6]

Prior to the consumption of grains, and certainly prior to widely broadcast advice to make grains the centerpiece of our diet, diabetes was uncommon. The weight and visceral fat loss you'll experience after eliminating grains, combined with the few additional strategies mentioned above, should make use of such supplements largely superfluous.

UNWINDING HYPERTENSION

As hypertension essentially parallels blood sugar for most people, all the efforts that help reduce high blood sugars will also, over time, reduce high blood pressure: That means you should take your vitamin D and magnesium and manage your bowel flora as discussed on page 190. In addition, omega-3 fatty acid supplementation of 3,000 to 3,600 mg per day, divided into two doses, allows blood pressure to drift downward.

There are several unique issues surrounding blood pressure.

- Reductions in blood pressure may be delayed by the flood of fatty acids and triglycerides unleashed into the bloodstream while experiencing active weight loss, so don't be discouraged if your weight is dropping and your visceral fat is shrinking, but your blood pressure is stubbornly staying high. A few weeks after your weight plateaus, blood pressure typically drops as fatty acid release slows.

- A few blood pressure medications cannot be stopped abruptly, but need to be reduced gradually. This is especially true for beta-blocker drugs and clonidine. You should wean off of these with the assistance of a knowledgeable health-care provider, as the feasibility and safety of removing them needs to be assessed. (The weaning process for someone taking a beta-blocker for hypertension may be different if coronary disease, angina, heart rhythm issues, or migraine headaches are also present.) Ridding yourself of beta-blockers and diuretics, such as hydrochlorothiazide and chlorthalidone, allows blood sugars to drop, HDL values to increase, triglycerides to drop, small LDL particles to drop, and long-term potential for diabetes to reduce by as much as 30 percent. Also, note that beta-blockers also block your ability to lose weight; removing them helps restore that ability.

- Achieving your ideal weight will maximize the likelihood of enjoying normal blood pressure and freedom from drugs. For some people, even a modest quantity of excess weight over ideal can allow high blood pressures to persist, especially if they carry the weight in their abdomen. Losing this bit of excess weight often yields outsize blood pressure–reducing benefits.

An occasional person will experience persistent hypertension despite doing everything right. This situation can usually be blamed on genetic variants that cause hypertension, suggesting that there may be benefits to managing hypertension with prescription agents, at least until newer insights into better and natural management of such genetic variants emerge.

Just as we should have zero tolerance for low blood sugar, we should also have zero tolerance for low blood pressure, or hypotension. While not as dangerous as hypoglycemia, hypotension can still, at its most extreme, cause you to pass out or even injure yourself. I tell my patients to report any light-headedness that develops and to monitor blood pressures daily. When light-headedness or blood pressure at or below 100 mmHg (systolic) develops, blood pressure medications need to be reduced or eliminated immediately. (Note that there may be exceptions due to the above precautions concerning certain drugs.) Also, fluid and salt intake need to be examined. Minus the fluid- and salt-retaining properties of grains, the majority of people need both vigorous hydration and modest salt use, which is the *opposite* of what applies to grain-consuming people.

Know that the majority of people taking one or more drugs for hypertension are simply taking drugs that address just one more manifestation of a grain-containing diet. Remove the grains, address common deficiencies that plague modern people, and most people are able to enjoy normal blood pressures at or below 120/80 again.

LEPRECHAUNS, NYMPHS, HIGH CHOLESTEROL, AND OTHER FANCIFUL NOTIONS

At the start of their grain-free journey, people often have concerns about losing the purported health benefits of grains while increasing their intake of fats, including saturated fats. They are worried that such a dietary change will "increase cholesterol" and thereby increase risk for heart disease.

Let's get this straight right from the start: Cholesterol in your diet does not cause heart disease any more than fat, saturated fat, or a voodoo doll pricked with pins by your worst enemy causes heart disease. Just because cholesterol is found in both particles in the bloodstream as well as in atherosclerotic plaque does not necessarily mean that one caused the other. Cholesterol, after all, makes up 25 percent of the fat content of *all* cells of the body. Cholesterol in the bloodstream does not cause heart disease but is a convenient way to measure your risk. Just as you would not blame the dipstick in your car for the engine failing to start, we should not blame this "dipstick" that measures particles of cholesterol in the blood for causing heart disease. Then why is there this astounding focus on something as blameless as cholesterol? Why have billions of marketing dollars been spent urging us to reduce consumption of it, why do armies of drug representatives and physicians dispense drugs to treat it, and why do media reports endlessly warn us of its dangers?

To understand this situation, we have to review how and why we got here, as well as what *really* goes on in the body that raises risk for heart disease. It may be a bit painful to follow this discussion, but I believe that the world of cholesterol will become crystal clear once you grasp these concepts.

A quick history lesson on cholesterol testing: Back in the early 1960s, William Friedewald, MD, and other research scientists at the National Institutes of Health (NIH) conducted sophisticated studies on the various components of the blood. They came to understand that fat-carrying proteins in the bloodstream (lipoproteins) appeared to gain access to the walls of arteries, such as those of the heart, thereby leading to accumulations of atherosclerosis and, eventually, heart attacks. They reasoned that quantifying lipoproteins in the bloodstream might offer a way to gauge long-term potential for coronary atherosclerosis. The NIH team also knew that when blood was spun (centrifuged) at high speed, it would separate lipoproteins in test tubes into various fractions: a high-density fraction at the bottom and low-density and very low-density fractions toward the top. In particular, the particles found in the low-density fraction appeared to be the most cholesterol-rich—and cholesterol was one of the compounds retrieved from arteries bearing atherosclerosis.

Each lipoprotein particle, regardless of which density fraction it comes from, shares various components, such as phospholipids, proteins, triglycerides, and cholesterol. Dr. Friedewald and his colleagues reasoned that, by choosing one component and measuring it, they could compare this one component across different individuals. Measuring one component in each density fraction thereby *indirectly quantified the amount of lipoproteins in each density fraction*: Higher levels of a component in one fraction correlated, albeit crudely, with greater numbers of lipoproteins in that fraction—a virtual dipstick of lipoproteins. They chose cholesterol as their indirect measure, since it was an important component in atherosclerotic plaque, was present in every density fraction, and could be easily measured using 1960s technology. So they measured the cholesterol in the unseparated blood (total cholesterol) and then in each density fraction: a high-density lipoprotein (HDL) fraction, a low-density (LDL) fraction, and a very low-density (VLDL) fraction. The amount of cholesterol in each fraction was used to compare the amount of cholesterol in one person versus another, and that allowed them to indirectly compare the number of lipoproteins in each density fraction.

Cholesterol was therefore a convenient component to measure. They could have chosen phospholipids, triglycerides, or some other component, but they chose cholesterol. Cholesterol was not measured because it *caused* atherosclerosis; it was simply a component of atherosclerotic plaque that could also be measured in the bloodstream. Dr. Friedewald and colleagues went a step further: Because the low-density fraction, in particular, was cumbersome to measure, they devised a simple equation that allowed laboratories to measure the cholesterol in the entire blood sample, the high-density and very low-density fractions, and then estimate the fraction in the low-density fraction through a crude calculation. This gave them a value that approximated the true measured value. Several assumptions were used to allow this calculation, including the assumption that everyone ate a fairly uniform diet.

Despite its admitted shortcomings, this was the birth of the conventional lipid panel of three measures—total cholesterol, HDL cholesterol, and VLDL cholesterol (now estimated by measuring triglycerides)—that's then used to calculate LDL cholesterol:

LDL cholesterol = total cholesterol - HDL cholesterol - triglycerides/5

(Triglycerides divided by 5 is an estimate of VLDL cholesterol.)

Such simple testing was widely adopted to gauge risk for coronary disease and heart attack, despite Dr. Friedewald and his colleagues' misgivings about its limitations, including the inaccuracies introduced when the high-density and very low-density values strayed from the assumed range. Accordingly, as lipid panels, including LDL cholesterol values obtained using the "Friedewald equation," expanded in clinical use, numerous objections were raised that such testing was crude, imprecise, and outdated.[7]

Beyond the fact that this assessment was crude and indirect and suffered from faulty built-in assumptions, it also had several other deficiencies. Because, for instance, it relied mostly on measuring or calculating the amount of cholesterol in the various density fractions of blood, it made no effort to decipher the actual shape, conformation, density, surface characteristics, duration of persistence, or other crucial aspects of lipoprotein behavior. Instead, it assumed that every lipoprotein particle within, say, the low-density fraction, was the same in every person regardless of age, sex, diet, weight, insulin or blood sugar status, presence or absence of diabetes, etc., because it was viewed only from the perspective of cholesterol content.

Fast-forward to the 1980s and 1990s, and a very clever way to cash in on this widely adopted, though flawed, method of testing was devised: Statin drugs that inhibit the liver synthesis of lipoproteins by blocking the HMG-CoA reductase enzyme were created. These drugs were billed as "cholesterol reducing" drugs because, by reducing liver production of cholesterol, lipoprotein production was also restricted.

Even though the dietary contribution to cholesterol synthesis from foods (such as egg yolks and animal fats) is small to negligible compared to the body's capacity to manufacture cholesterol, such foods got labeled as unhealthy, while foods low in cholesterol (grains, vegetables, and sugars) got labeled as healthy. Largely ignored was the contribution carbohydrates make to increasing cholesterol production by the liver.[8] Even worse, the potential for carbohydrates to provoke formation of excessive quantities of VLDL that cause dramatic shifts in the size, density, and composition of other particles (such as converting LDL particle size from large to small) was never acknowledged because the standard cholesterol panel does not reflect these phenomena.

Focus on the crude values yielded by cholesterol testing, especially calculated LDL cholesterol, also prompted national advice to reduce total fat, saturated fat, and cholesterol intake, a campaign that has failed to reduce total or LDL cholesterol in the United States.[9] Nationwide reductions in total and LDL cholesterol are only attributable to use of statin drugs, not diet. (Yes: Advise people to follow the wrong diet, then come to their "rescue" with prescription drugs.) We focus on only one component of lipoproteins, cholesterol, ignore the varied ways in which lipoproteins behave, then equate cholesterol in lipoproteins with cholesterol in atherosclerotic plaque: This is where we find ourselves in the early 21st century, having blundered our way here with hundreds of millions of people worldwide being treated for "high cholesterol."

Why Not Measure *Lipoproteins?*

We can't blame people like Dr. Friedewald for this blunder, as his intention was simply to provide a simple, widely accessible means of characterizing lipoproteins half a century ago. Not too many years after Dr. Friedewald and his colleagues completed their research, the technology to directly, rapidly, and easily measure lipoproteins in all fractions of the blood emerged, essentially making Dr. Friedewald and colleagues' methods unnecessary and outdated, much like Teletypes and mimeographs. Ultracentrifugation, electrophoresis, and nuclear magnetic resonance (NMR) all proved to be useful means of *directly* examining both the number and size of the various lipoprotein fractions—not the cholesterol within lipoprotein fractions, but the lipoproteins themselves, including assessments of size, surface electrical charge, density, triglyceride content, and other features. Such methods have been widely available for more than 20 years—widely available, but not widely used. (I have been using them for nearly that long.) Because medical practice requires 20 or more years for a conventional notion to give way to newer insights, even today the outdated and crude method of lipid, or "cholesterol," testing persists. This method is even further entrenched because of the enormous and unprecedented marketing push of the pharmaceutical companies who manufacture the eight available statin drugs that drive more than $20 billion per year in sales. Statins are among the most financially successful drug class in history.

There is no longer any lingering doubt: Lipoprotein assessments are substantially superior to cholesterol assessments. They are better predictors of the quantity of atherosclerosis, likelihood of heart attack, and cardiovascular mortality.[10] In fact, many analyses have demonstrated that total and LDL cholesterol are virtually no better than a roll of the dice when predicting risk for heart disease, performing among the *worst* of all examined markers of cardiovascular risk. People at low or no risk are prescribed statin drugs, while people at high risk are untreated, undertreated, or mistreated. Roll these dice and the only winner is the pharmaceutical industry.

The question that should be asked when addressing risk for coronary heart disease is, "Which fractions of lipoproteins appear to be associated with increased risk for coronary heart disease, and what can be done to modify those fractions?" We then discover that a number of lipoproteins emerge as culprits. For instance, increased numbers of VLDL particles and reduced numbers of large HDL particles (often called HDL2b) have been associated with increased risk. In particular, an increased number and percentage of small LDL particles has proven to be among the most powerful of risk markers.

Small LDL particles are more prone to oxidation and glycation (glucose modification), they persist many days longer in the bloodstream than large LDL particles, they're poorly cleared by the liver but more adherent to tissues in arteries and atherosclerotic plaque, and they're more potent triggers of inflammatory responses in arteries.[11] Long-lasting *glycoxidized*—glycated and oxidized—small LDL particles should be viewed as the number one culprit behind heart disease.

What triggers small LDL particles? Three things: grains, sugars, and cooked starchy legumes (in that order, from most to least responsible). Genetic predisposition also plays a role, as consumption of a standard quantity of amylopectin starch from grains can produce 1,500 nmol/L small LDL particles in one individual but 700 nmol/L in another. But the fact remains that these small LDL particles emerge from consumption of those three types of food.

Fats also play a role, but it's secondary: They increase the number of small LDL particles triggered by consumption of grains, sugars, or cooked starchy legumes. Fat consumption in the absence of these three carbohydrate sources rarely provokes formation of small LDL particles. (There are occasional genetic exceptions to this general rule.)

You can now appreciate that the common question, "Will this lifestyle change raise my cholesterol?" is too simplistic to answer effectively. Instead, the question should be, "What are the lipoprotein consequences of this lifestyle change?" These changes include:

- **Reductions in VLDL particles.** Dramatic reductions in the number of VLDL particles reflect the reduced conversion of amylopectin starches to triglycerides via reduced de novo lipogenesis in the liver (conversion of carbohydrates to triglycerides), as well as a marked reduction in after-meal (postprandial) lipoproteins that previously developed from digestion of grain amylopectins.[12] Reduced VLDL is crucial for reducing small LDL particles and small HDL particles, as well as for reducing blood sugar and allowing insulin responses to normalize, since VLDL formation is the first step in creating this array of effects.[13]

- **Reduced small LDL particles.** A typical reduction would be (in terms of a typical NMR panel) 1,800 nmol/L at the start to 200 nmol/L or even zero after grain elimination. A reduction in small LDL particles means that oxidation- and glycation-prone LDL particles that persist for extended periods are no longer present or are present at much reduced levels. A reduction in VLDL particles leads to reduced formation of small LDL particles. If grains are eliminated, there is less liver de novo lipogenesis, fewer VLDL particles are produced, and small LDL particles are reduced or eliminated—and risk for heart disease is reduced along with it.

- **Increased total HDL, increased large HDL (HDL2b), reduced small HDL (HDL2a).** The reduction in VLDL particles also results in reduced formation of the less-protective small HDL particles and an increase in the more-protective large HDL particles.

Observing the effects on VLDL and small LDL particles quickly teaches the observer some important lessons: Cutting fat in the diet exerts very little change in lipoproteins, while unrestricted carbohydrate and grain consumption causes massive disruptions, including substantial surges in VLDL particles and creation of small LDL particles. Conversely, eliminating grains and limiting sugars and cooked starchy legumes yields dramatic reductions in VLDL and small LDL particles.

Despite the limitations of the standard cholesterol panel, it does allow observation of changes that are fairly predictable and evident to the informed observer (though these changes generally underestimate the real underlying changes in lipoproteins). These changes include:

- **Reduction in triglycerides.** This effect can be dramatic, such as a drop from 600 mg/dl to 60 mg/dl. This occurs because cutting out the amylopectin of grains, as well as other sources of sugars (such as candy, soft drinks, and sugary snacks), cuts off the flow of sugars to the liver, which is no longer converting these carbohydrates to triglycerides. Reduced triglycerides also allow HDL to increase, blood sugar to drop, and insulin responses to improve.

- **Increases in HDL.** Because excess blood triglycerides lead to degradation and clearing of HDL, reduced triglycerides allow HDL to increase. Over time, this can lead to spectacular rises in HDL; a change from 39 mg/dl to 80 mg/dl would not be at all uncommon. (Personally, my HDL value rose from 27 mg/dl to 97 mg/dl, an increase of more than 300 percent.)

- **LDL cholesterol becomes moot.** Recall that LDL cholesterol is calculated using the Friedewald equation that assumes that everyone eats the same relatively high-carbohydrate and grain-rich diet and that everyone's triglyceride and HDL values fall within a narrow range. As we convert to a grain-free, limited-carbohydrate diet, the assumptions built into the Friedewald calculation are no longer valid: We no longer consume grain amylopectins that drive high triglyceride values, while triglyceride composition of VLDL and other lipoproteins is dramatically altered. Calculated LDL cholesterol was a crude and imprecise value to start with; it is essentially worthless with this lifestyle change. Accordingly, in a grain-free lifestyle, LDL cholesterol can increase, decrease, or remain unchanged, but usually has no real meaning.

- **Total cholesterol can go in either direction**. Because total cholesterol incorporates HDL (which goes up), triglycerides (which go down), and LDL cholesterol (which can do anything), you can't predict which direction your number will head in. Total cholesterol is, as a result of such mixed determinants, a worthless value. It's shocking that it's still even reported on lipid panels.

By now you can probably appreciate the very limited value and imprecise nature of cholesterol testing—imprecision that permits faulty conclusions such as "reducing saturated fat reduces cholesterol." While triglycerides and HDL on a standard cholesterol panel typically reveal dramatic improvements with this lifestyle, most physicians pay no attention to those values, choosing instead to focus on the value most flawed but most treated by the drug industry, calculated LDL cholesterol.

The way to solve this problem is to insist on a full lipoprotein analysis if your desire is true insight into your potential for cardiovascular disease. (See Appendix D for lipoprotein testing resources. They are widely available and are now widely covered by health insurance, though your doctor may not know this.) Bear in mind that you may need to find a better-informed doctor to help you interpret the results—a health-care practitioner who has invested the time and effort to pursue additional education and who, perhaps, has even come to understand the absurdly simplistic and profiteering nature of the "reduce your cholesterol" argument. The grain-free lifestyle yields dramatic improvement in lipid and lipoprotein values, but it requires a knowledgeable eye to understand the changes—not someone who only sees calculated LDL cholesterol, statin drug prescriptions, and the good-looking sales representative making promises of dinner and an all-expenses-paid trip to Orlando.

Additional Strategies to Improve Lipid and Lipoprotein Values

There are strategies beyond grain elimination that can yield additional improvements in the values recorded by lipid and lipoprotein testing. You may not be surprised to find that many of the same supplements and lifestyle changes discussed for other conditions also benefit lipid and lipoprotein profiles.

- **Restore vitamin D.** In addition to all the other wonderful effects of obtaining a favorable 25-hydroxy vitamin D blood level, restoration of this important hormone also, over many months, reduces triglycerides, raises HDL, and contributes to the reduction of small LDL particles.[14]

- **Supplement omega-3 fatty acids.** EPA and DHA from fish oil (but *not* from krill or linolenic acid sources such as flaxseed or chia) reduce both fasting and after-meal VLDL and triglycerides. The effect is dramatic, particularly when doses of 3,000 to 3,600 mg of EPA and DHA per day are used. (Note that the quantity doesn't refer to the amount of fish oil, but to the content of EPA and DHA listed on the label.)[15]

- **Normalize thyroid function.** Just as thyroid status has an impact on so many other aspects of health, it can also have major effects on lipid and lipoprotein values. Obtaining *ideal* thyroid status reduces LDL values, increases HDL, and reduces triglycerides. If achieving ideal thyroid status facilitates weight loss (which is common), the effects are even more significant.[16]

- **Feed your bowel flora.** Healthy bowel flora species, especially *Lactobacillus* and *Bifidobacteria* species, can exert substantial beneficial effects on LDL levels because these organisms participate in bile acid metabolism. Bile is released by the gallbladder to digest and emulsify fats. The bile acids are then reabsorbed through the intestine to become available to form cholesterol in the liver. *Lactobacillus* and *Bifidobacteria* species in the intestine perform a reaction called *deconjugation* that prevents bile acid reabsorption, resulting in reduced LDL values, modest increases in HDL, and reductions in triglycerides.[17] All the bowel flora strategies discussed above and in Chapter 9 (see page 190), including an initial probiotic supplement followed by long-term incorporation of prebiotic fibers and fermented foods, facilitate improvements in lipoprotein values.

- **Pursue weight loss.** Achieving an ideal weight exerts benefits above and beyond what's achieved by changes in diet, bowel flora, vitamin D, and thyroid function. Because visceral fat constantly releases fatty acids into the bloodstream, resulting in higher triglycerides, reduced HDL, higher blood sugar, higher insulin, and more inflammation, losing excess visceral fat reduces the flow of fatty acids into the bloodstream and reverses these effects.[18]

While much of the health-care world continues to dispense statin drugs after providing ineffective nutritional information, we flip this procedure: We begin with effective nutritional information, starting with elimination of grains; we then normalize multiple metabolic phenomena with the natural strategies just described. Only *after* adopting such natural and benign strategies should we even begin to ask whether drugs like statin agents are appropriate. In my experience, the majority of people who follow the simple strategies above obtain *superior* results, and thereby reduced cardiovascular risk beyond what is possible with drugs alone.

RED HOT: INFLAMMATION

Inflammation is the term used to describe the hundreds of responses designed to deal with bacteria, viruses, and other invaders, and to eradicate errant cells that could initiate the cancer process. It also describes situations in which there is an influx of inflammatory white blood cells; redness, swelling, and pain in the knees or wrists; itchy redness in the skin; or impaired "surveillance" of cancer cells before they have a chance to proliferate and spread. Inflammation is therefore *normal* to a degree, but not when it serves to incite abnormal health conditions.

Most modern people are boiling pots of inflammation: hot, steaming, churning cauldrons of disordered, chaotic inflammatory responses, much of them due to food choices that conform poorly to human dietary needs. Sit with people like this in an enclosed room and you can literally feel the room heat up. (I have endured countless hours of this in my office.)

Some signs of an excessively stimulated inflammatory response are:

- Increased c-reactive protein (CRP); any level above 1.0 mg/dl signals increasing levels of inflammation.

- Increased white blood cell (WBC) count; even values in the high normal range suggest an underlying inflamed state.

- Increased inappropriate sweating.

- Increased insulin or blood glucose, since inflammation blocks insulin, thereby raising blood sugar.

- Increased blood pressure, since inflammatory proteins cause constriction of arteries and other abnormal blood pressure–raising effects.

- Swelling, pain, or redness of any area of the skin, muscles, joints, or respiratory or gastrointestinal tract.

- An autoimmune process in any organ.

A complex web of intertwined inflammatory proteins is also involved, including tumor necrosis factor, various interleukins, and dozens, if not hundreds, of others. Given our present knowledge, it is impossible to measure and individually manage all of them.

Funny thing: If one marker in this complex web is activated to abnormally high levels, so are many others. For example, if interleukin-6 is increased, CRP is also increased, along with other interleukins, tumor necrosis factor, mitogen-activated protein kinase, nuclear factor-kappa B, and various matrix metalloproteinases. The interconnected nature of inflammatory responses acts as if an inflammatory skirmish in one system or body part activates the entire army.

If we tried to turn off this complex web of interconnected inflammatory responses one marker at a time, we would go crazy because of its complex and tangled nature. Thankfully, there are several strategies that exert broad inflammation-suppressing effects that reach across most, if not all, inflammatory pathways and result in reduction of many of the common markers we use for identification of inflammatory responses. Typically, people who eliminate grains and eat otherwise healthy food lose visceral fat and the excessive inflammation associated with it; witness drops in blood sugar, insulin, and blood pressure; experience relief from inflammatory rashes, joint pain, and swelling; obtain relief from inappropriate sweating; and see reductions in CRP (often to near zero even from high starting levels) and WBC counts. In other words, most of the signs of inflammation dramatically reverse with grain elimination.

To further reduce or eliminate excessive levels of inflammation, consider the same strategies suggested to facilitate correction of lipid and lipoprotein abnormalities, particularly vitamin D and bowel flora management. These are proving to be very powerful means of reducing inflammatory phenomena.[19]

Beyond those, there are two others to consider that may be helpful after all other avenues advocated in this book have been pursued.

Curcumin

The active polyphenol component of the spice turmeric, curcumin is proving to exert unexpectedly broad anti-inflammatory effects that include reduced markers such as tumor necrosis factor and nuclear factor-kappa B.[20] More than 50 clinical trials have been conducted with this food component, and more than 30 ongoing trials have been registered.

Clinical data have demonstrated promising effects of curcumin on cancer, inflammatory conditions, neurological disorders, diabetic kidney disease, and pain.[21] Effective curcumin doses have varied across a wide range, from 30 mg to 8,000 mg (8 g), though lower doses may be required when combined with piperine, which enhances absorption.

Taking up to several thousand milligrams (with piperine, preferably) per day as a nutritional supplement may augment the power of other anti-inflammatory strategies. If turmeric or curcumin is purchased as a supplement, note that the quantity of curcumin contained should be specified on the label.

You can also include turmeric spice in your foods; it's 2 to 8 percent curcumin by weight. Turmeric is in curry powder, so use that flavoring liberally. You can also use turmeric spice with garlic, onion powder, and peppers to spice up chicken, fish, cauliflower, Brussels sprouts, and other dishes.

Boswellia

As with curcumin, broad anti-inflammatory effects are being observed with the extract of frankincense, boswellia. Preliminary studies have suggested beneficial effects in the inflammatory processes involved in rheumatoid arthritis, gingivitis, inflammatory bowel diseases, and asthma.[22] Dosing regimens have not been well sorted out; typical dosing is 300 mg two or three times per day. Boswellia extracts are not easily absorbed, but absorption can be substantially magnified when it's taken along with a high-fat meal.[23]

"I'VE FALLEN AND I CAN'T GET UP!": OSTEOPOROSIS AND OSTEOPENIA

Perhaps nothing better portrays the helplessness and disability of osteoporosis and osteopenia (a milder degree of bone weakening than osteoporosis) than those commercials of elderly people who fall and are unable to obtain help. Given the bone-eroding effects of grains, falling is no longer the plight of elderly alone—middle-aged and even younger people are at risk. Because the technology to measure bone density, and thereby long-term potential for osteoporotic fractures, is now widely available, many people have been diagnosed with reduced levels of bone density, and most of them are offered prescription drugs to remedy the situation.

Almost as a rule, people with celiac disease develop osteoporosis or osteopenia during grain-consuming years. Removal of all gluten leads to improvement in the majority, though most people do not achieve normal bone density again and many are left with mild degrees of osteopenia or osteoporosis that increase the potential for hip and other fractures.[24] Following a gluten-free diet is therefore insufficient to correct reduced bone density in people with celiac disease.

Even outside of celiac disease, osteoporosis and osteopenia are common, accounting for two million fractures of the wrist, spine, hip, and pelvis in 2005 alone.[25] The process of progressive bone weakening gets its start at age 25 in women and age 40 in men.[26] Bone weakening is worsened by chronic consumption of grains, inadequate intake of green vegetables, carbonated soft drinks, hormonal changes accompanying menopause, and years of acid-base status disrupted by grains (chronic low-grade acidosis).[27] It is a common occurrence, particularly in postmenopausal women, and men are by no means spared from this issue, as they account for 29 percent of all osteoporotic fractures. While osteoporosis and osteopenia are often regarded as "just" bone diseases or deficiencies of calcium, like many other conditions, they represent the long-term result of metabolic distortions largely due to diet and other factors.

Given the widespread and chronic nature of osteopenia and osteoporosis and their long-term risk for fractures, it is no surprise that the pharmaceutical industry has gotten on board. Their business objective is to develop agents to treat chronic diseases of lifestyle, not acute illness, because lifestyle issues allow them to sell their drugs for years, not just a few days or weeks. This means that the average physician views osteopenia, osteoporosis, and long-term potential for hip fractures as situations that require drugs. And when it comes to osteoporosis and osteopenia, most physicians also pooh-pooh the value of diet and nutritional supplements other than calcium.

This is emblematic of the misdirected focus in health care. Why are doctors prescribing drugs, and even procedures, when nutritional or other natural strategies can be as or even more effective? Part of the explanation is that, when nutritional agents such as vitamins D or K_2 have been individually compared to osteoporosis drugs over comparable timelines, the nutritional agents have been shown to be effective, but not as powerful in reversing bone thinning as the drugs are. Physicians therefore interpret this to mean that drugs are preferred as first-line agents in treatment. What they fail to acknowledge is that when we can use benign, safe nutritional agents over many years to prevent, as well as reverse, osteoporosis and osteopenia, natural self-administered methods are preferable. They can be effective, and they lack the costs, side effects, and uncertain long-term potential of drugs. In addition, when used in combination, nutrients such as vitamins D and K_2 demonstrate increased effectiveness, often proving comparable to prescription drugs and sometimes even proving effective when the drugs have been unsuccessful.[28]

If you've been diagnosed with osteoporosis or osteopenia, or have had an incomplete bone density response to gluten elimination, or if you simply wish to prevent such bone health issues in your future, here are the steps to consider after eliminating the bone-destroying effects of grains.

Vitamin D: The Make-It-or-Break-It Factor

If there is one factor that has the potential to make or break a bone health program, it is vitamin D. Vitamin D is the master control over calcium metabolism and bone health. Correcting vitamin D deficiency holds considerable power for restoring normal bone density.

Humans were meant to obtain vitamin D from sun exposure and the modest quantities provided by seafood, shellfish, organs of land animals (especially their livers), egg yolks, and mushrooms. The problem is, in modern life we wear heavy clothes much of the year, work indoors even during sunny weather, and avoid foods like egg yolks and liver while only occasionally eating seafood. In addition, we lose the ability to activate vitamin D in our skin as we age; by age 40, most people have lost much of this ability and fail to achieve optimal levels even with a dark Florida tan.

Conventional "wisdom" includes advice for calcium supplementation. This outdated advice fails to incorporate more recent observations demonstrating that the intestinal absorption of calcium is doubled or quadrupled if vitamin D deficiency is corrected.[29] Cut out grains, especially gluten-containing forms, and urinary calcium loss is also substantially reduced.[30] This suggests that calcium intake never was the limiting factor in bone health; vitamin D deficiency and grain consumption were.

Unfortunately, the clinical trials examining the effect of combining vitamin D and calcium have used low doses of vitamin D—far below what's required to fully restore blood levels to ideal ranges. Most studies have thereby failed to demonstrate a reduction in hip fractures or increased bone density. Though commonly prescribed, the typical dose of 400 international units (IU) of vitamin D and 1,000 mg of calcium has been shown to have no effect on reducing hip fractures.[31] The best data we have comes from a recent exhaustive meta-analysis of more than 31,000 individuals. It showed a 30 percent reduction in hip fractures and a 14 percent reduction in other fractures with higher doses of vitamin D, in the 800 to 2,000 IU per day range; calcium appeared to play no role.[32]

Maximum suppression of bone reabsorption (which leads to osteoporosis) occurs when 25-hydroxy vitamin D levels are raised to 40 ng/ml, or perhaps even 60 to 70 ng/ml.[33] Based on such observations and the fact that young people who enjoy sun exposure naturally develop blood levels of 70 to 84 ng/ml or higher without adverse effect,[34] I advise patients to take 4,000 to 8,000 IU per day of oil-based vitamin D_3 (usually in gelcap form, for assured absorption); this dose is sufficient to achieve a blood level of 60 to 70 ng/ml. Ideally, blood levels should be reassessed every 6 to 12 months to ensure that you're still within the target range.

Is There Any Role for Calcium?

The proven importance of vitamin D has shown that taking calcium to improve bone health may be boneheaded. New data demonstrate that intestinal calcium absorption is increased when vitamin D is restored to healthy levels and urinary calcium losses decrease with grain elimination. Increased grain consumption causes a 63 percent increase in calcium loss through the urine (called calciuria).[35] Elimination of grains thereby decreases urinary calcium loss, while vitamin D enhances intestinal calcium absorption—a powerful net positive effect on calcium status *without* calcium supplementation.

While millions of women have been advised to supplement calcium for bone health, this may not be a benign practice. Several analyses have suggested increased heart attack and death from calcium supplementation, particularly with intakes of 600 mg or more per day.[36] It is not even clear that *any* amount of calcium supplementation is beneficial.

It has become increasingly clear that (1) calcium is either barely effective or ineffective at increasing bone density and reducing risk for osteoporotic fracture; (2) calcium probably increases risk for cardiovascular disease; and (3) calcium is normalized simply with grain elimination, vitamin D restoration, and eating healthy foods such as vegetables. Calcium supplementation is not only ineffective, it is potentially dangerous.[37]

In my view, calcium supplementation should not figure into your approach to bone health. Instead, rely on vitamin D supplementation and a healthy diet that reduces calcium losses and provides calcium from foods.

Vitamins K_1 and K_2: A Whole New Kan of Worms

The K vitamins, traditionally thought of as doing nothing more than assisting in the normal process of blood clotting, also play crucial roles in bone health. Low intakes of K_1 and K_2 may not be something we can blame on grain consumption, but other modern dietary habits, such as inadequate quantities of green vegetables in the diet and avoiding foods such as egg yolks, liver, and full-fat dairy from pasture-fed cows, have contributed to poor status for both.

Green vegetables are the most important sources of vitamin K_1. Vegetables also provide potassium, magnesium, and other bone-healthy nutrients.[38] Kale and spinach are exceptional sources of K_1, with 1,000 to 1,200 mcg in 1 cooked cup, compared to 97 mcg in 1 cup of leaf lettuce and 32 mcg in one broccoli spear.

Inadequate intake of vitamin K_1 is associated with reduced carboxylation (adding a carboxyl group) of the bone protein osteocalcin, which is necessary for creating strength in bone. Obtaining adequate vitamin K_1 allows carboxylation to proceed, reduces bone calcium turnover, and improves bone strength. The RDA for K_1 is 90 mcg for adult women and 120 mcg for adult men; however, the RDA may not represent the ideal intake to achieve full carboxylation. In one study, dietary intake of just a bit more, 109 mcg per day of vitamin K_1, was associated with reduced osteoporotic hip fracture.[39] Reduced fractures were not accompanied by increased bone density, even with a K_1 dose as high as 5 mg per day over 2 years, suggesting an effect independent of increased calcium in bone.[40] Vitamin K_1 may also require vitamin D to fully exert its benefits.[41]

Vitamin K_2 also plays a role in bone health, perhaps an even more important one than K_1. Like K_1, K_2 is essential for carboxylation of osteocalcin.[42] Interestingly, in Japan, vitamin K_2 is used as a prescription agent to treat osteoporosis (though it's available as a nutritional supplement in the United States). Vitamin K_2, obtained either through diet or supplementation, increases bone density and decreases osteoporotic fracture risk without side effects, even at the higher doses used to treat osteoporosis in Japan (as high as 45 mg per day).[43] Adding K_2 to other prescription drugs for osteoporosis further reduces fracture rates. Vitamin K_2 in combination with vitamin D has been demonstrated to have greater synergistic effects in increasing bone density than either supplement alone, with a nearly 5 percent increase in bone density over 2 years of combined treatment. This matches or exceeds improvements accomplished with prescription drugs.[44]

Doses of the short-acting vitamin K_2 form, MK-4, as low as 1.5 mg (1,500 mcg) per day exert healthy bone effects.[45] For the longer-acting form of K_2, MK-7, 100 to 180 mcg has been show to increase bone density over 1 to 3 years.[46]

K_2 can be obtained through diet. Egg yolks, hard cheeses, beef, chicken, and organ meats are the most plentiful sources, though other meats and dairy products contain lesser quantities. And nothing tops the K content of natto, or fermented soybean, but most people find it inedible.

Bowel flora play a role in converting vitamin K_1 to K_2, but the implications of this are uncertain. It is clear that prior antibiotic use dramatically reduces liver stores of K_2.[47] My prediction: Vitamin K_2 will prove to be yet another one of those deficiencies that develops as a result of mistakenly avoiding foods rich in K_2, a deficiency made worse by distortions of bowel flora that impair conversion of K_1 to K_2. Explorations of K_2 and bowel flora are growing rapidly, so I bet we'll have our answer in the near future.

Magnesium: Mortar for the Bones

We all need magnesium, which provides structural integrity to bone and reduces levels of parathyroid hormone (PTH) that, if increased, cause calcium to be extracted from bone.[48] Widespread and common deficiencies add to osteoporosis, worsened by grain consumption and several modern trends that lead to deficiency.

The RDA for elemental magnesium is 320 mg per day for adult women and 420 mg per day for adult men. Most Americans obtain only 245 mg per day—far less than the RDA.[49]

Women who supplemented with magnesium demonstrated a 1.8 percent increase in bone density over 1 year, compared to a reduction in bone density in women not taking magnesium.[50] In a study using a combination of nutrients for bone health, 25 mg of elemental magnesium was a component of a panel of nutrients that improved bone density by 4 percent over 1 year, more than that achieved by prescription alendronate.[51]

See page 174 for dietary sources of magnesium and dosage information for supplementation. Note that if you are tracking RBC levels of magnesium, full restoration can require several years of supplementation.

Vegetables, Fruit, and the Potassium Advantage

Vegetables and fruits are a cornucopia of bone-healthy nutrients: They have vitamin K1, potassium, and magnesium, plus an alkalinizing effect that reduces formation of metabolic acids that pull calcium from bones. Phytonutrients may also exert beneficial effects.[52]

Some of the benefits of vegetables and fruits are due to their rich potassium content, so potassium supplementation with the bicarbonate or citrate (alkaline) form may provide an alternative method of ensuring sufficient quantities and reaping even more of potassium's benefits. For instance, in one study a nearly 1 percent increase in bone density was observed over 1 year with potassium citrate supplementation (but not potassium chloride, the most common prescription form of potassium), along with a reduction in urinary calcium and phosphate loss. This benefit was similar to that achieved with prescription drugs.[53]

Exercise: Gotta Build Muscle

Aging is accompanied by loss of muscle. It is not uncommon to lose 15 to 20 pounds of muscle between the ages of 20 and 70 and with it, bone density. The situation is worsened if you have experienced substantial weight loss, since muscle is inevitably lost, compounding the potential for loss of bone density, as well as impairing future weight loss potential.

Thankfully, muscle can easily be rebuilt to youthful levels. Strength training and other efforts that build or maintain muscle mass therefore play an important role in increasing bone density and reducing risk for osteoporotic fracture. This is in contrast to aerobic efforts, such as walking, biking, or swimming, which are of little to no benefit to bone health.[54] (They provide cardiovascular and metabolic benefits, but not bone benefits.) Jumping, aerobics, and other high-impact movements increase bone density, but to a lesser degree than strength training.[55]

Strength training can achieve dramatic increases in bone density—as much as 8.8 percent over 3 years.[56] Bone health is affected in both younger and older people, with results obtained in as little as 6 months and further increasing over longer periods. So dust off those old weights in the basement, join a facility with strength training equipment, or at least engage in heavy lifting or other manually stressful work, and your bone health will improve substantially.

Sex Hormones: Juju for Bones?

Along with hair, libido, and the urge to dance, a number of hormones recede with aging, and that contributes to reductions in bone density. While both men and women are affected, women experience an especially precipitous reduction in bone density during their menopausal years.

In women, restoring hormones is one way of maintaining or restoring bone density, but the benefits come with risks because of the pharmaceutical industry's reliance on nonhuman hormone preparations. Premarin, an estrogen replacement drug made from horse estrogens, increased bone density and reduced osteoporotic fractures but was accompanied by adverse effects. In the Women's Health Initiative Trial, the incidence of osteoporotic fractures was reduced by 30 percent over 7 years, but this was accompanied by increased heart attack, stroke, deep vein thrombosis, and breast cancer.[57] For these reasons, the use of nonhuman estrogen supplementation has fallen out of favor.

"Bioidentical" hormones—hormones identical to those occurring naturally in humans—have therefore been offered as a logical solution. Unfortunately, the effectiveness of bioidentical estrogens, with or without progesterone, to prevent osteoporosis has not been adequately studied, though preliminary data demonstrate that blood glucose, triglycerides, and perceived feelings of well-being are all improved with bioidentical topical creams, suggesting beneficial physiological effects.[58] Restoring progesterone levels with bioidentical hormone replacement may increase bone density by increasing the activity of osteoblast cells that build bone.[59] However, it is not clear whether progesterone administered alone effectively increases bone density or whether it must be administered along with estrogens. Nonetheless, given the other positive effects of progesterone supplementation, such as facilitation of weight loss and improved mood and sleep, bioidentical replacement may be worth considering for any woman interested in maximizing bone health.

Bone health in men may improve with testosterone replacement. In men with low testosterone levels, testosterone replacement increases bone density in as little as 6 months.[60] Likewise, 25 to 50 mg per day of the adrenal testosterone-like hormone dehydroepiandrosterone, or DHEA, increases bone density in the lumbar spine by as much as 2.5 percent over 1 to 2 years in both men and women, with larger benefits in people who start with lower levels of DHEA.[61]

GRAINLESS METABOLISM: MINUS THE "-ITIS"

You likely noticed that the strategies to reverse diabetes, hypertension, "high cholesterol," and osteoporosis are largely the same, overlapping in many, if not most, ways. The same is true of other metabolic distortions that can lead to cancer, colitis, prostatitis, pancreatitis, hepatitis, cholecystitis, thyroiditis, dermatitis, and the multitude of other forms of "-itis" that afflict humans. This is because distortions of metabolism and inflammatory phenomena are almost never confined to one rash, joint, or inch of intestine, but are body-wide issues and must be remedied that way.

CHAPTER 11

THE ANNOYED THYROID: BOOBY TRAP FOR WEIGHT AND HEALTH

You are no bigger than the things that annoy you.
—Jerry Bundsen

THE THYROID, SITTING quietly and unnoticed on the front of the neck, day in and day out, would very much like to do its job: silently turn out quantities of thyroid hormone sufficient to sustain the metabolic rate of the body. But modern influences in our lives disrupt such simple ambitions. Disruption of the thyroid is so common and carries such enormous implications for health and weight that it gets an entire chapter of its own. It is, for example, among the most common reasons that weight-loss efforts fail despite valiant attempts at diet and exercise.

While it may seem that such an extended treatment of the topic is more than is necessary, I can reassure you that when you come to understand the issues surrounding thyroid health, you can address the solutions more confidently. And if you're thinking that this chapter may not apply to you, remember that even if you don't have a thyroid condition now, thyroid dysfunction is becoming part of the lives of many people; it will be useful to recognize what it looks and feels like should you develop the condition in the future. If you don't educate yourself, you risk exposing yourself to the neglect or indifference common in health care today—dismissals that can go on for years before the condition is recognized. Get your thyroid issues tackled properly, and you have accomplished yet another big step toward total health.

GO FOR THE THROAT

The thyroid gland is like the ultra control freak at work who pays attention to every aspect of everyone's behavior and responds with over-the-top ranting and raving if something is just a teensy weensy bit off. The thyroid performs the crucial function of modulating metabolic rate. It fine-tunes the function of virtually every tissue in the body, from the lowly cells responsible for creating fingernails to the nerve cells in the brain that guide memory and thought.

The world has changed. Few people write letters with pen and paper, affix a stamp to an envelope, and then wait a couple of weeks for a reply. Likewise, the world surrounding our endocrine glands has become unrecognizable. From the perspective of thyroid health, we have been living in a world increasingly contaminated by thousands of industrial chemicals. Many of these compounds get into the human body and have the peculiar capacity to disrupt the function of endocrine glands. Endocrine gland functions are complex, interconnected webs that are normally under tight control. But the same complexity and interconnectedness that make the human body such a splendid and highly adapted organism are also a vulnerability in a modern life filled with chemicals that disrupt the delicate workings of this system. This is a situation never before encountered by *Homo sapiens* and unique to the modern industrialized world.

Welcome to the world of *endocrine disruption*. This new age was created by the cavalier attitudes of industry, which dismissed the hazards of thousands of chemicals introduced into the environment and our bodies. They get in through foods, herbicides and pesticides, the coatings on cooking utensils, contaminants in the water supply, flame retardants on carpeting and clothing, and plastics that are everywhere and in everything, from cars to the lining of canned foods to water bottles. They are even in the rainwater and air. Nobody—and I truly mean *nobody*—alive today has avoided exposure to these ubiquitous chemicals. The Environmental Working Group tested blood from the umbilical cords of newborns and uncovered 287 different industrial compounds, including mercury, 21 different pesticides, and components of industrial lubricants— this was in newborns, not 60-year-olds who had worked a lifetime in factories or other contaminated environments.[1] Endocrine disruptive industrial chemicals can be detected in hair, urine, blood, liver, kidneys, and just about any other bodily fluid or organ. One recent study assessed individuals for the presence of perchlorates, a residue of synthetic fertilizers. Of 2,800 people tested, all 2,800 had detectable levels of perchlorates in their bodies.[2] You've heard that saying about death and taxes? Well, add industrial chemical exposure to the list of things unavoidable during life. (I will discuss this further in Chapter 12.)

Marginal or mild thyroid dysfunction, in particular, is among the most common forms of endocrine disruption. (Neuroendocrine, adrenal, ovarian, and testicular disruptions are other common forms.) It is also the one that has the greatest relevance in the grain-free experience, as even marginal degrees of thyroid dysfunction—which are very common—can impair capacity for weight loss. Thyroid issues can also block your return to total health, since impaired thyroid function disrupts other physiologic phenomena, leading to higher levels of LDL cholesterol, higher triglycerides, higher blood pressure, high blood sugar, low energy, disrupted bowel health, and water retention. Correction of even subtle degrees of thyroid dysfunction can help aim you in the direction of full control over your health. It can also make you feel happier and be more energetic, as well as help you fit into that size 4 dress you've been eyeing.

Unfortunately, there is no "detox" program that has been shown to reduce perchlorates or polychlorinated biphenyls from the thyroid gland or remove perfluorooctanoic acid residue from the adrenals. You can't unwind the effects of fungicides like vinclozolin just by taking some purging supplement or submitting to four enemas per day. While there are lots of discussions about the health benefits of "detoxification" programs that may indeed have merit, none have been shown to undo or protect us from endocrine disruptive effects.

Because we cannot undo such effects, we have to deal with the downstream endocrine consequences. It may not be the perfect system, but it's the best we've got.

The Grain-Fried Thyroid

Too many people who are hoping to sprint through life are kept hobbling and limping, slowed by a thyroid gland that has been beaten, battered, and deep-fried by the forces set on disrupting it. Those who follow the advice to consume more "healthy whole grains" may unmask the potential for autoimmune thyroid disease if they are genetically susceptible. Imagine giving the general public advice to drink as much alcohol as you want, ignoring the development of alcoholism in a genetically predisposed minority: It would be unthinkable. But it seems that nothing is beyond the scope of ill-conceived advice in the world of grains.

By removing grains, you remove a great disrupter of endocrine gland function. Removing grains removes the prolamin proteins responsible for triggering the first step in autoimmunity: self-targeting of the immune system that can inflame and damage the thyroid and other glands. Going grain-free removes lectin proteins that also exert inflammatory effects on the thyroid.[3] The autoimmune thyroid diseases Hashimoto's thyroiditis and Graves' disease can start with the bagels, pretzels, or rye bread that you thought were harmless to eat. Antibodies aimed against the prolamin proteins in wheat, rye, and barley have been identified in more than 50 percent of people with Hashimoto's thyroiditis, the most common cause of hypothyroidism.[4] Yes, autoimmune thyroid disease is largely a disease of grain consumption, so removing grains is step one in regaining control over thyroid health.

Although the prolamin proteins in wheat, rye, and barley are triggers of autoimmune thyroid inflammation, it is uncommon to experience improved thyroid function with their elimination, as the thyroid is not very effective at recovery after enduring an inflammatory beating. Efforts to monitor thyroid function are therefore recommended, especially if you are taking thyroid hormone replacements, such as levothyroxine or Armour thyroid.

THYROID HEALTH: "NORMAL" MAY NOT BE NORMAL

After grain elimination, the next step in regaining thyroid health is to assess thyroid status. You allow your thyroid gland to heave a sigh of relief after you cease the beating it has been taking from grains, and like a victim pulled out of the pummeling he was receiving, your thyroid may or may not be left unscathed.

Hypothyroidism, or deficiency of active thyroid hormones, is the most common situation that persists after removing grains. It's been known for decades that when hypothyroidism is severe, signs of it are obvious and allow even heart failure and death to occur. More recently, we've recognized that even mild degrees of hypothyroidism can contribute to poor health—even degrees typically regarded as "normal" as assessed by thyroid blood tests. Mild hypothyroidism is also proving to be far more common than was previously suspected. Because it is less dramatic, mild degrees of hypothyroidism can go undetected for years. Stories of struggling with weight, low energy, hair loss, depression, unexplained constipation, escalating cholesterol values, high blood pressure, etc., are often dismissed as just "getting old" or the consequences of laziness and gluttony. Subtle degrees of hypothyroidism can be tricky (though by no means impossible) to diagnose. Add to this the debate within the medical community over the boundary between normal and abnormally low thyroid function, and many people endure varying degrees of hypothyroidism for many years, culminating in substantial health problems.

Before we get to *how* to gain control over thyroid health, let's first talk more about the forms of thyroid dysfunction and why they develop.

It's Your Thyroid Gland Talking

Knowledge is power, particularly when it comes to recognizing when the thyroid gland is not operating properly. Understanding the language of the thyroid will also empower you in discussions with your health-care provider. If you can discuss thyroid issues knowledgeably, you will be more likely to be taken seriously in a world in which thyroid dysfunction is typically overlooked, minimized, or dismissed. It's tough to ignore someone who says, "I am convinced that my free T3 level is low because I have persistent hypothyroid symptoms despite taking levothyroxine. Perhaps I'm suffering a form of endocrine disruption. I believe my free T3 level should be assessed." Only the most negligent practitioner or control freak could ignore such a plea.

Though it bridges the trachea and is located just beneath the surface of your skin, you should not be able to feel a normal thyroid. An enlarged thyroid gland can be felt, however, and signals that something is wrong.

T4, the relatively inactive form of thyroid hormone, accounts for 80 percent of the hormones produced by this gland. It is converted to the active form, T3, via the action of deiodinase enzymes throughout the body that remove—deiodinate—one iodine atom. (The 4 and 3 refer to the number of iodine atoms per thyroid hormone molecule.) T4, which persists in the blood for several days, acts as a reservoir, providing the body with a continual supply of the much shorter-lived T3. T3 controls metabolic rate at the cellular level by modulating the rate of energy consumption in virtually every tissue in the body. The thyroid produces only small amounts of T3 (15 to 20 percent of body requirements), relying mostly on conversion of T4 to T3 in various organs (primarily the liver and kidneys). T3 is a particularly powerful hormone, such that the body requires only one trillionth of a gram per liter of blood to function properly.

Conversion of T4 to T3 is therefore a crucial step in determining thyroid status, and it's a step that can be disrupted by factors that block the 5'-deiodinase enzyme. Critical point: Many industrial compounds block this step. Examples include polychlorinated biphenyls (PCBs, used in thousands of industrial processes and products, including electronics), polybrominated diphenyl ethers (PBDEs, used in flame retardants, polyurethane, and textiles), triclosan (used in antibacterial soaps, hand lotions, clothing, kitchenware, and toys), and "Red Dye #3" (erythrosine), a common food coloring.[5] This is only a partial list, which means that all of us, without exception, have been exposed to chemicals that block the conversion of T4 to T3. If you breathe, drink water, eat food, walk on carpeting, wash your hands, or have watched at least one episode of *Walking Dead*, you have been exposed to compounds that block deiodination.

Many new insights into health are obtained by bridging disciplines that often fail to talk to one another and share findings. For instance, some of the most important insights into the effects wheat and grains have on human health originated with insights obtained by talking to agricultural scientists. But physicians rarely ever speak to agricultural scientists, and vice versa. In the world of thyroid health, endocrinologists rarely speak to toxicologists or toxicologists to endocrinologists. This means that, in a world in which awareness of endocrine disruptive chemicals is mandatory, most endocrinologists have *no* understanding of this area of health. That leads them to dismiss many of the abnormal health phenomena caused by endocrine disruption as inconsequential, or to fail to recognize them. They don't recognize that blocked conversion of T4 to T3 can be caused by household compounds like the triclosan in hand soap. This lack of knowledge leads to statements such as, "I don't know why you're so cold all the time, depressed, and can't lose weight. Why don't you take an antidepressant?" Failure to recognize this as a blatant example of endocrine disruption occurs because there has been little to no cross-discipline discussion.

The deiodination process also has the potential to create what is known as reverse T3 (rT3), which is structurally similar to T3 except that the iodine molecule is removed from a different location. The two hormones are indistinguishable on most diagnostic tests, but rT3 binds to the same tissue receptor sites as T3, thereby blocking the action of "real" T3. While rT3 can be directly measured, it often is not, which means doctors fail to identify a cause for hypothyroidism symptoms that's not apparent from the usual tests.

T3 and T4 hormones are only active when not bound to blood proteins and in their free forms. Reflecting their impressive potency, less than 1 percent of all T3 and T4 are present in their free state, and it's that form that we are most interested in. For this reason, when we assess thyroid hormone status, among the important tests we run are free T3 and free T4.

The thyroid gland is under the control of the pituitary gland in the brain; the pituitary, in turn, is under the control of the hypothalamus. The pituitary produces thyroid-stimulating hormone (TSH) to stimulate production of T4 and T3. If tissue levels of T4 and T3 are low, the pituitary responds by increasing TSH; consequently, the higher the TSH level, the greater the degree of hypothyroidism. The TSH level is therefore the most common blood test used to diagnose hypothyroidism. The level of TSH that should be regarded as "abnormal" has been debated for years, dropping from 10 mIU/ml, to 7.5, to 5.5, to 4.5. Most recently, the American Thyroid Association (ATA) asked whether 2.5 mIU/ml or lower should become the new target.[6]

Despite its considerable shortcomings, TSH remains the primary method of confirming that symptoms may be attributable to hypothyroidism. The standard (though disputed) TSH ranges from the ATA are listed below.

0.0–0.4 mIU/ml	Hyperthyroidism
0.4–2.5 mIU/ml	Normal range
2.5–4.0 mIU/ml	At risk; repeat TSH test at least once a year
4.0–10.0 mIU/ml	Subclinical (mild) hypothyroidism
Above 10.0 mIU/ml	Hypothyroidism

This categorization tends to underestimate the impact of rising levels of TSH. New studies, such as the 25,000-participant Norwegian HUNT Study, suggest that an ideal TSH level may be as low as 1.5 mIU/ml or less (judging by coronary heart disease mortality, an association most powerful in women).[7] In my experience, genuine, total health only occurs when TSH levels are in this low range of 1.5 mIU/ml or less.

One major problem with diagnosing and treating a thyroid issue is that endocrine disruption can also affect the hypothalamus and pituitary, not just the thyroid gland itself. Many of the same industrial compounds that block conversion of T4 to T3 also block the hypothalamus and pituitary. PCBs, perchlorates, pesticides, PBDEs, and bisphenol A (BPA) are among the dozens of compounds that have demonstrated effects in impairing thyroid function via hypothalamic or pituitary gland disruption. These effects can even be exerted on a fetus in utero and persist into childhood and adult life.[8] This raises another fundamental problem that challenges the conventional notions of diagnosing thyroid dysfunction: Thyroid status that is disrupted at the hypothalamic or pituitary level cannot be diagnosed with the usual screening methods because in these cases the TSH level (normally the only lab test used to assess thyroid function) is typically normal—even if substantial hypothyroidism is present. In practical terms, this means that a woman with years of progressive weight gain, depression, water retention or edema, hypertension, thinning hair, disrupted bowel function, peculiar rashes, and a host of other health issues will go undiagnosed for years, life and health impaired due to inadvertent exposure to plastics, flame retardants, or hand cleaners—all while being advised that her thyroid function is fine.

The failure of the endocrine community to fully integrate the issues unique to this new age of endocrine disruption is among the most important health issues of our time. But don't expect John Q. Endocrinologist to have even an inkling of what you are talking about if you raise such questions.

Hypothyroidism: Life in the Slow Lane

Disorders of the thyroid can be broken down into two general categories: hypothyroidism (underactive thyroid) and hyperthyroidism (overactive thyroid). Hypothyroidism is far more common and more insidious, often evading diagnosis for years. Because hypothyroidism is, by a long stretch, the most common form of thyroid dysfunction, we will confine our discussion to this condition.

Hypothyroidism is a condition in which the thyroid produces inadequate amounts of the thyroid hormones T4 and T3, resulting in a slowed metabolic rate no matter how meticulous or careful your diet, no matter how vigorous your exercise program. Hypothyroidism, even of a mild or subtle degree, can thereby completely impair a weight-loss effort and can even result in weight gain, despite your best efforts. But the consequences of hypothyroidism don't end at impaired weight loss. Hypothyroidism can have serious long-term consequences, including an increased number of LDL particles, high triglycerides, higher blood pressure (particularly diastolic hypertension), and increased risk for heart disease and heart attack, carpal tunnel, and depression.[9]

People diagnosed with Hashimoto's thyroiditis or Graves' disease, both of which can be initially triggered by the autoimmunity activated by grains, can be left with hypothyroidism due to injury incurred during the inflammatory flare. That means that the injured thyroid gland is no longer capable of producing sufficient thyroid hormone to suit your body's needs. Iodine deficiency (discussed below) is another cause for hypothyroidism, as is endocrine disruption from exposure to industrial chemicals.

Hypothyroidism usually shows itself through one or more symptoms, including:

- Reduced energy, fatigue, increased need for sleep
- Inappropriately cold hands and feet, reduced or absent sweating

- Dry, itchy skin

- Dry, brittle hair; hair loss or thinning hair

- Difficulty losing weight or weight gain

- Short-term memory impairment, slowed thinking

- "Pins and needles" in hands and feet

- Constipation

- Puffiness around eyes, edema of hands or ankles

- Carpal tunnel

- Heavier or more frequent menstrual periods, worse cramps, worse premenstrual symptoms

- Depression

- Goiter (enlargement of the thyroid)

- Higher diastolic blood pressure (the bottom value)

- Iron deficiency anemia, low ferritin (iron storage protein measured as a blood test)

Diagnosing hypothyroidism by symptoms alone can be tricky, as many of the symptoms are not specific to hypothyroidism or may be vague (though the presence of inappropriately cold hands and feet and impaired weight loss are two very reliable signs). Because symptoms are not absolutely specific to hypothyroidism, blood tests are useful when making a diagnosis. And symptoms do not have to be present: For unclear reasons, some people have no symptoms despite mild to moderate degrees of hypothyroidism.

The frequency of hypothyroidism increases with age, and though estimates vary due to differing cutoffs for "normal" TSH, most cite a range of 2 to 4 percent of people developing it early in life and as many as 15 to 20 percent developing it later in life, with greater prevalence in women.[10] However, with more strict criteria, the percentage of people with more subtle degrees of hypothyroidism is likely 25 to 30 percent, which makes it not at all uncommon. This means that as many as 25 to 30 percent of people who follow a nutritional program perfectly will fail at weight loss because of hypothyroidism. Aging also plays a role: One study demonstrated that the increase in TSH with low thyroid function is 75 percent less compared to younger people, making TSH an increasingly unreliable index of thyroid function as we age.[11]

Beyond TSH, other commonly used laboratory tests to gauge thyroid function include free T4 and free T3. Reference ranges for free T4 and T3 should be provided by the testing laboratory, with ideal ranges generally falling in the upper half of the reference range. Low free T3 is another common signifier of hypothyroidism. T4 can also be low, but this is uncommon. There are a number of other thyroid tests, such as T4 uptake and T3 uptake, that have been replaced by direct measurement of free T4 and free T3; they are outdated and should therefore not be used.

Autoimmune thyroid inflammation, which can be responsible for both hypo- and hyperthyroidism, can be identified by measuring antibodies against the thyroid components thyroid peroxidase antibody (TPOAb) and thyroglobulin antibody (TgAb). Approximately 90 percent of people with Hashimoto's thyroiditis will test positive for elevated TPO antibodies, and approximately 60 percent of Hashimoto's thyroiditis sufferers will test positive for elevated thyroglobulin antibodies.[12] Testing positive for *both* TPO and thyroglobulin antibodies increases the likelihood of Hashimoto's thyroiditis to 95 percent.[13] More than half of people with Hashimoto's thyroiditis also test positive for antibodies against the gliadin protein of wheat. It is helpful to obtain the above antibody tests as, if elevated, they can suggest that ongoing thyroid inflammation is present and that thyroid status may change after the removal of wheat, rye, and barley. This means that periodic reassessment will be necessary to gauge any shifting thyroid replacement needs.

The diagnosis of hypothyroidism can be especially troublesome when exploring mild or borderline degrees of underactive thyroid function. As you can appreciate, being diagnosed with hypothyroidism can depend on the opinions and judgment of the health-care practitioner who is conducting the evaluation. The following practical guidelines are worth understanding to help you obtain reliable and useful information about your thyroid status.

- Symptoms, especially inappropriately cold hands and feet, low energy not attributable to other causes (such as sleep deprivation), and impaired capacity for weight loss despite the dietary guidelines provided here, are fairly reliable signs of hypothyroidism, or at least sufficient to justify assessment. They are not foolproof, but they should be regarded as hypothyroid symptoms until proven otherwise.

- The higher the TSH, the more likely hypothyroidism is present. A TSH of 5 mIU/ml, for instance, is virtually guaranteed to represent hypothyroidism. A TSH of 2.5 mIU/ml probably represents hypothyroidism, especially if symptoms such as inappropriately cold hands and feet, low energy, and impaired weight loss are present. TSH values of 1.5 mIU/ml and below are much less commonly associated with hypothyroidism, though they can be if there is endocrine disruption or dysfunction at the hypothalamic or pituitary level or impaired conversion of T4 to T3.

- The combination of a somewhat high TSH and low free T4 is suggestive of iodine deficiency. For example, a TSH of 3.5 mIU/ml and a free T4 near the bottom or below the quoted reference range nearly always improves with iodine supplementation (see below). Correction can require several months of iodine supplementation. If a goiter (enlarged thyroid gland) is present, both the goiter and the TSH and free T4 values nearly always improve or completely normalize with iodine.

- Free T3 in the bottom half of or below the reference range (regardless of TSH levels) can suggest 5'-deiodinase impairment from exposure to industrial chemicals that block this enzyme. However, note that ongoing active or recent (within the previous several weeks) weight loss can transiently cause a low free T3 value and even a modest increase in TSH. If these levels are due to weight loss, they will correct themselves within a few weeks. Also, chronic low free T3 should not be confused with something called *low T3 syndrome*, in which free T3 levels are low during an acute illness, such as pneumonia, sepsis, cancer, or a heart attack. T3 replacement in this situation is unnecessary and may be detrimental. The low T3 level of low T3 syndrome corrects itself with resolution of the acute condition.[14] However, this unrelated situation is the source of reluctance on the part of some physicians to replace T3 in chronic situations. (See page 257 for more discussion on low T3.)

Another useful do-it-yourself-at-home tool to assess and track thyroid status is to take your oral temperature immediately upon arising. Normal oral temperature is 97.3°F. Temperatures consistently below this suggest hypothyroidism. (See "Thyroid Health: Check Your Thermostat" on page 254.)

When diagnosing hypothyroidism, judgment and experience on the part of your health-care practitioner are priceless. Insist on full explanations for your symptoms, not dismissals such as "You're just getting older" or "Your thyroid is fine." Demand a full discussion of the rationale (or lack of) for your diagnosis. If you are convinced that you have hypothyroidism but your health-care practitioner refuses to evaluate or to correct it (which is, unfortunately, common), then find someone who will. The champions in this area are functional medicine practitioners, naturopaths, and open-minded medical physicians—but rarely endocrinologists.

IODINE: WATER TO A THIRSTY DOG

Just as a dog, hot and panting from an afternoon of playing outdoors, will lustily lap up water, so your thyroid takes up iodine, which is essential for its function. Iodine is necessary for health. It is the primordial antibacterial, essential for single-celled organisms on up. Without it, life ceases. Don't let anyone tell you that iodine is not important; it is crucial. Simply meeting the Recommended Daily Allowance (RDA) of 150 mcg per day ensures that you won't develop a goiter (an enlarged thyroid from lack of iodine, felt as fullness on the front of the neck). However, a greater intake may be required for ideal thyroid function and total health. (See Chapter 6 for information on how and why iodine deficiency develops, especially in the modern age.)

If symptoms of hypothyroidism are present, such as inappropriately cold hands and feet or failed weight loss after grain and sugar elimination, iodine deficiency should be near the top of the list of potential causes. Recall that, on a basic thyroid panel, free T4 at the low end or below the reference range, along with a TSH of 2.5 to 3.5 mIU/ml or slightly higher, suggests iodine deficiency. If there is any indication of iodine deficiency or hypothyroidism, most people benefit by increasing iodine intake to the 500 to 1,000 microgram (*not* milligram) per day range, preferably from an iodine supplement such as kelp tablets. That's the form that approximates the natural, ocean-derived source and which can accelerate recovery of thyroid function if the underlying cause is iodine deficiency. Iodine is also available from health food stores as potassium iodide drops, capsules, and tablets. Also note that there may be a mild increase in TSH for several months after iodine is initiated, but it drifts back down over time.[15]

If hypothyroidism or a goiter is present, iodine intake should be determined and thyroid status monitored by your health-care provider. Rarely, someone with hypothyroidism or goiter will develop an abnormal thyroid response to iodine. This occurs because of iodine deficiency or other factors present *before* correction that can lead to the formation of abnormal nodules of tissue in the thyroid. Adding iodine can actually unmask the presence of abnormal thyroid nodules or another condition and result in hyperthyroid symptoms, such as nervousness, sleeplessness, and heart palpitations. Stopping the iodine reverses these effects but should prompt further evaluation of the thyroid.

Iodine replacement is therefore best undertaken alongside monitoring of thyroid function by your health-care provider. Alternatively, some people have success by increasing the dose of iodine gradually, starting at the RDA of 150 mcg per day and building up by 50 to 100 mcg increments gradually over 6 months until the desired dose, 500 mcg per day, is achieved. Anyone with a history of Hashimoto's thyroiditis, Graves' disease, thyroid cancer, or thyroid nodules should also supplement iodine only under the supervision of a knowledgeable health-care provider.

Thyroid Health: Check Your Thermostat

The regulation of body temperature, or thermoregulation, reflects the body's capacity to maintain body temperature within a narrow range. If not for our ability to regulate our own body temperature, we'd have to bask in the sun like turtles and alligators do. Deviations from this normal range thereby suggest disruption of internal control. Measuring your oral temperature with a home thermometer can therefore be a useful tool to help assess your thyroid status. It is another measure, like blood pressure or blood sugar, that's a simple assessment you can perform on your own and track over time.

Body temperature normally fluctuates within a range. Studies conducted over the last 70 years suggest that normal oral temperatures range from 96.3°F to 99.9°F and vary predictably with the time of day.[16] This is contrary to the widely held view that a normal temperature is 98.6°F no matter what time of day—an outdated relic of 19th-century observations of human temperatures.

External environmental extremes can overwhelm temperature control, as can factors that disrupt internal control. Anyone who has experienced hypothermia from cold exposure or a fever of 104°F knows that just a few degrees of deviation in either direction is uncomfortable, and even life-threatening. Body temperature also undergoes predictable circadian variation. Over a 24-hour cycle, the highest temperature occurs at around 8:00 p.m. and the lowest at around 4:00 a.m. It is the temperature *low* that is most reflective of thyroid status, and this is best approximated by an oral temperature reading obtained immediately upon awakening.[17] Low body temperature signals hypothyroidism, while increased body temperature suggests hyperthyroidism (as well as other conditions, including ovulation in women, exercise, and fever). Any oral temperature taken immediately upon arising that's consistently less than 97.3°F is suggestive of hypothyroidism; the lower the temperature, the more likely it represents hypothyroidism. A temperature of 94.7°F, for instance, is more strongly suggestive of hypothyroidism than a temperature of 97.1°F.

Long-time adherents of this practice cling to the original notion of measuring axillary (armpit) temperatures to assess body temperature. This is outdated. Axillary temperatures are unreliable and are susceptible to variation based on external ambient temperature, the amount and composition of clothing, sweating, whether the right or left arm is used (there can be a variation of up to 2.0°F from right to left), and other factors. We are interested in tracking internal temperatures most accurately; axillary temperatures can vary by as much as 1.8° to 2.7°F within several minutes and therefore should not be used.[18]

Because nobody wants to put a thermometer in their backside first thing in the morning, we use oral temperatures to approximate internal ("core") temperatures. Taking your oral temperature is useful when identifying hypothyroidism, particularly when laboratory values are borderline or equivocal, when symptoms are unusual or atypical, or when you are considering whether you should pursue the question further with your healthcare provider or ask about blood tests. Low temperature may suggest low thyroid status even when all other measures, including TSH, are normal. Temperature can also be useful to follow trends over time, which allows you to gauge the adequacy of thyroid-correcting efforts, such as iodine supplementation or thyroid hormone replacement.

There are several lessons to keep in mind when temperatures are used to assess thyroid status.

- Oral temperatures are best used as a gauge of thyroid status alongside symptom assessment and thyroid lab tests that include TSH, free T3, free T4, and, ideally, reverse T3.

- Oral temperatures should be assessed immediately upon awakening, before getting out of bed, and before drinking water or other liquids or eating anything; alcoholic beverages should be avoided the evening prior. Temperature should not be assessed during calorie restriction, fasting, or sleep deprivation.

- If an oral temperature is taken upon awakening at 8:00 a.m., it will be higher than the true low, which for most people occurs between the hours of 3:00 a.m. and 6:00 a.m.—usually around 4:00 a.m. Waking temperatures later than 6:00 a.m. can be adjusted to the "6:00 a.m. equivalent" by subtracting 0.18°F for every hour that's passed since 6:00 a.m.

- Women of childbearing age should take oral temperatures during the first 7 days after beginning menstrual bleeding (the follicular phase), which does not show the exaggerated increase in temperature triggered by ovulation or a surge in progesterone.

THYROID REPLACEMENT IN THE AGE OF ENDOCRINE DISRUPTION

Modern life during the latter half of the 20th and early 21st century has meant that reality TV dominates our attention, social media has emerged as the social interaction of choice, and chicken nuggets are the preferred food for millions of children. Even more widely pervasive are the industrial chemicals that disrupt endocrine gland function. The thyroid gland is, for many of us, the weakest link.

Because we cannot extract or undo the effects of a lifetime of industrial chemical or grain exposure, we do what is second best: supplement thyroid hormones. Most people are happier—they experience better mood, increased energy, an improved tolerance to cold, better bowel function, thicker hair, and more successful weight loss—when both T3 and T4 are included, either as combination tablets (such as Armour thyroid or NatureThroid) or as two separate tablets of liothyronine (T3) and levothyroxine (T4).

Contrary to popular opinion in the medical establishment, synthetic T4 (levothyroxine, or Synthroid) is *not* sufficient to resolve the symptoms of hypothyroidism in a substantial proportion of people with hypothyroidism. That's because not everyone converts T4 to active T3 with equal efficiency in this new age of endocrine disruption. T3 supplementation has positive effects on the psychological symptoms of hypothyroidism, with several studies showing that well-being, mood, and cognitive function are improved; weight loss is also greater with added T3.[19] T3 supplementation tailored to symptom relief, such as relief from fatigue or inappropriate feelings of coldness, can also address the issue of reverse T3 by providing an external source of this active hormone.[20]

Replacement of T3 remains controversial, however, because of confusion surrounding low T3 syndrome (see above). T3 replacement in critically ill people with low T3 syndrome provides no benefit or results in harm.[21] But low T3 syndrome is distinct from the chronic situation of someone who is not critically ill but who is experiencing long-term hypothyroid symptoms due to low free T3. This confusion, however, has made some health-care practitioners reluctant to address T3 issues, or even adamantly opposed to prescribing it. I believe this is a serious mistake. T3 replacement for people with chronic symptoms of hypothyroidism who show low levels of free T3, high reverse T3, or persistent symptoms while on T4 replacement alone typically demonstrate wonderful reversal of all hypothyroidism phenomena with correction of T3.

It's not uncommon for someone who is prescribed only levothyroxine to struggle with depression, fail at weight loss (or gain weight), lose hair, experience constipation, have inappropriately cold hands and feet—all the symptoms of hypothyroidism—despite having a TSH value at or near the desirable range. The vast majority of these people experience complete reversal of all hypothyroid symptoms when a T3 preparation is added or levothyroxine is replaced with a T4 plus T3 combination tablet. If your doctor will not discuss this issue or refuses to conduct a deeper assessment, find a doctor who will. *This aspect of thyroid health is crucial and can be sufficient to make or break your overall health and weight-loss efforts.* Another handy way to identify an enlightened practitioner is to contact a compounding pharmacy in your area (pharmacies that mix, or "compound," special prescription preparations) and ask for the names of practitioners who prescribe compounded thyroid preparations tailored to individual needs. That level of attention is a sign of a careful and knowledgeable thyroid practitioner.

Not everybody feels better with added T3. An occasional person will develop symptoms of hyperthyroidism, such as anxiety, palpitations, or sleeplessness, whether the extra T3 is taken as one of the combined thyroid preparations or alone. This is a person who is likely to do fine on T4 alone. They are in the minority, but they do exist.

Getting your thyroid status "just right" is important. Some simple rule-of-thumb measures that suggest that thyroid status is perfect include:

- TSH of 1.5 mIU/l or less, but preferably no lower than 0.1 mIU/ml
- Both free T3 and free T4 in the upper half of the reference range
- Reverse T3 within the reference range
- Good energy, good mood, freedom from excessive and inappropriate coldness—a general feeling of well-being
- Oral temperature of at least 97.3°F immediately upon awakening

Correction of hypothyroidism that includes T3 and factors in the possibility of endocrine disruption at the pituitary or hypothalamic levels comes to the rescue of people who claim, "I stopped eating all grains and didn't lose weight. This doesn't work!" It does work, but hypothyroidism so commonly gets in the way that thyroid status must be addressed before the weight loss and other health benefits of grain elimination are able to do their work.

VITAMIN D AND THYROID INFLAMMATION: A SPECIAL RELATIONSHIP

Vitamin D deficiency has implications for thyroid health (and other auto-immune conditions) that include greater potential for inflammation, including inflammation caused by autoimmunity.[22] As many instances of thyroid dysfunction have their basis in autoimmune inflammation pro-voked by grain consumption, it would logically follow that vitamin D defi-ciency may play a role.

Indeed, that is true: People with Hashimoto's thyroiditis—the auto-immune destruction of the thyroid—have a high likelihood of vitamin D deficiency, with more than 90 percent of people having 25-hydroxy vita-min D levels of 30 ng/ml or lower.[23] (Also worth noting: Hashimoto's starts with grain consumption in more than 50 percent of sufferers.) The association also applies to children, with vitamin D deficiency detected in 73.1 percent of children with Hashimoto's thyroiditis but only 17.6 percent of children without it.[24]

This suggests that achieving favorable levels of vitamin D may help you avoid developing autoimmune thyroid inflammation. It also suggests that achieving a favorable level of vitamin D may be a crucial factor in stopping or reversing autoimmune inflammation. (See Chapter 8 for more on achieving optimal levels of this important nutrient.)

UP TO YOUR NECK

Hypothyroidism is the prototypical example of endocrine disruption in our time. Unfortunately, mainstream health-care practices allow much thyroid dysfunction to be dismissed, ignored, misdiagnosed, or mistreated, and the proliferation of endocrine disrupting grains and industrial chemicals all around us isn't even acknowledged. You've been advised to eat more "healthy whole grains" and told, "You don't need iodine," "You need an antidepressant," and "Your thyroid is just fine" as you struggled to get by, thyroid gland sputtering and backfiring.

It shouldn't be this way; you shouldn't have to be neck-deep in thyroid problems before you are taken seriously. It is therefore crucial to your overall health and the success of your weight-loss efforts that you recognize when serious consideration should be given to thyroid questions. Don't wait for more serious health conditions to develop before you press for answers.

CHAPTER 12

ENDOCRINE DISRUPTION: TROUBLE IN THE GLAND SCHEME OF THINGS

Sam, your hormones have staged a coup d'état on your brain.
—Diane Chambers, *Cheers*

THE ENDOCRINE GLANDS produce hormones. Not just sex hormones, like estrogen and testosterone, but hormones charged with regulating metabolic processes, hunger, body temperature, blood sugar, blood pressure, and growth and maturation, all the way from birth to our last breath. The effects of endocrine glands are so far-reaching that they affect virtually every facet of human health. Leave them alone and they follow a script written in our genetic code, timing and tempo masterfully orchestrated, no conscious effort required.

The thyroid gland is not the only endocrine gland that can be disrupted. Mess with these glands and their hormonal tightrope walk, and it undermines some of the most fundamental processes that define human life. In children, this can stop growth or cause organ systems to mature at different rates. It can be responsible for premature development of adult sexual characteristics at age 8 or 9. As adults, it can account for increased stimulation of breast tissue that leads to breast cancer. It can result in such wide-ranging symptoms as fatigue; depression; difficulties in regulating body temperature, blood sugar, and blood pressure; reduced libido; inappropriate hunger or thirst; and numerous other body processes that are ordinarily meant to operate automatically. Chaos, lawlessness, rioting in the streets . . . this is not Tahrir Square or Baghdad. It's the pandemonium that erupts when the endocrine system encounters something that upsets its fragile balance.

The endocrine system is open to disruption by anything nonhuman that looks vaguely like a human hormone. Many compounds, both natural and synthetic, resemble human hormones. Chlorinated pesticides and estrogen-like molecules in plastics, for example, can mimic thyroid hormone and estradiol or activate human genes in ways that are unnecessary, disruptive, and outside the usual order. Given its weblike complexity, a disruption at one point in the endocrine system ripples, or sometimes belly flops, throughout the entire system. Disruption of just one pituitary signal by a small quantity of one of these hormone impostors, for instance, can result in lower body temperature and feelings of inappropriate coldness, thinning hair, constipation, high cholesterol, high blood pressure, water retention, infertility, and fatigue by interrupting a signal to the adrenal gland, ovaries, testicles, and liver.

When it works, it is truly a grand design that operates like clockwork, quietly doing its duty. When it's disrupted, just about anything can happen. Because this topic is huge and has many implications for health, I will confine our discussion to aspects that are of special importance from the standpoint of the grain-free experience.

AIN'T GLANDS GRAND?

If the network of endocrine glands were an orchestra, the conductor would be the hypothalamus, a cashew-size collection of specialized tissues buried deep within the brain. The hypothalamus orchestrates the tempo (metabolic rate and circadian rhythms) and the tune (hunger, fatigue, sleep, sweating, or shivering), and it decides who should play when, such as the pituitary gland, thyroid, adrenals, ovaries, and testicles. Just as a conductor hears the music as his musicians play, each organ sends signals back to the hypothalamus, a back and forth interaction that allows the conductor to maintain various functions within their desired ranges.

For the orchestra to play beautiful music, both the conductor and the musicians need to do their jobs correctly, playing with proper pitch and volume at the right moment. If, say, one of the cello or trombone players is out of tune, comes in late, or loses his place, the entire production suffers. If the conductor himself flubs, the whole production comes tumbling apart. The same applies to the endocrine gland system: Dysfunction can occur at the level of the hypothalamus or the next-in-line pituitary, resulting in dysfunction of multiple different glands, as well as any individual organ.

Imagine that some people start blowing horns and banging drums chaotically, out of sync with the orchestra, ignoring the direction of the conductor. The beautiful music of the orchestra is reduced to a painful cacophony of sounds, thanks to the many disruptions to the finely balanced interconnections between rhythm and melody. You might recognize the tune, but it's hardly the same. So it goes with disruption of the endocrine system. Of course, the consequences of disrupting the endocrine system are far greater than just making bad music.

Endocrine disrupters are everywhere: They're in air, water, soil, mother's milk, hand creams, soaps, shampoos, hair conditioners, cosmetics, prescription drugs, plastic containers, tin cans, pots, pans, and food. You can try to minimize exposure, but as long as you breathe, drink water, eat food, shower, and engage in ordinary day-to-day activities, you will be exposed to endocrine disruptive chemicals to one degree or another. Many such disrupters of the endocrine system have been identified, including those listed below.

- **Plastics, plasticizers, and the compounds that elute from them:** bisphenol A (BPA), phthalates, dioxin, styrene, vinyl chloride

- **Pesticides and fungicides:** vinclozolin, chlordecone, cyfluthrin, permethrin, tetramethrin, fenthion, hexachlorobenzene, malathion, parathion, heptachlor, beta-hexachlorohexane, gamma-hexachlorohexane, p,p'-DDE, tributyltin, triphenyltin

- **Fertilizers and herbicides:** perchlorates, imazamox, glyphosate, dioxin, methoxychlor, chlorpyrifos, chlornitrofen, chlomethoxyfen, methyl bromide, atrazine

- **Industrial compounds:** polychlorinated biphenyls (PCBs), polybrominated diphenyl ethers (PBDEs), 4-methylbenzylidene camphor,

3-benzylidene camphor, benzophenone-3, benzophenone-4, isopentyl 4-methoxycinnamate, octyl methoxycinnamate, homosalate, octocrylene, benzyl salicylate, phenyl salicylate, octyl salicylate, para-aminobenzoic acid and octyl dimethyl paraaminobenzoate, dichlorostyrene, benzotriazole

- **Heavy metals:** cadmium, arsenic
- **Household products:** triclosan (hand sanitizer, antibacterial soaps), perfluorooctanoic acid (Teflon-coated cookware), dithiocarbamates (cosmetics), parabens (cosmetics)

All of the compounds listed above have been associated with endocrine disruption in clinical studies.[1] While some are used as pesticides, fungicides, or herbicides, contaminating our vegetables, fruits, and water, others come to us through common household products, such as hand sanitizers, soaps, Teflon, and cosmetics. And even if you don't spread herbicides on your lawn, your neighbors might, which means those chemicals are leaching into your soil, seeping into your groundwater, and getting carried into your house through the air. The amount of time such compounds reside in the soil or groundwater is measured in years, and sometimes even a decade or longer.[2] Likewise, some compounds, once they enter the body, stay in those tissues for years.

Grains figure prominently among the many endocrine status–disrupting factors in our world. Wheat germ agglutinin (WGA), the lectin of wheat, rye, barley, and rice, mimics the hormones insulin, insulin-like growth factor-1, leptin, and cholecystokinin (CCK), leading to weight gain, failure to suppress appetite despite meeting nutritional needs, and disrupted digestive function, as well as increased risk for cancer growth.[3] Gliadin and related prolamin proteins disrupt endocrine function indirectly. If autoimmune destruction of the thyroid (Hashimoto's thyroiditis or Graves' disease) is triggered, both hyper- and hypothyroidism can result.[4] Autoimmune destruction of insulin-producing beta cells of the pancreas triggered by gliadin and related prolamins disrupts endocrine function by killing off the capacity to produce insulin, resulting in type 1 diabetes.[5] Likewise, antibodies to the adrenal cortex, which is responsible for producing the hormones cortisol, DHEA, and aldosterone, can be triggered, causing adrenal dysfunction.[6] Grains also add to endocrine disruption by promoting the growth of visceral fat.

Remove grains, of course, and you remove an inciting cause for endocrine disruption, although hypothyroidism, diabetes, disrupted digestive function, dysbiosis, type 1 diabetes, adrenal dysfunction, and other phenomena can persist and may need to be specifically addressed. In type 1 diabetes, for instance, beta cells that have been destroyed do not grow back and a lifelong need for insulin persists. Likewise, failed recovery of response to the digestive hormone CCK may account for persistent indigestion, bloating, and dysbiosis, even though CCK-blocking lectins are no longer present.

Nonetheless, grain removal is one assured way to reduce your exposure to factors that disrupt endocrine status. Unfortunately, removing the industrial chemicals, pesticides, herbicides, and other chemicals that disrupt endocrine gland function is not as easy, given their ubiquity and their persistence once they're in the environment and the body. Is there a detoxification process that allows you to remove such industrial chemicals? The only strategies that have been demonstrated to provide such protection (and only partial protection at that) are consumption of isothiocyanates obtained from cruciferous vegetables, such as broccoli, cauliflower, kale, and Brussels sprouts, and consumption of phytoalexins from tomatoes, garlic, and beans, both of which activate liver enzymes that clear toxic chemicals. This likely provides a partial explanation for why enthusiastic consumers of vegetables experience reduced cancer incidence.[7]

Iodine can also protect us from many endocrine disruptive chemicals. If you recall the periodic table of elements from your high school chemistry class, you may remember that the next-to-last column on the right contains the halogens: iodine, bromine, chlorine, and fluorine. This means that chemicals that contain a halogen, such as polychlorinated biphenyls, perfluorooctanoic acid, and perchlorates, can be partially blocked from accessing your organs in the presence of sufficient quantities of iodine. This is especially true for the iodine-rich thyroid gland.

Let's now consider several prominent consequences of endocrine disruption.

Adrenal Disruption: Cortisol Wherewithal

Like the thyroid gland, the adrenal glands can be disrupted directly, at the hypothalamus, at the pituitary, or at any of the signaling places in between. This most commonly results in fatigue, poor sleep, and difficulty with weight loss. Because of the unique circadian cycling of adrenal cortisol release, symptoms of adrenal disruption typically occur in predictable patterns every day: every morning, every afternoon, every night.

As discussed in Chapter 5, there are several components in grains that can disrupt adrenal function. The same industrial chemicals that disrupt hypothalamic and pituitary signals to the thyroid can do the same with signals to the adrenal glands, resulting in increased or decreased release of the adrenal hormones cortisol, DHEA, and adrenaline. Because disturbances of cortisol, in particular, are common and are the most relevant to our grain-free discussion, that is what I will focus on.

Major chronic stress also plays a role in disrupting adrenal function, provoking a peculiar resistance to cortisol called *glucocorticoid resistance*. This causes reduced responsiveness to cortisol, potentially resulting in symptoms of reduced cortisol but with normal or high cortisol levels.

The most characteristic symptoms of disrupted cortisol release include low morning energy, exaggerated afternoon fatigue and sleepiness, inappropriate surges in energy at night (resulting in insomnia), depression, inability to lose weight, and, less commonly, low blood pressure, salt cravings, or light-headedness. These symptoms should prompt the question of whether adrenal dysfunction and disrupted cortisol circadian cycles are to blame. This can be investigated by creating a cortisol curve that reflects the levels of active cortisol released over the course of a day. This is readily achieved by assessing salivary cortisol levels, a simple way of indirectly tracking blood levels.[8] This simply involves obtaining a salivary cortisol test kit (see Appendix D for sources) and collecting four samples: upon awakening, at midday, at dinnertime, and at bedtime. The samples are sent to a lab and a cortisol curve is constructed. A normal curve shows the highest level upon awakening (since one of cortisol's duties is to create arousal), followed by a drop to the noon value and a plateau to dinner, then a further decline toward bedtime (which permits normal sleep).

Among the most common abnormal patterns are:

- Abnormally low morning cortisol and an abnormal surge at night, associated with low morning energy and inappropriate high nighttime energy and insomnia

- Low energy throughout the day associated with abnormally low cortisol over the entire 24 hours

- Excessively high morning levels with an abnormally precipitous drop-off, resulting in afternoon fatigue and sleepiness, typically associated with chronic stress

This evaluation is best undertaken with the assistance of a health-care provider with experience and insight into adrenal and cortisol issues, such as a functional medicine practitioner or naturopath.

The solution to your cortisol problem depends on the pattern revealed by your 24-hour cortisol curve. Very low morning cortisol, for instance, responds to supplemental (prescription) oral hydrocortisone, which restores energy. An excessive morning surge followed by a sharp afternoon drop-off responds to addressing the source of stress that initiated the process, along with a low dose of hydrocortisone in the late morning. Inappropriate nighttime surges in cortisol that disrupt sleep are among the toughest variations to address, but efforts may include taking the nutritional supplements phosphatidylserine and high-dose melatonin at bedtime.

An informed practitioner who also factors in the possibility of hypothalamic and pituitary disruption, as well as glucocorticoid resistance, can be important. This is especially true when obesity, diabetes, stress (including post-traumatic stress disorder), or depression are present, assessed with additional measures, such as the level of adrenocorticotropic hormone (ACTH) that provides a measure of pituitary function. After grain elimination, solutions will often include addressing the major stressors that cause or worsen adrenal dysfunction, such as inadequate sleep, unhappy relationships, or unrewarding work.

In short, adrenal dysfunction and cortisol circadian disruptions are somewhat complex issues for which there is no one-size-fits-all solution. But, if they're addressed properly by an informed health-care practitioner, you will be rewarded with additional improvements, such as better energy and mood, improved sleep, and weight loss, even after grains and endocrine disruptive chemicals have done a major hatchet job on your health.

SEX EDUCATION: TESTOSTERONE, PROGESTERONE, AND DHEA

We've discussed how grain consumption, as well as the excess visceral fat that develops from grain consumption, are sex offenders who disrupt sex hormone status. Women develop high estrogen and prolactin, as well as high testosterone, while men develop high estrogen and prolactin and low testosterone. For women, this results in infertility or repetitive miscarriages, low libido, and increased risk for breast cancer; for men, it means depression, low libido, and enlarged breasts—fairly offensive effects in anybody's book, and all due to "healthy whole grains." Grain elimination starts the process of reversal, with benefits compounded by weight loss. Women experience a reduction in abnormally high estrogen and prolactin, restoration of fertility, increased potential for carrying a baby to full term, improved libido, and a reduced risk for breast cancer. Men experience reductions in estrogen and prolactin, accompanied by a rise in testosterone, improved libido, and receding breast size.

That's what *typically* happens. Unfortunately, that's not what *always* happens, and various disruptions of hormonal status can persist. Here are the most common forms of persistent sex hormone disruption that, once addressed, provide benefits in addition to those obtained through grain elimination.

1. **Low testosterone.** Women normally have a low level of testosterone—certainly lower than men. But the lower level does not mean inconsequential levels. Low testosterone in women is associated with low energy, low libido, difficulty with weight loss, and depression. Should low testosterone develop after grain elimination, weight loss from visceral fat, and restoration of vitamin D (which can occasionally raise testosterone), then assessment and correction may be in order. In men, low testosterone shows itself as low energy, irritability, difficulty with weight loss or difficulty maintaining muscle mass, and low

libido. Men and women should both aim to keep testosterone levels in the upper half of the reference range for their sex, as quoted by the laboratory, since values in the lower half are typically inadequate for full relief of symptoms. Also, testosterone is most easily and inexpensively obtained through compounding pharmacies, which are specialized in filling individualized prescriptions tailored to your health-care practitioner's specifications. Testosterone can be prescribed as a cream rubbed on the chest, arms, or neck, either alone or in combination with other hormones, including progesterone for women and DHEA for men and women.

2. **Low progesterone.** Progesterone starts its decline in a woman's late 30s, with a sharp drop-off occurring during the menopausal years. Low progesterone is typically signaled by low energy, foggy thinking, an impaired ability to lose weight, disrupted sleep, reduced libido, and irritability. As with testosterone, progesterone is readily assessed and replaced using a cream applied to the skin in a dosage specified by your doctor and based on blood or salivary levels of progesterone. Women who have progesterone replaced typically report improved mood and reduced irritability, increased libido, better sleep, clearer thinking, thicker hair, smoother skin, and a restored ability to lose weight. Progesterone is not accompanied by the risks that come with the use of horse estrogens (Premarin), provided that bioidentical progesterone is prescribed, rather than a synthetic progestin loaded with awful side effects.[9]

3. **Low DHEA.** DHEA has a multitude of effects in the body. As with many hormones, DHEA levels decline over a lifetime and present symptoms that overlap with those of low testosterone and, to a lesser degree, low cortisol. DHEA is easily assessed and replaced, though low doses are best (5 to 10 mg per day). Higher levels are safe, but they tend to be associated with aggressive behavior and facial hair in women and aggression in men. However, when low levels are corrected, most people experience a modest improvement in energy and mood, a modest improvement in the capacity to lose visceral fat, and improved libido.[10]

Get your hormonal house in order. After removing the disrupters of hormonal health—grains and visceral fat—address any residual dysfunctions that persist in your effort to acquire total health. It may require some agitating on your part to get your health-care practitioner to do the right thing and explore your hormonal status, but the rewards will be worth the effort.

CHAPTER 13

END THE SELF-DEFEAT: RECOVERING FROM AUTOIMMUNITY

Friendly fire . . . isn't.
—Murphy's Law of Combat

AUTOIMMUNITY: A GENUINE perversion of nature.

Like a mother hamster consuming her young or a traitor that's infiltrated the ranks of soldiers, autoimmunity—the misguided immune attack against organs in your own body—conjures up disturbing feelings of mistrust and betrayal. Treachery, treason, Benedict Arnold, Judas: It is disloyalty and double-crossing that undermine the normal order of things.

Your lungs are your lungs, your thymus gland is your thymus gland, your brain is your brain—and none of these organs should be confused with the proteins of some bacteria, virus, or fungus, nor should they be confused with the proteins in foods.

Why would your own immune system, handily defeating bacteria, fungi, and viruses for many years, suddenly turn on the body it lives in, destroying, for instance, the pancreas (autoimmune pancreatitis, type 1 diabetes), liver (autoimmune hepatitis), thyroid (Hashimoto's thyroiditis, Graves' disease), tissues covering the brain and nervous system (multiple sclerosis, dementia, cerebellar ataxia), or skin (psoriasis, alopecia areata, dermatomyositis, scleroderma, vitiligo)? Why would a complex system of surveillance and attack direct antibodies, inflammatory proteins, and lymphocytes against its former friends?

Autoimmunity is not so much an act of betrayal as it is an act of misrecognition: Mistaking friend for foe, it is the friendly fire of health. It means mistaking, for instance, the synovial tissues of joints for the proteins in a virus. It means mistaking the iris of the eye for proteins from the herpes simplex virus that causes cold sores. It means mistaking the tissues of the ileum for intestinal bacteria, as in Crohn's disease. Every protein in every organ in the body is a potential target for the misguided attacks of autoimmunity. It is truly an unsettling thought that such serious conditions can be launched without any health wrongdoing on your part; it just happens.

Or does it? Think about it: Autoimmunity is entirely counterintuitive, counteradaptive, and counterrevolutionary. It would seem to be a self-correcting process: If you were struck with, say, rheumatoid arthritis while living in the wilderness, foraging for your food, and defending yourself against violent predators, joint pain and disfigurement would be a substantial disadvantage and, sooner or later, you would perish. Likewise, the neurological impairment of multiple sclerosis and the ruined digestion of ulcerative colitis both compromise survival.

So what could have entered the lives of *Homo sapiens* recently enough, in evolutionary terms, that it has not had sufficient time to exert maladaptive effects on survival? And why are autoimmune diseases on the rise, breaking records with each passing year? It is estimated that 5 to 10 percent of the population of Northern Europe and North America are now afflicted with some form of autoimmune disease, with numbers increasing for autoimmune thyroid disease, inflammatory bowel diseases, type 1 diabetes, and multiple sclerosis.[1] Pharmaceutical industry executives salivate over the autoimmune disease market, now topping $40 billion annually and growing, since the diseases of autoimmunity are a drugmaker's dream come true: chronic conditions requiring years of treatment that often involve biological agents, such as antibodies and peptides, that cost thousands of dollars per month.

Something has clearly changed. It might be some stealth virus affecting millions of humans worldwide. It might be those darned industrial chemicals that provoke endocrine disruption and lead the immune system astray. Some autoimmunity may be due to modern lifestyle mistakes, such as reduced reliance on breast-feeding or exposure to immune-disturbing toxins in cigarettes. And, of course, consumption of "healthy whole grains" plays an underappreciated role in this drama. At least some autoimmunity can be blamed on the process of molecular mimicry, in which the structure of some foreign protein closely resembles the structure of a human protein. The foreign protein can originate with a virus, bacteria, or fungus. Such molecular mimics have been found in strains of the herpes simplex virus and the *Streptococcus sanguinis* bacterium, which trigger the autoimmunity of Behçet's disease; the *Neisseria meningitidis* bacterium, the causal factor in bacterial meningitis, which mimics numerous proteins in the liver, testicles, and skin; and *Campylobacter jejuni*, which causes gastroenteritis but triggers Guillain-Barré syndrome (autoimmune damage to the nervous system). We have more in common with primitive organisms than we'd like to think.

Molecular mimics can also come from food, especially foods that we are not fully evolutionarily adapted to consuming. The products of bovine mammary glands—dairy products—added to the human diet at about the same time that grain consumption became a part of the human experience, trigger human antibodies against dairy proteins, such as bovine serum albumin, casein, and bovine insulin. These antibodies have the potential to launch a misdirected immune attack against pancreatic beta cells, resulting in some cases of type 1 diabetes.[2] Likewise, proteins in the seeds of grasses can fool the body's immune system due to their resemblance to human proteins. The gliadin protein of wheat, with identical proteins in rye and barley, and a similar protein in corn, is the model for this process of molecular mimicry from grains.

Certainly not everybody develops diseases of autoimmune misrecognition, as genetic predisposition is clearly part of the picture. People predisposed to ankylosing spondylitis, for example, nearly always have a gene for the immune system HLA-B27 protein variant. Conversely, only 5 percent of people with the HLA-B27 gene actually develop the spine inflammation that characterizes ankylosing spondylitis, telling us that while genetics play an important, permissive role, there are other factors that unmask genetic predisposition.

Nutritional deficiencies are increasingly recognized as being among the factors that allow autoimmunity to develop. Vitamin D deficiency, in particular, is proving to be a huge factor in allowing the misrecognition of "self" as invader, as is omega-3 fatty acid deficiency. Deficiencies of either or both allow misguided immune behavior, but both are easily addressed and corrected. Factors that disrupt bowel flora also play a role in autoimmunity. In particular, excessive growth of unhealthy species can increase intestinal permeability, or "leaky gut," which allows foreign substances, including bacterial by-products, to enter the bloodstream and reach the organs.

Autoimmune destruction of one organ can, not uncommonly, be associated with autoimmune destruction of other organs. Type 1 diabetes, for example, is often accompanied by celiac disease, Hashimoto's thyroiditis, or rheumatoid arthritis. Misrecognition of the components of one organ can therefore be followed by misrecognition of the components of other organs.

There's not a lot you can do to remove your prior exposure to streptococcus or to change your HLA immune recognition protein genetics. But there is plenty you can do to remove immune-stimulating grains from your diet and to help correct the common deficiencies that allow an autoimmune condition to emerge.

GRAINS START THE AUTOIMMUNE BALL ROLLING

The prolamin proteins of grains—the gliadin of wheat, secalin of rye, hordein of barley, and zein of corn—initiate the small intestinal process that gets the fires of autoimmunity burning. And they do so in more than one way. You could even argue that prolamin proteins are perfectly crafted to create autoimmunity.

Prolamin proteins of grains are masters at molecular mimicry. The prolamin proteins have been found to trigger immune responses to a number of human proteins, including the synapsin protein of the nervous system; the transglutaminase enzyme found in the liver, muscle, brain, and other organs; the endomysium of muscle cells; and the calreticulin of virtually every cell in the body.[3] If sequences in foreign proteins resemble sequences in a protein of the human body, a misdirected immune attack can be launched, sending antibodies, T lymphocytes, macrophages, tumor necrosis factor, and other weapons of the immune apparatus against the organ. Some targeted human proteins, such as transglutaminase and calreticulin, are ubiquitous and can therefore be associated with autoimmune inflammation of just about any organ of the body, from brain to pancreas.

Molecular mimicry is not the only means by which grains provoke autoimmunity; they also do so by increasing intestinal permeability. We've discussed how prolamins can resist digestion. When they remain intact, they bind to the intestinal lining and initiate a unique and complex process that opens the normal intestinal barriers to the contents of the intestines, such as food components, and to bacterial components and by-products, such as bacterial lipopolysaccharide—a potent driver of inflammation. The multistep process initiated by grain proteins was worked out through elegant investigations performed by Alessio Fasano, MD, and his team at the University of Maryland (see page 67), extraordinary work that makes the confident connection between the diseases of autoimmunity and grains. Grain prolamins increase the expression of the zonulin protein that, in turn, opens up the normal barriers—"tight junctions"—between intestinal cells, allowing unwanted peptides and bacterial components into the bloodstream, where they can trigger an immune response.[4] Besides gliadin and related prolamins, the only other trigger of this form of intestinal permeability are intestinal infections, such as cholera or dysbiosis.

This means that gliadin and related proteins of grains are the first step in initiating autoimmunity, a mechanism that has nothing to do with gluten sensitivity or celiac disease. Susceptibility to various autoimmune diseases can also be determined by genetic patterns, but in a staggering proportion of cases, the initiating event boils down to a single factor: consumption of grains.

Autoimmunity: Turning the Titanic

Many conditions respond to grain elimination within days. For instance, joint pain in the fingers and wrists, acid reflux, and the bowel urgency of irritable bowel syndrome typically disappear within 5 days of your final pancake. Not so with the phenomena of autoimmunity. The swelling, joint pain, stiffness, and disfigurement of rheumatoid arthritis is going to take longer to respond to grain elimination, typically weeks to months, and occasionally even longer.

Perhaps this should come as no surprise, as the complex mechanisms of autoimmune inflammation develop over years. Likewise, changes in lymphocyte responses, clearance of antibodies, reductions in fluid, localized inflammation, and a wide range of other phenomena reverse themselves over time. The key is to eliminate all grains, and then wait; don't declare the effort a failure if 2 weeks pass and nothing has happened. Patience is key. That's why I liken the reversal of autoimmune conditions to slowing a locomotive or turning an ocean liner—neither occurs quickly, but they both happen with time.

It is also important to correct the other abnormal phenomena that make autoimmunity worse. The majority of people with autoimmune conditions fail to address factors that play an important role in permitting or sustaining autoimmunity; by addressing these factors, you stack the odds of complete relief from autoimmunity in your favor, which we'll discuss next.

Vitamin D: Master Immune System Modulator

Vitamin D plays a critical role in immune regulation, protecting against viruses, bacterial infections, cancers, and autoimmunity. The seasonal variation in conditions such as the flu and other viral infections, multiple sclerosis, heart attacks, and cancer—higher incidence in winter, lower in summer—make sense in light of the seasonal variation of sun exposure, which activates skin vitamin D. Many diseases also increase in incidence the farther you get from the equator, due to the diminishing intensity of sunlight. Our modern lifestyles, which keep us from obtaining sufficient sun exposure, coupled with our aversion to consumption of vitamin D–rich organs of animals, such as liver, have allowed vitamin D deficiency to reach epidemic proportions and autoimmune conditions to rise in the wake of this deficiency. Vitamin D deficiency is proving to be a powerful "permissive" factor in allowing autoimmunity to develop,[5] and it tends to be worse in people who develop autoimmune conditions. Vitamin D deficiency has also been associated with worse symptoms of autoimmunity, such as pain, swelling, and neurological disability.

Type 1 diabetes, an autoimmune response that can be triggered by the gliadin and related proteins of grains and which results in damage to the beta cells of the pancreas, is among the best studied of autoimmune diseases. Therefore, it illustrates the role vitamin D restoration can play. Children diagnosed with type 1 diabetes have substantially lower 25-hydroxy vitamin D blood levels compared to children without type 1 diabetes.[6] Multiple studies have shown that supplementation with vitamin D reduces the incidence of type 1 diabetes by between 30 and 78 percent, with higher doses (2,000 international units, or IU, per day) resulting in a greater success rate.[7] Because a substantial proportion of type 1 diabetes cases are triggered by exposure to the prolamin proteins of grains, elimination of all grains—combined with restoration of vitamin D status—is a powerful means of preventing the autoimmunity that leads to type 1 diabetes.

The list of other autoimmune conditions associated with vitamin D deficiency includes primary biliary cirrhosis, alopecia areata, multiple sclerosis, Behçet's disease, vitiligo, autoimmune hepatitis, Sjögren's syndrome, systemic lupus erythematosus, Hashimoto's thyroiditis, pemphigus vulgaris, immune thrombocytopenic purpura, and inflammatory bowel diseases (Crohn's disease and ulcerative colitis).[8] It is not entirely clear just how vitamin D is best restored among these conditions and how many people under each autoimmune category will respond, as clinical trial data are incomplete. (This is common with nutritional issues, as they do not enjoy the sort of vigorous funding that drug studies enjoy.) However, having assisted many thousands of people in correcting vitamin D, I believe there is virtually no downside to vitamin D restoration when an autoimmune condition is present or as part of a broader effort to maintain health and prevent autoimmune and other conditions. In fact, correction often results in a broad range of health benefits. (The one relative contraindication to correction of vitamin D deficiency is sarcoidosis; correction in this condition requires monitoring blood levels of 1,25-dihydroxy vitamin D and should only be attempted under the supervision of a health-care provider knowledgeable in this area. However, this situation is unique to sarcoidosis.)

Vitamin D is readily restored using oil-based gelcap forms of cholecalciferol, or vitamin D_3, the naturally occurring human form of vitamin D. Because maximum advantage should be sought when an autoimmune condition is present, and because some autoimmune conditions involve impaired nutrient absorption, 25-hydroxy vitamin D blood levels should be tested every 6 months, as dosage needs can vary widely and can change over time. While the target blood level is a topic of debate, I have used 60 to 70 ng/ml as a target with excellent results and no toxic effects. This blood level is generally achieved with 6,000 to 8,000 IU per day of D_3 in the form of a gelcap when intestinal absorption is normal, higher when absorption is impaired. I base this target level on epidemiological observations that demonstrate that diseases across a broad spectrum, including cardiovascular disease and cancer, drop sharply in incidence in this range, and because it is a range easily achievable by healthy young people who maintain the capacity to activate vitamin D with plentiful sun exposure of the skin, which suggests that it's a physiologically appropriate level. See page 175 for more information on vitamin D.

Omega-3 Fatty Acids: Part of the Solution

Omega-3 fatty acids (EPA and DHA) have demonstrated modest effects on reducing the inflammation associated with autoimmune conditions.[9] Rheumatoid arthritis is the best studied among them, with several studies demonstrating that doses of at least 2,000 mg per day of EPA and DHA (combined total) exert positive effects, reducing joint pain, stiffness, and swelling.[10] Not surprisingly, clinical trials concerning other autoimmune conditions showed mixed results when low doses of omega-3s were used without addressing issues such as grain consumption and vitamin D deficiency.

Omega-3 fatty acids are insufficient on their own to cause remission, but they play a complementary role to other efforts, especially grain elimination, vitamin D restoration, and altering bowel flora composition (see below). Between 3,000 and 4,000 mg of combined EPA and DHA per day is required to take full advantage of this effect.

Bowel Flora: Snug as a Bug

While it is clear that bowel flora are altered in unhealthy ways in people with autoimmune conditions, it is not clear whether this develops before the expression of the disease or whether it is a consequence of the disease. Nonetheless, once it develops, alterations in bowel flora compound the inflammation of autoimmunity, worsening symptoms such as the joint pain of rheumatoid arthritis, the bloating and diarrhea of ulcerative colitis, and the muscle weakness of polymyositis.[11]

Celiac disease, in particular, is associated with major disruptions of intestinal bacterial populations, with decreased healthy populations of Bifidobacteria and dominance of unhealthy bacteria such as *Escherichia coli* and Bacteroides species.[12] Preliminary evidence in experimental models of type 1 diabetes suggests that bowel flora play a role in the development of the disease, such as increased Bacteroides species in animals developing the condition.[13] People with inflammatory bowel diseases experience changes in bowel flora similar to those seen in celiac disease.[14]

Prolamin proteins induce an increase in intestinal permeability and molecular mimicry, both of which serve to initiate autoimmunity, and the changed bowel flora yield greater quantities of lipopolysaccharide (LPS), a component of the cell walls of unhealthy bacteria such as *E. coli.* Taking advantage of the increased intestinal permeability, LPS enters the bloodstream, providing another powerful instigator of inflammation and turning up the volume on autoimmune inflammation.[15]

Attention to gastrointestinal health in general and bowel flora in particular can therefore be an important part of recovering from various autoimmune conditions. Do everything else right—eliminate the initiating factor in autoimmunity, correct vitamin D and omega-3 fatty acid deficiencies—but neglect bowel health and the restoration of desirable bowel flora, and a return to full health and relief from autoimmunity may be compromised.

As discussed in Chapter 9, the full Monty for restoration of bowel flora involves a period of probiotic supplementation, along with lifelong intake of prebiotic fibers to help sustain the renewed population of healthy bacteria and enhance production of butyrate. The consumption of fermented foods is also beneficial. Make your bowel bugs happy and they will serve you well.

Heavy Metals: More Than Head Banging

The increasing human exposure to heavy metals, particularly mercury, lead, cadmium, and arsenic, has the potential to trigger the misguided responses of autoimmunity. Experimental data clearly show that there are distortions of T lymphocytes, in particular, that play a role in the autoimmune response. What is not clear is just what percentage of people with various autoimmune diseases have toxic levels of these metals and whether improvement can result after their removal.

Heavy metal exposure, like exposure to industrial chemicals, is an increasing hazard in modern life. For example, we're exposed to methyl-mercury from consumption of fish; cadmium from cigarette smoking and the increasing reliance on this metal for nickel-cadmium batteries; lead from prior use in leaded gasoline; and arsenic from food (especially rice) and drinking water.[16]

Levels of these metals in blood, hair, or nails can be clinically measured, and all can be reduced or removed using various chelating or binding agents that are administered intravenously, orally, or rectally. As in many other areas of health, most primary care physicians are ill-equipped for such issues; if you want to pursue chelation, you are likely to have greater success with a functional medicine practitioner or naturopath.

Other Food Sensitivities

Immune sensitivities to foods other than grains can involve dairy, eggs, peanuts, nuts, and meats, among other common foods. While data are preliminary, it appears that some people who express higher levels of antibodies against the components of such foods may obtain health benefits, including a reduction in autoimmune responses, by identifying and eliminating such triggers.[17]

There is controversy over how to identify such sensitivities. A number of methods are available, including elimination diets, in which a diet of neutral foods is consumed and other foods are added back one at a time to gauge the body's response. It's typical to wait several days after each addition to allow for the development of delayed responses. Skin testing, blood testing for antibodies against various foods, assessment of lymphocyte responses to foods, and stool testing are among the other methods available. Unfortunately, there has been insufficient comparison of such methods to make meaningful judgments about their relative values.

While it is certain that there are people who have autoimmune and other conditions triggered by immune responses to different foods, what is not yet clear is what proportion of people with autoimmune diseases can be expected to have such sensitivities and what proportion can be expected to experience improvement with removal of the offending food. The key, if you suspect that you have a food sensitivity or if you experience continued symptoms of autoimmunity despite taking all of the above steps, is to identify a practitioner skilled in the use of one or more forms of food sensitivity testing.

AUTOIMMUNITY: DRUG ABUSE

The conventional medical approach to autoimmune diseases ignores disturbances of intestinal permeability, molecular mimicry, immunomodulation by vitamin D and omega-3 fatty acids, composition of bowel flora, exposure to industrial chemicals or metals, and the notion that various foods can initiate and perpetuate an immune system gone wrong.

Instead, modern health care chooses to focus only on turning off the immune responses with drugs. Some treatments are imprecise and nonspecific drugs, such as steroids like prednisone, which, by shutting down the entire immune system, also make us susceptible to infections. Other treatments are more specific, such as tumor necrosis factor blockers like Enbrel and Humira. These intravenous agents only work occasionally with incomplete success, are extraordinarily expensive, and are accompanied by the potential for tuberculosis, viral and bacterial infections, liver damage or failure, and activation of viral hepatitis. They even allow other autoimmune diseases to develop—an imperfect solution, to say the least.

The wonderful thing about addressing the potential contributors to autoimmune processes, such as eliminating grains, restoring vitamin D, and correcting disruptions of bowel flora, is that they help restore health in many ways, not just by reducing inflammation or autoimmunity. Eliminate grains, for instance, and depression can lift, blood sugars drop, visceral fat is lost—and autoimmunity can recede. Raise vitamin D blood levels to 70 ng/ml and your thinking becomes clearer, bone density increases, insulin levels drop—and autoimmunity can recede. And such interventions are safe and inexpensive, costing little compared to the thousands of dollars per month you'd spend on autoimmune drugs.

Take natural steps appropriate for a non-grass-consuming member of the species *Homo sapiens*, and allow your immune system to distinguish friend from foe.

CHAPTER 14

WHAT IF THE WEIGHT DOESN'T COME OFF?

People say their weight is genetic. But it turns out that people
who are overweight don't just have overweight kids.
They also have overweight pets. That's not genetic.
—Dr. Mehmet Oz

"HEALTHY WHOLE GRAINS" are not healthy, nor do they help you control your weight. In fact, the opposite is true: Grains are a powerful means of gaining weight. Those studies that purport to show that "healthy whole grains" help you control or lose weight do nothing of the kind, but actually demonstrate that whole grains cause less weight gain than white flour products do. In the Nurses' Health Study of 74,000 women tracked over 12 years, for example, those who consumed the least whole grains (and thereby more processed grains) gained an average of 10 pounds compared to those who consumed the most whole grains, who gained an average of 9 pounds, proving that refined grains make you fat and whole grains make you slightly less fat.[1] It sounds absurd when put into these terms, but that is the flawed brand of reasoning used to justify eating grains in nutritional "science" and conventional dietary advice today.

What if you've taken all the steps articulated so far, yet you encounter a "wall" in weight loss? You had visions of showing off in a size 4 bikini on a beach in the Caribbean, but you find yourself no better off 8 weeks into your grain-free life than you were before, and you're still sucking in to zip up your jeans. You did your best, even enduring the emotional and physical tumult of withdrawal and annoying family and friends with fatigue, headaches, and bad humor. But weight loss eludes you. Or maybe you lost something like 10 pounds, only to have weight loss stop for an extended period, stranding you on a frustrating weight plateau lasting weeks or months, with another 50 or 100 pounds to lose before you can confidently claim that you've succeeded. You've read all of those wonderful success stories and seen all of those eye-popping "before" and "after" photos here and on Wheat Belly social media sites. You've seen evidence of astounding weight loss successes, people boasting about 30, 50, 150 pounds lost, and now you're asking why a strategy that yields rapid and often astounding weight loss in the majority of people does not work for you.

The weight-loss experience of grain elimination can indeed vary from individual to individual. While the majority of people who follow the grain-free lifestyle lose 5 pounds the first week, 15 to 18 pounds the first month, and continue experiencing losses over the subsequent months that can total 70, 100, or even more pounds over the course of a year, experiences can vary across a range. (Follow the discussions on Wheat Belly social media, such as the Facebook page, and you will witness the daily flow of stories, most wildly successful, some modestly successful, and some unsuccessful.) The pace of weight loss differs in men versus women (men lose faster), is dependent on how overweight you are to begin with (the more overweight you are, the faster you lose in the beginning), varies with age (younger people lose faster), and is influenced by muscle mass (greater muscle mass allows more rapid loss of fat). This last issue becomes a factor for people whose weights have yo-yoed over the years, as each episode of substantial weight loss is accompanied by loss of muscle mass. Regain the 30 pounds that you lost and it is all fat, not muscle. You are now heavier but have less muscle, making weight control even harder. (More on this to come later in this chapter.)

Could failed weight loss mean that wheat, rye, barley, rice, corn, and other grains are actually good for you, that you are somehow different from other members of our species? Could it mean that you escaped the inflammatory effects of prolamin proteins, the digestive disruption caused by lectins, the allergic effects, the high blood sugars of grain amylopectins, oral and bowel flora changes, provocation of small LDL particles, and the unexpected diagnoses of autoimmune conditions? Is eliminating grains therefore of no benefit to you, as demonstrated by its failure to yield the weight-loss benefits that most people enjoy?

No, absolutely not. Weight loss or not, you are still exposed to all the other adverse effects of grains.

A failure to lose weight means that there is something impeding weight loss success, that there is some factor or factors that, despite grain elimination and an otherwise perfect diet, are blocking the capacity to lose excess fat weight. Like figuring out why your car doesn't run quite right despite a tune-up, those factors need to be identified, one by one. These are factors that, no matter how hard you try, no matter how many calories you cut, no matter how long you exercise, will continue to shut down your capacity to lose weight. By losing weight, you are really trying to regain *health*, as excess weight is just one aspect of an unhealthy metabolism. If you encounter stalled weight loss, then there is something wrong with your health, and those unhealthy factors must be identified and corrected for weight loss to proceed, often accompanied by benefits in other areas of health beyond weight. Each and every one of these factors needs to be addressed and cast out of your way before weight loss will proceed as you'd hoped.

In this chapter we'll consider the impediments to weight loss despite grain elimination and discuss how to correct them, one by one.

DON'T REPLACE A PROBLEM WITH ANOTHER PROBLEM

In Chapter 7 we discussed the need to avoid gluten-free foods made with "junk carb" ingredients like cornstarch, potato flour, tapioca starch, and rice flour, but it bears repeating, as so many people continue to hear the Wheat Belly message as a "gluten-free" message. The majority of gluten-free foods sold in stores pack on the pounds and impair your ability to lose weight. Just because they lack gluten does not make them healthy. Eating gluten-free breads, pastas, and muffins is like eating bags of jelly beans and wondering why you can't lose weight. Lose the jelly beans—they have no place in a weight-loss effort. And the weight you gain from gluten-free junk carbs is the worst weight: inflammatory visceral fat within the abdomen. Nobody should eat gluten-free processed foods made with these ingredients. Sometimes, people with celiac disease or gluten sensitivity will say, "But I have to eat gluten-free foods!" They do not understand the issues: Yes, they need to meticulously avoid all gluten sources, but they do not need gluten-free junk carbohydrate ingredients in their place. This is the sort of self-destructive thinking encouraged by the gluten-free food industry. Nobody should be consuming gluten-free breads, biscuits, or rolls—nobody.

"Low-carb" bars, pasta, breads, muffins, etc., are another weight-loss impediment. Some of these items may indeed be low in carbohydrate content, but other unhealthy ingredients are often included. There is a popular line of "energy" bars, for instance, that are low in carbohydrate content but contain a concentrated form of gluten, and therefore gliadin, which degrades to appetite-stimulating opiates, adding to weight gain. They should be called "Weight Gain Bars," not energy bars. And a line of low-carb pasta claims that their product does not raise blood sugar as high as conventional pasta due to the addition of several ingredients, including added wheat gluten, and therefore it can be a healthy part of a low-carb weight-loss effort. Combine this with the trivial reduction in blood sugar this product affords, and you have a food that causes a net weight gain.

Consumption of diet soft drinks sweetened with aspartame, neotame, and sucralose does not result in weight loss (when compared to consumption of sugar-sweetened soft drinks), and it may even be responsible for weight gain.[2] Diet soft drinks sweetened with these ingredients therefore potentially impair your capacity to lose weight and should be eliminated completely.

We once again return to the basic advice to consume real, single-ingredient foods to minimize the hazards. Eat cucumbers, zucchini, peppers, meats (with the fat), fish, poultry (with the skin and fat), raw nuts and seeds, mushrooms, and berries. Only when you are confident with this approach is it time to venture back into the world of some processed foods made with ingredients you know are safe.

PUNCH, KICK, AND SMACK INSULIN

Insulin is the hormone of fat storage. It causes glucose to enter cells and be converted to fats, prevents the degradation of fats into energy, and thereby makes you fat. At the start of a weight-loss adventure, most people have high blood levels of insulin. In a fasting state, ideal levels of insulin are near zero, and certainly no higher than 7 to 8 mIU/ml. Many people embarking on a weight-loss effort begin with insulin levels of 30, 40, or 50 mIU/ml, levels sufficient to completely turn off weight loss by stimulating fat deposition and inhibiting fat mobilization. Elimination of grains results in a reduction in insulin, but it may not be enough. This situation must be corrected in order for weight loss to occur.

Carbohydrates stimulate insulin far more than fats and proteins do. We therefore get rid of the foods that stimulate insulin the most: grains and carbohydrates. There is no longer any remaining debate: Restricting carbohydrates is more effective than restricting fat for losing excess weight.[3] This is one of the reasons I condemn gluten-free foods made with rice flour, cornstarch, tapioca starch, and potato flour; these foods ensure high insulin and, in my view, should never be consumed. Beware of many low-carb processed foods that are no better and are sometimes worse, including low-carb breads and pastas.

Most people can reenergize their weight-loss efforts by reducing carbohydrates to a level that's no higher than 15 grams (g) net carbs per meal (total carbs minus fiber), or around 45 g net carbs per day (though not eaten in a single meal but spread out throughout the day). There are a number of smartphone applications that provide nutritional analyses of foods and can help make this an easy process, especially in restaurants or other settings outside the home. There are also many Web sites that list the nutritional composition of foods. (Search for "nutritional analysis.") Technology makes carb counting ridiculously easy. If you don't have a smartphone or computer, an old-fashioned handbook listing the nutritional info for various foods works fine.

You will discover, for instance, that a ripe, medium banana (not to be confused with a low-in-carbohydrate, high-in-indigestible-prebiotic-fiber green unripe banana) contains 29 g of total carbohydrates and 4 g of fiber, thereby providing 25 g net carbohydrates—more than enough to provoke insulin (and blood sugar) to levels sufficient to impair weight loss. A whole banana therefore does not fit into this approach. (Cut the banana in half or eat it unripe, instead.) People are frequently surprised at their carbohydrate intake, often consuming much of it in foods they thought were healthy, such as oatmeal, baked potatoes, or excessive quantities of legumes such as kidney beans. It is important to obtain modest quantities of prebiotic fibers from lentils, chickpeas, hummus, and legumes to nourish bowel flora, but limit your intake to 15 g of net carbs per serving. One-quarter cup of hummus, for instance, contains 10 g net carbs while providing prebiotic fibers. (This restriction does not apply to inulin, unripe green bananas, or raw potatoes, as they contain nearly all indigestible fibers that do not add to the digestible carbohydrate count. See Chapter 9 for further discussion.)

If this easy approach fails to work after 4 weeks, then let me introduce you to what I call "the most effective weight-loss tool ever invented": a glucose meter. Monitoring and managing blood sugar is an exceptionally effective way to manage carbohydrates more closely and thereby gain control over weight. (See the extended explanation of how to check blood sugar in Chapter 7.) Check blood sugars immediately prior to and then 30 to 60 minutes after the start of each meal, and aim for *no change* in blood sugar. Allowing no change in blood sugar virtually ensures that there is no excessive provocation of insulin.

If your blood sugar increases from, say, 90 mg/dl to 140 mg/dl 30 to 60 minutes after eating, then reexamine the foods you ate to identify the culprit. The answer will be found in some hidden or underappreciated source of carbohydrates. Cut back on your portion size or eliminate that food. Once a meal has been demonstrated to be safe without raising blood sugar, there is no need to retest that meal in the future, unless you add or change one or more components. After just a few weeks of this, you will know which foods cause blood sugar trouble, and testing will only be necessary when you're introducing unfamiliar foods. Monitoring blood sugars to maintain no change pre- and postmeal works wonders for many people who find they can finally snap out of a stubborn weight plateau. Blood sugar checks can be conducted in concert with counting carbohydrates, to help you establish your personal carbohydrate tolerance.

An occasional person will need to go the full low-carb mile and require a ketogenic state to achieve weight loss—all carbohydrates will have to be eliminated in order to metabolize fats. In its most extreme form, a ketogenic diet, in which there is near-zero (less than 20 g net carbohydrates per day) intake of carbohydrates with high fat intake to quell hunger, diverts metabolism toward mobilization of body fat, resulting in ketone formation, or ketosis.

You can detect ketosis by the fruity odor on the breath. However, the most assured and precise method is to assess blood levels of ketones with a finger stick, just like checking blood sugar. The tips on page 146 for checking blood sugars also apply to checking ketones with a finger-stick testing device. The only difference is in timing, as ketone checks can be performed at any time, unlike the after-meal checks for blood sugar. Most people test ketones first thing in the morning, which approximates the highest value for the day. At the moment, the Abbott Precision Xtra is the only device that allows testing for both blood sugar and ketones by using test strips designed for either test. To maintain a ketogenic state to accelerate weight loss or break a weight-loss plateau, aim for a ketone level of 1.0 to 3.0 mmol/L, and maintain that for as long as you desire accelerated weight loss. If you fall below this cutoff, it means that continuing carbohydrate consumption is preventing conversion to a ketogenic state.

Note that urine can be tested using a dipstick for ketones, such as Ketostix, but these can only detect ketones in the higher range, as are experienced by type 1 diabetics during diabetic ketoacidosis. Urine monitoring is therefore less sensitive for identifying the subtler levels of ketosis experienced physiologically, which makes it inadequate for weight-loss purposes.

Maintaining ketosis is not just a means of accelerating weight loss, but also of enhancing mental and physical performance. You'll experience this yourself, with heightened mental clarity, energy, and endurance in a ketotic state. (See the recipes in Appendix A for a few foods, such as Fat Blasters, that can help you achieve or maintain ketosis with a hefty dose of fat.)

Physicians and dietitians often warn people that ketosis is dangerous and can lead to kidney damage. This is not true. They are confusing ketosis, a natural adaptation to periods when carbohydrates are unavailable (which is a common seasonal situation for hunter-gatherers), with diabetic ketoacidosis, a dangerous condition that develops in type 1 diabetics who, when deprived of insulin, develop extremely high levels of blood glucose and a high level of ketones sufficient to generate a life-threatening drop in blood pH. None of this occurs in physiological ketosis generated by carbohydrate restriction in people without type 1 diabetes. Critics also argue that ketosis can damage the kidneys due to high protein intake. This is not true; the clinical data does not demonstrate any deterioration in kidney function with high intakes of protein in people with normal kidneys.[4] Additionally, ketosis does not necessarily require an increase in protein intake over the usual levels, but rather an increase in fat intake, which has no effect on kidney health.

Attention should still be paid to intake of prebiotic fibers, which do not impact blood sugar or ketosis. In my view, making sure that you obtain sufficient prebiotic fibers is crucial to maximizing the benefits of a keto-genic state. (See Chapter 9 for more on prebiotics.)

This important step of managing carbohydrates, glucose, insulin, and ketones would likely have been unnecessary during any other era of human history, when food consumption more closely matched human needs for survival. But the industrialization of food has made heightened awareness of carbohydrates, due to their cheap, commoditized nature, a necessity.

NO WHEY

The problem with dairy is not fat; it's the whey fraction of protein and, to a lesser degree, the lactose sugar. Ironically, we've spent the last 50 years worrying about the fat content of butter, cream, whole milk, and other fatty dairy products, steering people toward low-fat dairy, while the healthiest component of dairy products has always been the fat. But there remains a potential problem with dairy protein.

Some people are susceptible to the insulinotropic action of whey that triggers a tripling of insulin output by the pancreas, a situation that stalls weight loss in some people. The solution: Avoid all dairy products. (Note that this includes whey protein sold as a powder since, well, it is whey protein.) The only practical way I know of to identify whey as the culprit causing stalled weight loss is a trial of elimination. To determine whether this is an issue for you, commit to a 4-week trial of complete dairy elimination. If your weight drops, say, 10 pounds, then you can safely conclude that you are sensitive to the insulin-provoking effects of dairy; if nothing happens, then this effect likely does not apply to you and resuming dairy will likely have no effect on your weight, good or bad. Eliminating dairy does, however, make a grain-free diet very restrictive, so you may want to do this only for as long as you are trying to lose weight. Once you achieve your goal and are adding dairy back into your diet, focus mostly on cultured cheeses (most of the whey is removed during the process of creating the cheese), butter, and ghee (which contain small or negligible quantities of whey).

If you choose this path, coconut milk products (canned and carton), as well as goat and sheep milk products, are useful substitutes.

MOVE TO FAT CITY

This is a common mistake made by people who eliminate grains: They remain fearful of fats and oils. But you shouldn't be.

The outdated arguments, sloppy studies, misrepresentations, misinterpretations, and fairy tales that led to the low-fat argument for the prevention of heart disease have now crumbled. It is now clear that total fat and saturated fat have nothing to do with heart disease risk.[5] It took 40 years and much reanalysis of the data originally interpreted to associate fat intake with cardiovascular risk, but it has become clear that, not only has cutting fat on a nationwide scale failed to reduce the incidence of cardiovascular disease, it has actually contributed to the overweight, obesity, and diabetes crises. This was a big mistake. Forget about cutting fat, saturated fat, and cholesterol. The majority of us do not have to cut fat for cardiovascular benefit.

Fats and oils are satiating. They turn off appetite and reduce our desire for sweets. Liberal fat intake, contrary to conventional wisdom, does not make you fat; it helps make you skinny. After you have eliminated grains and slashed carbohydrates to dodge their insulin-provoking effects, you must increase fat and oil intake to make up for the calorie loss and deal with your hunger.

The last 50 years of dietary misadventures brought to us by Big Food have also created a collection of oils and fats that really should be avoided—these aren't naturally occurring fats and oils, but man-made forms that have no business being consumed by humans. The fats to avoid are hydrogenated (trans fats), partially hydrogenated, and any fat used to fry foods (due to changes in fat structure that occur at high temperatures). It's also important to avoid overexposure to processed polyunsaturated seed oils like corn, mixed vegetable, safflower, sunflower, grapeseed, soybean, and canola. This will help you avoid overconsumption of the omega-6 fatty acids, linoleic and arachidonic acids, which is common. While linoleic acid is an essential fatty acid that you cannot do without, most of us are overexposed to omega-6 fatty acids, given their ubiquitous presence in processed foods and seed oils.

A useful strategy is to add healthy fats and oils to foods, such as 2 to 3 tablespoons of extra-virgin olive or coconut oil to scrambled eggs or soups. Safe oils include extra-virgin or extra-light (to remove vegetal flavor for baking) olive oil; coconut oil; avocado oil; macadamia oil; flaxseed oil; and, to many people's surprise, lard and tallow—but only if you make them yourself or purchase them nonhydrogenated and without unhealthy additives such as BHT.

Some people even choose to consume coconut oil straight off a spoon, mixed into coffee, or blended into a low-carb smoothie, thereby providing rapid satiety, as well as a healthy source of fatty acids. Fat Blasters (see page 334) are little snacks that provide a wallop of fat for anyone who needs quick satiety on the run or a fat boost to encourage ketosis. And to get serious about embracing the notion of fat consumption, eat the fat on your beef, pork, lamb, and poultry; ask for the liver or other organs; boil the bones to make soup or stock, and then don't skim off the gelatin or fat when it cools. If dairy is a part of your diet, choose full-fat products—cream, whole milk, full-fat cheese, etc.—not skim, low-fat, or 1 percent. It's important to not be hungry: If you are experiencing hunger, then it's likely you've failed to increase fat and oil consumption.

Members of the *Homo* species have consumed animal fat for the last 2.5 million years. Don't let agencies give you silly, misguided advice that such evolutionary adaptations are all wrong just because agribusiness and Big Food have asked them to.

LIFE IN THE RAW

Raw foods are inefficiently digested foods.

We're not talking about eating raw foods for their purported health effects, as some people do. I am talking about consuming as many foods in their raw, uncooked state as possible and putting inefficient digestion to work for you. The process of heating—baking, roasting, sautéing, frying, steaming—increases the digestibility of proteins and carbohydrates. Conversely, eating an exclusively raw diet makes it difficult to obtain sufficient calories and nutrients, reflected in abnormally low bone density, high incidence of amenorrhea (absence of menstrual cycles), and malnutrition in people who rely on raw foods completely.[6] In a wild setting, where food may intermittently fall short of need, there is no advantage to the inefficient digestion of raw foods, and heating to increase digestibility is preferred for survival. But in our world of access to limitless energy and excess weight, we can use their indigestibility to our advantage.

Eating mostly or entirely raw foods is therefore meant to be a short-term strategy for weight loss, not a long-term strategy for health. Eat vegetables raw. Consume potatoes raw (see Appendix A). Eat meat rare, whenever possible, since modern people don't like the idea of consuming raw meat (and because domesticated livestock and modern meat processing can introduce pathogens, particularly into pork and chicken, and they should therefore be consumed only fully cooked). If you're into sushi and Japanese food, sashimi (raw fish) is another good choice. Once you have achieved your weight-loss goal, however, fire up the stove, oven, and microwave and cook your food for increased digestibility.

IS IT YOUR THYROID?

Thyroid dysfunction is an issue that takes center stage when you expect to join the legions of people who have enjoyed spectacular weight loss with grain elimination but you find yourself left helplessly behind. The thyroid is to blame in many of these instances, or more precisely, prior grain consumption, exposure to industrial chemicals, and iodine deficiency are to blame, leaving your thyroid (the innocent victim) unable to perform its job of maintaining metabolic rate. For weight-loss purposes, we are talking only about hypothyroidism, or low thyroid status. (Thyroid dysfunction is so common and exerts such a powerful influence over health that it is the subject of all of Chapter 11.)

About 20 percent of people with hypothyroidism can blame their underactive thyroid status on iodine deficiency. This nearly always responds to simple supplementation with 500 to 1,000 mcg of iodine per day from kelp tablets or iodine drops. You could use iodized salt, but be aware that the iodine is essentially gone from the canister 4 weeks after you open it. Supplementation is therefore a more assured means of gaining control over iodine intake. Supplementing iodine is no more dangerous than salting your food with iodized salt; and adverse reactions, such as anxiety or nervousness due to an overly excessive response to iodine, are rare. However, if a hyperthyroid response occurs (anxiety, palpitations, sleeplessness) it should be explored to rule out issues such as Hashimoto's thyroiditis and active thyroid nodules (which are occasionally cancerous). These conditions can be silent until they're unmasked by appropriate levels of iodine that allow such responses to occur.

Most people find that supplementing iodine for at least 3 months is required to fully regain their capacity to lose weight, though improvements can begin within the first few days of supplementation. If you have a known thyroid condition, consult with your health-care practitioner before initiating iodine; however, don't be surprised if you are advised by your doctor that iodine is unnecessary or dangerous. If this happens, find a health-care provider who is knowledgeable about iodine and thyroid health, such as a functional medicine practitioner or naturopath.

One problem with a diagnosis of low thyroid status, or hypothyroidism, is that most health-care practitioners treat it by prescribing the T4 thyroid hormone only (Synthroid or levothyroxine), while failing to address T3, even if it is abnormally low (though it is usually not even measured). Chapter 11 explains in detail why this is a big mistake and why the majority of people do better supplementing with a mix of T3 and T4 for weight loss and for health. What is the ideal TSH that allows weight loss to proceed? A value of 1.5 mIU/ml or less, perhaps even 1.0 mIU/ml or less—not the 3.5 or 4.0 mIU/ml many doctors are content with.

Even marginal thyroid dysfunction, or undertreated hypothyroidism, can completely block success at weight loss. Correct thyroid status to ideal levels and weight loss proceeds for most people. It's really very simple, though you may have to push your current doctor aside to resolve this issue.

CORTISOL: GET BACK IN RHYTHM

Disruption of weight control is not so much about excess cortisol as it is about disruptions of circadian rhythms, though excessively high levels of cortisol can also occur. Cortisol levels should follow a predictable circadian rhythm under the control of signals from the hypothalamus and pituitary glands. Normally, the adrenal gland receives a signal from the pituitary to release an early morning surge of cortisol to arouse you from sleep and prepare you for action. Levels decline to a midday plateau and then drop to lower levels in the evening to allow normal, recuperative sleep. (Cortisol and adrenal issues are discussed at greater length in Chapter 12.)

This natural circadian cycling is lost in many people; some experience a flip-flopping of the pattern, with low levels in the morning (associated with inappropriate morning fatigue) and high levels at bedtime (associated with insomnia), which can result in stalled weight loss or weight gain. Other people have excessively high levels in the morning or throughout the entire day, a situation that can mimic the effects of taking the drug prednisone, and anyone who has taken prednisone knows that it causes an explosive increase in appetite and weight gain. High cortisol can mimic this effect, stalling weight loss or causing weight gain.

The most common cause for such disruptions is unrelenting emotional or physical stress. In addition, the same processes that disrupt thyroid function (exposure to the autoimmune effects of grains, exposure to industrial chemicals, inflammatory signals gone haywire due to weight gain, visceral fat accumulation) can be blamed for disruptions of cortisol.[7] Persistently high cortisol levels are especially destructive to a weight-loss effort, as higher cortisol levels tend to result in diminished muscle mass and higher insulin levels, which encourage fat deposition and halt weight loss.

Cortisol status therefore needs to be assessed, usually with a salivary cortisol assessment. See page 266 for details on how to do this and what steps can be taken to correct your individual cortisol issue.

While it may involve some effort and expense, correcting an adrenal issue involving cortisol and circadian rhythms can finally break a frustrating weight plateau, much as stopping prednisone stops weight gain.

Correcting cortisol patterns can also help restore health in other areas by helping reduce visceral abdominal fat, blood sugar, and blood pressure; achieve better quality sleep; and increase daytime energy. Getting cortisol status back in the proper circadian rhythm can help you be happier, more energetic, better rested, and more slender. Yup: night and day.

STRESS: THE GREAT WEIGHT-LOSS SPOILER

Chronic stress caused by relationships, work, financial worries, and other major life issues can block weight loss. This occurs due to higher levels of cortisol, inflammatory responses, and our tendency to lose control over impulsive and comforting food choices when we're stressed. If sustained over a long period, this can lead to further disruptions in cortisol's circadian rhythmicity and even greater loss of control over weight, as well as fatigue and depression.

Unfortunately, chronic stress is probably the toughest item to control on this list of weight-loss impediments, as the solution is to try the best you can to remove the source of stress or remove yourself from the situation. I know that this is not always possible; you can't exactly remove yourself from an aging parent with dementia or an autistic child whose care you provide. It is therefore impossible to offer easy, pat solutions to the many complex situations that can lead you here. Suffice it to say that it helps to know that chronic stress, regardless of the source, impairs health, and the stall in weight loss is just one expression of the metabolic distortions that stress has provoked. Realize this and, over time, try to craft solutions that minimize your involvement in the stress-provoking situation, if possible.

DRUGS BLOCK WEIGHT LOSS

A number of commonly prescribed drugs can block your ability to lose weight, no matter how serious your nutritional efforts. The "drug for every condition" mentality that applies in modern health care means that even if you have to endure weight gain or impaired weight loss, you will still be prescribed a drug. We are not talking about rare, exotic drugs; we are talking about common drugs used to treat common conditions, such as hypertension, depression, and diabetes. We are talking about tens of millions of people who take such drugs, all suffering with the side effect of weight gain. Beta-blockers, such as metoprolol, atenolol, carvedilol, and propranolol; antidepressants, including amitriptyline (Elavil), doxepin, paroxetine (Paxil), and trazodone, as well as others; Lyrica for fibromyalgia and pain; valproic acid (Depakote) for seizures; Actos and Avandia for prediabetes and diabetes; and insulin have all been associated with weight gain or failure to lose weight when attempting weight loss.

It's no surprise that injectable insulin, being the hormone of fat storage, is an especially powerful drug that impairs weight loss or causes weight gain. I've seen patients gain 20, 30, even 50 or more pounds within several months of initiating long-acting insulin preparations. It's easy to reduce insulin by eliminating grains, along with other carbohydrates and sugars. It is critical to avoid hypoglycemia when doing so, and reductions in insulin doses (injectable or continuous by pump) of 50 percent are typically needed during the first few days, and sometimes even within the first 24 hours. Identifying a health-care practitioner with interest and knowledge in reversing diabetes is extremely helpful and makes this process safer. This is such an important issue that it is discussed at greater length in Chapter 10. Reducing, then eliminating, the need for insulin is typically associated with a renewed ability to lose weight.

There are many other drugs that impair weight loss. Obviously, attempts to reduce or eliminate these drugs should be undertaken with the knowledge and cooperation of your health-care provider, as no prescribed medication should just be stopped. Discuss how and why you would like to wean off of or discontinue these drugs. If you encounter resistance, ignorance, or a refusal to discuss or answer questions, find a health-care practitioner who will work with you; they are out there.

GET ADEQUATE ZZZZ'S

You must sleep. All mammals need it. All lower creatures need it. If you don't get it, you can die. And if you compromise on quantity or quality, you cannot lose weight.

Sleep deprivation has major implications for health, with inadequate sleep increasing risk for high blood pressure, asthma, arthritis, diabetes, heart disease, and stroke. It also carries implications for weight.[8] Lack of sleep increases cortisol and insulin, impairs sensitivity to insulin, and increases appetite, all of which add up to stalled weight loss or weight gain. And the less sleep you get, the worse it gets. This occurs with even a single night of reduced sleep. While there is some debate over the details of just why and how sleep deprivation adds to weight, including uncertainty over effects on appetite-regulating hormones such as leptin and ghrelin, it is clear that inadequate sleep increases appetite and triggers increased calorie intake of 300 to 559 calories per day.[9] Interestingly, increased calories tend to come not from increased portion sizes at meals, but from an increase in snacking.[10] Just several days per week of poor sleep can therefore have a substantial impact on appetite and calorie intake, especially if increased calories come in the form of grains or sugars. If we do the arithmetic, three nights per week of poor sleep can add 22 pounds of added weight over the course of a year. Compound the increased appetite and calorie intake with the overlapping effects of opiates from grains, and you have a powerfully effective way to gain a substantial amount of weight very quickly. Adequate sleep after grain elimination is therefore crucial to gaining control over hormonal status and appetite and allows weight loss to occur.

How much sleep is enough? This obviously varies from individual to individual, but most people require 7½ hours to prevent the effects of sleep deprivation. After several days of reduced sleep, a "sleep debt" accumulates that magnifies the metabolic distortions that contribute to both weight gain and unhealthy effects. One full night of sleep does not completely undo the impact of the sleep debt. Several days of sleep beyond the usual 7½ hours (usually 9 hours or more per night) are required to normalize glucose, insulin, cortisol, and leptin distortions.[11]

You may have noticed that normal, uninterrupted sleep occurs in 90-minute "packages" (for example, a full night could be 7½ hours or 9 hours). These durations allow your brain to completely cycle through all of the sleep phases, from light sleep to the deepest phases, including rapid eye movement (REM), which is sleep accompanied by dreaming. Because it's best to adhere to this normal cycling of sleep, set your alarm to a quantity of time that honors this physiologic phenomenon; it helps with alertness and mood and may even contribute to health. There are also several devices now available that can wake you gently at the set time using either increasingly bright light; a soothing, nonjarring sound; or vibration. Smart phone apps are also appearing, often coupled with a device (such as the Lark Un-Alarm Clock and Sleep Sensor or the UP system by Jawbone) to gently awaken you after tracking your sleep behavior and quality over the preceding night.

Sleep apnea, a condition where the airway becomes obstructed during sleep, causing the person to partially arouse from the deepest phases of sleep, can be a real wrench in the works if you're trying to improve sleep quality and achieve weight-loss success. Such "partial awakenings" can occur dozens or hundreds of times per night and are associated with many of the same metabolic distortions of sleep deprivation—but worse. People with visceral obesity and blood sugars in the prediabetic or diabetic range have as much as a 60 percent likelihood of having sleep apnea.[12] Snoring, inappropriate daytime sleepiness (even after a full night's sleep), depression, and restless legs all suggest the presence of sleep apnea. While weight loss can be curative for the majority, the accumulated sleep debt can be so severe that weight loss does not occur as readily as it does for other people. In these cases, a sleep study is needed to document the sleep apnea's severity and distinguish from some other conditions. Diagnosis is often followed by use of a continuous positive airway pressure (CPAP) device. This, of course, needs to be pursued with the help of your health-care provider.

Natural Sleep Aids

There are two natural sleep aids that I believe are superior to prescription drugs in that they help you "reset" your circadian rhythm and can even improve the architecture of sleep. This causes, for instance, lengthening of the most restorative, deep REM phases. And neither are habituating.

Melatonin

Melatonin is the natural hormone of sleep and circadian rhythmicity; its release is activated with exposure to dark and inhibited with exposure to light. (Sleeping in complete darkness, with no or minimal exposure to a bathroom light when going to the bathroom, is therefore a natural way to increase melatonin release.) Melatonin supplementation can accelerate the onset of sleep, deepening sleep and discouraging early awakening, making it very useful for restoring the normal circadian rhythmicity of sleep. Melatonin also has substantial effects in reducing blood pressure when taken as a sustained-release preparation.[13] Melatonin has been proven safe, even with long-term use.

People who have tried melatonin often declare that it doesn't work, but a little finesse in its use can go a long way toward obtaining a positive effect. For instance, if difficulty falling asleep is the issue, taking it approximately 2 or 3 hours before your desired bedtime can be helpful. It is not a sleeping pill, it is a sleep hormone; it simply makes your body more receptive to sleep. If staying asleep is your issue, then taking it at bedtime may work better to discourage early awakening; also, consider a time-release preparation for a more sustained effect. It also helps to experiment with different doses. While some people have wonderfully restful sleep with just 0.5 milligrams (mg), others require 3, 5, 10, or even 20 mg to obtain the same effect.

Melatonin's effects are enhanced by combining it with exposure to bright light in the morning, as this also helps reestablish day and night cycles. If bright sunlight is not an option, some people find it helpful to purchase high-intensity lighting (3,000 to 10,000 lux) for morning exposure, such as in the kitchen over breakfast; this also helps enhance mood and treat seasonal affective disorder.

5-Hydroxytryptophan

In addition to its helpfulness in reducing cravings during grain withdrawal, 5-hydroxytryptophan (5-HTP) can also be used to enhance sleep. Supplementation has been shown to extend deep REM sleep, suggesting that sleep is deeper and more restorative with its use.[14] As with melatonin, dose needs vary; most people take between 25 and 200 mg at bedtime. Note that 5-HTP should not be used in combination with antidepressant medications, as an excess of serotonin can result. It can, however, be used in combination with melatonin.

FAST INTERMITTENTLY

Intermittently fasting—not eating while getting plenty of water for, say, 15 to 48 hours—can be a wonderful way to break a weight-loss plateau. However, this should only be undertaken after you've confidently removed all grains and concluded your withdrawal experience. Fasting for more than 4 hours before grain elimination is absolute torture, as it means that you provoke the opiate withdrawal phenomenon every time you attempt it. For that reason, it is best to get the withdrawal process over and done with and lose the appetite-stimulating effect of grain prolamins, amylopectin, and lectins. Once you're grain-free, intermittent fasting should become an effortless, painless, seamless experience that occurs simply because you are no longer hungry.

Fasting can follow a number of patterns. For instance, you could have a healthy breakfast and then have nothing until the next day. Or you could skip breakfast, skip lunch, and then have a healthy dinner. Helpful fasts can be as brief as 15 hours or as long as weeks. Just be sure to stay well hydrated during that time.

Intermittent brief fasts can improve health in a number of ways, as has been proven by various groups who incorporate fasting for religious purposes, such as Seventh-Day Adventists, members of the Greek Orthodox Church, and Christians practicing the Daniel fast from the Bible. All practice intermittent fasting in one form or another and enjoy reduced risk for cardiovascular disease, diabetes, hypertension, and cancer.[15] You can re-create many of these benefits with intermittent fasting conducted outside of religious practice.

I'm guilty of repeating myself, but be sure to hydrate vigorously, as dehydration is the most common reason for experiencing symptoms such as light-headedness, nausea, and unexplained fatigue. Intermittent fasting should not be confused with the habitual skipping of meals, such as always skipping breakfast; habitually skipping meals in a consistent pattern causes weight *gain* due to a compensatory reduction in metabolic rate. If you skip meals, do so in an unpredictable and random pattern, so that your body does not adjust and ratchet down its metabolic rate.

People who should not practice intermittent fasting include pregnant women, those who are ill for any reason, individuals with uncorrected hypothyroidism or adrenal dysfunction, and people with type 1 diabetes. Anyone with type 2 diabetes, hypertension, or other medical conditions that require medication should discuss the possibility of temporarily stopping certain medications, especially insulin, oral drugs for blood sugar (specifically glimepiride, glyburide, and glipizide), and blood pressure drugs during the fasting period, particularly if it will be conducted for longer than 24 hours. The help of a knowledgeable functional medicine practitioner, naturopath, or other enlightened professional is priceless when dealing with this issue.

I believe that, more than the pound or so lost per day during every 24-hour fasting period, it is the renewed appreciation for food and the reawakened sense of taste that are responsible for the benefits of intermittent fasting. You will rediscover what food tastes like and enjoy every bite, every mouthful, as you become more mindful of eating.

MUSCLE THE FAT AWAY

Ever notice how many people, having lost a substantial quantity of weight, have abnormally skinny arms and legs, and saggy skin? This is partly due to loss of muscle.

Many people embarking on their grain-free adventure have previously lost weight, then regained it, yo-yo dieting many times. Each time you lose weight, approximately 30 percent of the lost weight is muscle.[16] A 30-pound weight loss, for instance, means losing 10 pounds of muscle—a substantial amount. When the weight is regained, it is virtually entirely fat, without replacement of the muscle. You are therefore worse off metabolically with weight regain than you were before you lost weight initially. This effect worsens with aging, as muscle is lost with the aging process, resulting in a state of excessive fat and depleted muscle, a condition some call "sarcobesity" (sarcopenia, or muscle loss, combined with obesity).[17]

Because muscle is a metabolically active tissue that makes a major contribution to the body's overall metabolic rate, reduction in muscle mass means reduced metabolic rate, which impairs future efforts at weight loss. Many people have noticed, for instance, that each weight-loss effort gets tougher and tougher; blame this on the relative reduction in muscle mass.

You can rebuild muscle mass and counteract this effect. This involves strength training efforts, which can increase muscle mass by many pounds when practiced consistently over months and years. Strength training provides other benefits, as well, such as reduced blood sugar, improved insulin response, improved sense of well-being, improved bone density, and reduced potential for falls later in life.[18] In my view, *everyone* should engage in strength training and develop this as a lifelong habit. In addition to strength training, engage in other muscle-building activities such as climbing stairs, performing heavy yard work or housework, or learning some yoga moves, all of which add to muscle.

If you gauge results by the scale, however, you may be disappointed initially. Because building muscle adds weight, the pounds will not drop off as quickly as you might like, though fat is indeed being reduced. Better ways to gauge your efforts while adding muscle include measuring waist size, measuring percent body fat using a body fat meter, or just looking in the mirror. Good muscle volume is suggested by erect posture, firm arms and legs, and a strong gait.

PROSECUTE SEX OFFENSES

Grain consumption is not sexy. If anything, grain consumption is the great disrupter of sex hormone status, turning normal hormone regulation into a swampy, murky mess. Getting rid of grains begins the process of reversing this situation, but you may need to take it further when achieving your ideal weight is among your goals.

We've discussed how correcting disruptions of insulin, cortisol, and thyroid hormones is important when you're trying to regain control over health and weight. Correcting imbalances in the sex hormones testosterone, estrogen, and progesterone can be similarly important. Overweight women typically have higher levels of estrogen, which can impair a weight-loss effort and forever banish you to a life of plus sizes.[19] The best solution to a high estrogen level is to lose the visceral fat that caused the high level of estrogen in the first place, rather than blocking or removing the excess estrogen (which requires toxic prescription drugs). As weight drops, levels of estrogens in the bloodstream and tissues decline—a normal and natural process.

Progesterone is another story. In women, this hormone declines naturally beginning in the late thirties and is associated with depression, disrupted or more difficult menstrual cycles, dry skin, thinning hair, impaired sleep and insomnia, and weight gain. Unfortunately, progesterone has undeservedly acquired a bad reputation due to the adverse effects observed in clinical trials when synthetic forms of progesterone (progestins) were used, resulting in an increased risk for breast cancer. Supplementing with the naturally occurring or bioidentical form does not appear to be associated with such adverse effects, at least based on preliminary observations.[20] Progesterone used all by itself will not result in much weight-loss success, but progesterone in addition to grain elimination and the other efforts discussed in this book will provide a considerable advantage.

Progesterone supplementation can help restore a more youthful capacity for weight loss and give you a feeling of well-being, thicker hair, and smoother skin. It can also reduce glucose levels, triglycerides, and inflammatory markers.[21] Progesterone can be taken orally or transdermally via creams mixed by compounding pharmacies and applied to the regions specified by your practitioner. A health-care practitioner knowledgeable about the hormonal issues unique to women and who has an interest in bioidentical hormone replacement can help you assess your progesterone status and devise a regimen appropriate for your stage of life (perimenopausal, premenopausal, menopausal, or postmenopausal).

Women may also benefit from a more extended evaluation that includes testosterone and DHEA, an adrenal hormone that is much like testosterone in effect. While many overweight women have high testosterone levels, an occasional woman has a low level that can impair weight loss, especially if it's combined with depression. Women with low testosterone tend to struggle with weight, libido, strength, and mood; correction of low testosterone results in increased muscle mass (which facilitates weight loss), increased strength, and increased sexual desire.[22] Because women convert DHEA to modest amounts of testosterone, some practitioners choose to supplement DHEA to enhance testosterone. DHEA can be taken orally, or testosterone and/or DHEA can be added to compounded cream preparations mixed by a compounding pharmacy. DHEA supplementation in doses ranging from 5 to 25 mg per day, rarely higher, can yield a more modest increase in testosterone and testosterone effects, if that is desired. Under proper supervision, such hormonal manipulations can yield dramatic improvements in mood, energy, and sleep quality, as well as improved control over weight. Just be careful with DHEA doses greater than 5 to 10 mg; they can be associated with increased mustache hair and aggressive behavior in women.

In men, excess visceral fat is associated with low levels of testosterone, due to both low testosterone production in the testicles and increased conversion of testosterone to estrogen by the abnormally active aromatase enzyme in visceral fat. Loss of visceral fat reduces aromatase activity, thereby increasing testosterone levels, not uncommonly *doubling* blood levels.[23] Low testosterone levels may therefore correct themselves with weight loss. DHEA can be added to a weight-loss effort, though the effects tend to be modest. Doses of up to 25 mg, and occasionally 50 mg, may be required, but beware of increased aggression at higher levels.[24] Management of both testosterone and DHEA are best undertaken under the supervision of a knowledgeable health-care practitioner. However, if weight refuses to drop after a reasonable effort, consider having free and total testosterone levels assessed, and supplement testosterone if levels are low (especially 350 ng/ml or less; the lower the level, the more likely it is a factor impairing weight loss). Testosterone is available as a prescription cream, patch, or gel, and in injectable forms. Creams or gels mixed by compounding pharmacies cost a fraction of what's charged for patches and gels supplied by pharmaceutical manufacturers. Locate a compounding pharmacy in your area by searching online; most states now have several.

HYDRATION FIXATION

The effect of vigorous hydration is small, but it can make a modest contribution toward losing weight.[25] An occasional person, especially one with a weak thirst-warning mechanism and who often confuses dehydration with hunger, can experience a more substantial weight loss benefit because attention to hydration can preempt this confusion.

Gauging the adequacy of hydration is tricky. I am not a fan of simple rules that involve gauging need by body weight or other measures, as individual variation in the way we handle fluids is too wide. The ability of our kidneys to concentrate fluid, the water content in our stool, our use of diuretics (caffeine and prescription drugs), exposure to varying ambient temperatures and humidity, type of clothing worn, tendency to sweat, and intensity of physical activity all affect how much liquid we really need. The hydration needs of a resident of Miami who spends plenty of time outdoors, walks and bikes while wearing shorts and a T-shirt, and drinks three cups of coffee per day will be very different than the hydration needs of a Minnesota resident who wears many layers of clothing, has little exposed skin, lives a sedentary lifestyle, and drinks no coffee. One person's adequate fluid intake may mean someone else's dehydration.

Simple methods to gauge the adequacy of fluid intake include urinating at least every 4 hours and passing nearly clear urine, never dark yellow or amber. (Note that B vitamins that contain riboflavin and some drugs can influence urine color.) Some people even use dipsticks (available in pharmacies) to check the specific gravity, or the relative concentration, of their urine; maintaining a level of 1.010 or less is desirable. If urine specific gravity is consistently, say, 1.020 or 1.030, that signals inadequate hydration (assuming normal kidney function).

Water is, by far, the best hydrating fluid. Coffee and tea, while they fit into a grain-free lifestyle, cause modest dehydration through their diuretic action. Carbonated beverages, even if they're unsweetened, are not the best due to the net acidifying action of the carbonic acid that provides carbonation. Dilute forms of coconut milk (in cartons, not cans; canned coconut milk is primarily useful for baking) and coconut water are excellent sources of fluid, as they are rich in electrolytes like potassium and are even useful for athletes. (See Appendix A for simple recipes to make a basic electrolyte solution helpful for hydration, including a useful beverage to sip during weight-loss efforts.) Note that improved hydration can add a pound or two that has nothing to do with body fat; it's just the weight of the fluid you've ingested.

OTHER FACTORS

There are some factors that make a small contribution to weight loss. None of these will, on their own, make the difference required to lose, say, 30 pounds, but they can help you lose the last few pounds of visceral fat or compound the weight-loss effects of all the other strategies you adopt.

Bowel Flora

The connection between bowel flora and weight is proving to be complex. Bowel flora composition undergoes a marked change as diet transitions from grain-based to grain-free. Are there any advantages gained by manipulating bowel flora with, say, probiotics or other supplements?

So far, the only strategy that has proven modestly effective in accelerating weight loss through bowel flora is the addition of prebiotics, fibers that are indigestible by humans but digestible by bacteria that dwell in our intestinal tracts (see Chapter 9). Inulin and fructooligosaccharide forms of prebiotic fibers, in particular, have been shown to modestly accelerate loss of abdominal fat.[26] Effective doses range from 10 to 20 g per day, with higher doses yielding undesirable gas and bloating. In addition to inulin sold in powder form at health food stores, you can find inulin and fructooligosaccharide fibers in some foods and nonnutritive sweeteners. (See Appendix D for a listing.)

Drink Coffee and Tea

This is by no means a big effect, or else all coffee and tea drinkers would be skinny. But thanks to caffeine and other components, such as chlorogenic acid, 2 to 3 cups per day of caffeinated or decaffeinated coffee or green, oolong, or white tea can yield modest weight-reduction effects. These drinks also provide other health benefits, including reduced potential for diabetes and Parkinson's disease.[27]

Stop the Alcohol

The ethanol in alcoholic beverages slows the mobilization of fatty acids from fat stores, essentially turning off weight loss.[28] For this reason, many people have observed that weight loss proceeds as expected, only to grind to a complete halt when they drink an alcoholic beverage. The weight-loss impairing effect of alcohol is compounded by the generous carbohydrate content of beers and some flavored drinks, not to mention the prolamin protein residues in alcoholic beverages, especially beers brewed from wheat, barley, rye, and corn. These yield appetite-stimulating opiates that are sure to derail your weight-loss efforts.

A single serving of alcohol will partially slow weight loss, but two or more drinks will turn off weight loss completely, potentially even causing modest weight gain. If you desire an alcoholic beverage during an ongoing weight-loss effort, then recognize that it is best to choose from the lowest carbohydrate forms, such as red wine, low-carbohydrate nonwheat beers (Michelob Ultra or Bud Light), or clear spirits (vodka, gin, or rum).

Other Food Intolerances

Occasionally, an intolerance to foods other than grains can cause weight gain or failure to lose weight, likely via an inflammatory mechanism. Most commonly, this involves dairy, eggs, peanuts, soy, shellfish, and sea-food. One way to tackle this question is to eliminate each of these foods, one at a time, for 4 weeks. Observe the effect; if you lose weight, you have fingered the culprit. Alternatively, there are a variety of tests that can identify food intolerances (see Appendix D). The science behind this approach is preliminary, so put this strategy at the bottom of your list.

DON'T WASTE YOUR TIME

While the items to consider when encountering a weight-loss plateau make a somewhat lengthy list, notice what I did not include.

- **Exercise more.** An occasional person can indeed experience accelerated weight loss with aerobic forms of exercise, but most people obtain only modest advantage, if any at all. There is no question that exercise is good for overall health, but it generally provides minimal to no advantage for weight loss. Exercise for health and, should you lose a few extra pounds, consider it a bonus. (This is to be distinguished from exercise that grows muscle, which *can* provide weight-loss advantages; see the discussion above.)

- **Eat less or cut calories.** Not only is calorie reduction misery, it can jeopardize your efforts because your metabolic rate will eventually drop, turning off your ability to lose weight.

- **Cut fat intake.** Cutting fat does not cut weight. This is part of the outdated notion of "calories in, calories out," an idea you should leave behind with shoulder pads and velour tracksuits.

- **Reduce portion sizes.** We eat until we are satisfied, and to avoid hunger and its impulse-eroding effects. We don't reduce portion sizes for the same reasons that we don't cut calories.

- **Various nutritional supplements.** You don't need *Irvingia gabanensis*, green coffee bean extract, white bean extract, hydroxycitric acid, or many others. Clinical data here tend to be relatively weak and real world experience tends to yield disappointing results. In general, such supplements are very costly ways to lose—best-case scenario—a pound or two.

SHOP IN THE PETITE SECTION

It is a rare individual who, after following a diet free of grains, eating healthy foods as discussed in this book, and checking off each and every one of the strategies offered, fails to obtain the weight loss they desire. Recall that what you are really trying to do is regain health while losing weight along the way. Excess weight is just one outward manifestation of something amiss in health; weight loss is a reflection of having corrected it.

One last thought: Attitude counts. I have watched many people approach weight loss by saying something like, "There's no way this will work for me." Or, "Nothing has ever worked before." Or, "I've always been fat and I will probably always stay that way." Such attitudes tend to be self-fulfilling. If you expect to be overweight, you will be. You will find ways to undermine your success.

On the other hand, if you fully expect to fit into that size 4 dress or jeans 6 inches smaller in the waist, even going so far as to purchase the new clothes you plan to wear, you are far more likely to achieve your goal. Set yourself up for success and, more often than not, you will hurdle over the obstacles that get in your way.

CHAPTER 15

CLEARER, SMARTER, FASTER: GRAIN-FREE PERFORMANCE

It wasn't a new training program that took me from being a very good player to the best player in the world in just 18 months. It wasn't a new racquet, a new workout, a new coach, or even a new serve that helped me lose weight, find mental focus, and enjoy the best health of my life. It was a new diet.
—Novak Djokovic

I HOPE THAT, by now, you recognize the power of removing grains from your diet. You can take an antibiotic to treat an infection or a drug to make you sleep or relieve back pain. But no drug or other health practice provides the breadth of health benefits achieved with grain elimination. No single drug can reduce blood sugar, get rid of skin rashes, reverse inflammation and autoimmunity, reduce appetite, provide relief from joint pain, elevate mood, and reverse hormonal distortions. Sure, there are drugs that address one issue at a time, for a substantial cost and accompanied by side effects. But there is no single drug that can even begin to match the power of grain elimination.

But improve human performance? Can elimination of grains do more than just free you from the health-impairing effects of the seeds of grasses, but actually unleash physical, mental, and life performance?

Yes: Grain-free people are more optimistic, smarter, learn more effectively, make better athletes, and make better lovers. We are not grain-free supremacists; we are people who have removed the yoke of impairment placed on us by the easy, accessible, and addictive products of the seeds of grasses. We choose to cast off this burden and revert back to life and performance the way they were supposed to be.

Improvements in performance apply to just about every setting and situation that you can imagine, from the classroom to the office, from the tennis court to the golf course, from the basketball court to the football field, and even to the bedroom. Grain-free performance means that you can be freed from common impediments to performance such as joint pain, swelling, bloating and gas, water retention, and mind fog, leaving you able to run longer, jump higher, think more clearly, and focus longer and more effectively. It can also mean renewed libido and erectile capacity for men, less bothersome menstrual cycles and menopausal symptoms for women, as well as reinvigorated libido. You name it, and there can be enhanced performance in that sphere of human endeavor.

In sports, we are hearing about more and more athletes shunning all things gluten (wheat, rye, barley), including tennis player Novak Djokovic, golfer Sarah-Jane Smith, New Orleans Saints quarterback Drew Brees, and Olympic runner Andrew Steele. Djokovic's first year without wheat and gluten was his best year ever; he won three Grand Slams and 50 of 51 matches. I propose that wheat and gluten elimination will raise the bar for performance standards in sports, setting a higher level that other athletes will need to work to reach. Being grain-free will become a requirement for performing at high levels and competing effectively.

You don't have to be a professional athlete, of course, to enjoy the performance benefits of grain elimination. Even if the only competition you engage in is trying to win at bingo in church, you can still enjoy substantial benefits by going grain-free.

LIFE IN THE GRAIN-FREE FAST LANE

How might grain elimination enhance human performance? The reasons behind improved performance for the ungrained constitute an impressive list. Let's put aside that grain elimination offers relief from countless health conditions, which we've discussed in the earlier chapters of this book. Instead, let's focus on why reverting back to the grain-free lifestyle that humans were supposed to follow results in being a more capable and effective human being.

Increased Energy

Among the most common observations reported by the newly grain-free is a surge in physical and mental energy. Comments such as, "I have more energy than I've had in years" and "I've turned the clock back 20 years and feel 30 years old again" are everyday events. Greater energy translates into higher levels of work, school, and life performance. Tackling a new project, writing a lengthy report, building a shed, cooking dinner for six—it's all less daunting, less burdensome, and more easily accomplished. You no longer have to make excuses: You don't have to tell the kids you don't have the energy to play ball, you don't have to tell your partner that you're too tired or disinterested to have sex, and you no longer have to bow out of activities because of pain and stiffness.

Unfortunately, energy is not something formally assessed through clinical studies, so there are no such data to cite. But it would not be a far leap to speculate that the removal of the mind-clouding effects of exorphins derived from gliadin and related grain proteins, reductions of blood sugar and inflammation, improved sleep duration and quality, and correction of hormonal distortions would all add up to the wonderfully increased energy levels experienced by the grain-free.

Exercise used to be a chore.

Now, without the carbs and wheat, I crave the workout. Now I feel as good as and perform like I am in 9th grade. Absolutely amazing. I was running today on the treadmill. I had to get off the treadmill at 60 minutes *only* because someone else was in line to use it, not because I wanted to.

My peers are all sluggish, and they say I am like a broken record: "Get off the wheat, get off the carbs." But they sound like broken records, too: "I hurt here," "I can't do this or that," "My headaches are back," "I need new pants because these are tight," "I'm sleepy at midday."

My athleticism is increasing at a phenomenal rate. I've done several half marathons, and I'm looking at a full marathon this year.

Wayne, Woodstock, Georgia

Improved Sleep

Deeper sleep means better restorative sleep, during which you may experience more vivid, colorful dreams—the kind you had as a child. Dreams may involve flying, dragons, monsters, and showing up in class unprepared to give your speech, but that's good, because it signals more time spent in the deepest, most restorative, phases of sleep, phase four and rapid eye movement (REM) sleep.

Many people also experience relief from the sleep-disruptive effects of restless leg syndrome. Weight lost from visceral fat experienced with grain elimination can provide relief from the sleep disruption of sleep apnea, reducing snoring and the need for corrective measures, such as a continuous positive airway pressure (CPAP) device or throat surgery. This also reverses the many health consequences sleep apnea can bring, such as hypertension, diabetes, heart disease, depression, and the need for medication.

Longer and deeper restorative sleep means that daytime functioning is improved: You'll experience freedom from the impediments of sleepiness, such as irritation, inattention, and impaired recall, while enjoying greater alertness, better mood, and improved capacity to learn. It can also contribute to a reduced need for medications for alertness, hypertension, high blood sugar, and depression.

Heightened Mental Clarity and Alertness

Getting rid of grains means you are no longer being doped. Getting rid of the morphinelike by-products of gliadin and related prolamin proteins from grains means you no longer have to contend with the mind fog, distractibility, difficulty sustaining attention, and diminished alertness that they bring. Once grain withdrawal is over, clarity, ability to concentrate for extended periods, and easier data acquisition and recall are common observations. We see this in children with attention deficit disorder and autistic spectrum disorder, and we see it in kids without these conditions. We see it in adults who have struggled because they're unable to sit, read a book or report, and recall and understand what they have read; once grain-free, they are able to sustain attention, understand, and retain in detail. We see it in the classroom setting with sustained concentration, improved recall, and improved capacity to synthesize and create, and we also see it in the work setting with capacity for sustained focus, sharpened delivery of information, and easier adaptation to challenges.

The roller-coaster ride of moods is reduced or eliminated after you lose the prolamin protein–derived exorphins. Moods are smoother and more appropriate to the situation; they're not the wild and inappropriate moods responsible for regrettable conversations, unjustified anxiety, angry outbursts, and tearful confrontations of the grained.

Amped-Up Metabolism

Consumption of grain amylopectin starches impairs physical performance. Failure to recognize this simple truth has thrown a generation of marathon runners, triathletes, and other endurance athletes off course. It has sidelined countless tennis, soccer, and football players, not to mention misguided weekend warriors and amateur athletes. It has created a world of athletes and wannabe athletes who, on the evening prior to an event, load up on pasta and other carbohydrates ("carb-load"), then eat bread, cookies, and energy bars and drink sugary drinks immediately before and during the event. This practice was based on studies that demonstrated that when athletes (or soldiers, or others experiencing various forms of deprivation) are deprived of carbohydrates, their performance suffers. When carbohydrates are added back, their performance improves.[1]

There is no doubt that elimination of carbohydrates, including amylopectin starches from grains, reduces performance during, say, running, biking, or combat—for the first 4 to 6 weeks in people who have come to depend on them for metabolism. Deprive the liver of dietary carbohydrate sources to produce glycogen (the energy storage form of glucose), and less glycogen is available to convert to glucose for muscle energy. But the process changes over time after carbohydrates are removed from the diet. Improved physical performance does not appear until 4 to 6 weeks after the body has moved away from reliance on liver glycogen and toward reliance on metabolizing fatty acids. This means that many studies of carbloading that demonstrated improved physical performance with restoration of carbohydrates were conducted for too short a time to allow for the energy conversion process to occur. After the initial 4 to 6 weeks are over, when glycogen reliance has been replaced with fatty acid metabolism, performance capacity then returns.

But it gets even better. If grain elimination—and thereby elimination of amylopectin starches—is carried out for even longer, physical performance is *improved* over that experienced during grain-consuming days. Stephen Phinney, MD, PhD, has been the pioneer in documenting and studying this effect. In his first study, overweight, untrained volunteers exercised on a treadmill before the diet change, then 1 week into an extreme low-carbohydrate (grain-free, near-zero-carbohydrates, or ketogenic, diet) effort, then again after 6 weeks on the low-carb restriction. While performance decreased during week 1, performance was spectacularly improved at week 6, with participants demonstrating 48 percent better endurance before exhaustion set in. Even more incredibly, because participants had lost an average of 22 pounds over the 6 weeks, during the 6-week endurance test each participant was required to wear a backpack that contained a weight equivalent to what they'd lost.[2] Dr. Phinney conducted a similar study with trained bicyclists. In spite of their superior health at the start of the study, they still saw minor weight loss and modest increases in performance. Also, the energy they consumed during exercise came almost exclusively from fat.[3]

This means that athletes will have to endure 4 to 6 weeks of diminished performance when eliminating grains and ceasing practices such as carb-loading, but they'll be rewarded with increased performance over a longer period. And by eliminating grain amylopectins, they'll also avoid the long-term joint and cartilage destruction that they provoke via inflammation and glycation that can result from the destructive practice of carb-loading.

Note that living without grain amylopectins also translates into greater reliance on burning fat stores. While the liver can store around 60 grams of energy as glycogen, which is enough to supply energy for 30 to 40 minutes of continuous exertion, even slender people have pounds of stored fat to draw on for energy, a virtually limitless source compared to what we get from glycogen. And burning fat is how you maintain a healthy weight, not by adding to it with the blood sugar and insulin effects of grain amylopectins.

Reduction or Elimination of Joint Pain and Stiffness

Mobility and flexibility are typically improved with grain elimination, providing obvious advantages in physical performance. Because removing grains removes the excess inflammation brought about by prolamins, lectins, allergens, and the effects of visceral fat, joint inflammation recedes, allowing you to bend, kneel, stand, walk, run, jump, or return a tough tennis serve more easily and with less or no pain.

Interestingly, many athletes and other hard-playing people also report faster recovery after eliminating grains. The soreness and stiffness that many people feel for as many as several days after a day of yard work or 20 minutes of strength training are reduced to a barely perceptible level, if they happen at all.

Increased Muscle Mass

Though gains vary from person to person, grain elimination results in increased muscle mass and increased muscle strength. People who strength train typically find that they can handle greater amounts of weight with less effort. They also maintain muscle mass and strength longer, even during periods when they don't strength train.

This gain in muscle can be experienced as a substantial reduction in waist and hip size unaccompanied by a commensurate loss of weight. To gauge this effect, you can track your body fat percentage and lean muscle mass (using a body fat analyzer device), or you can just appreciate the developing changes you see in the mirror (though not necessarily on the scale).

Increased muscle has many health benefits, including reduced potential for falls and injury; sustained youthful coordination and balance for walking, climbing, and jumping; improved insulin responses; and less potential for osteoporosis. Extra muscle also helps maintain a youthful appearance, as well as a feeling of youthfulness.

Less Gastrointestinal Distress

Surely nobody likes an attack of gas and bloating during a meeting, while sitting in class, or during a romantic evening. Being freed of the discomfort, bloating, gas, constipation, and diarrhea of irritable bowel syndrome (IBS) and other common grain-related gastrointestinal conditions is liberating. Not only are you spared the pain and distraction of these conditions, you are also spared the need to anticipate unexpected urgencies. You no longer have to plan trips, even those in your own neighborhood, based on the availability of a public toilet. This alone changes lives.

If an athlete has IBS, which 25 percent of the population suffers from, they can have disruptive and embarrassing bouts in the middle of a swim competition or baseball game. If you aren't an athlete yourself, it may be hard to understand the importance of this. However, if you could ask someone how the discomfort and inconvenience of IBS affected his or her performance, or talk to a distance runner who has had to deal with explosive bowel movements around mile 12, you'd understand. No human, athlete or otherwise, was meant to endure the uncomfortable, inconvenient, and distressful gastrointestinal disruption associated with the consumption of the seeds of grasses.

Enhanced Libido

Saying "no thanks" to the basket of bread at the start of a romantic dinner is better than any aphrodisiac. Because wheat elimination reduces estrogen and raises testosterone in men and reduces abnormally high estrogens in women, libido is increased. Increased libido is associated with enhanced sexual performance and drive, which translates into improvements in other spheres of life, including the health of your relationship.

I predict that, in the future, the advantages in performance achieved with grain elimination will be so sharp that we will be able to distinguish the grained from the ungrained, the underperforming grain-consumer from the highly performing grain-avoider. Go ahead, choose your side.

A HIGH-PERFORMANCE CHECKLIST

Many of the strategies that extend beyond grain elimination, but nonetheless have an impact on overall performance, have been discussed throughout this book. But viewed from the perspective of performance, these important strategies include:

- **Restoring vitamin D.** Vitamin D, restored to healthful levels (in my view 60 to 70 ng/ml) is an absolute requirement; it is second only to elimination of all grains if you want to achieve high levels of performance. Vitamin D alone increases mental clarity, improves mood, and reduces the potential for seasonal affective disorder. It also improves energy, deepens sleep, and leads to better memory. (Vitamin D is discussed in greater detail in Chapter 8.)

- **Achieving ideal thyroid status.** Thyroid dysfunction impairs bodily functions at just about every level. Correcting hypothyroidism is crucial if you want to achieve your highest levels of performance, as well as health and weight control. The degree of improvement will depend on the degree of thyroid dysfunction at the start of your journey, with the greatest benefits seen by those beginning with the greatest degree of dysfunction. Restoration of the T3 thyroid hormone, in particular, can be associated with perceptible improvements in mental clarity, concentration, and mood. (The process for identifying and correcting thyroid dysfunction is discussed in greater detail in Chapter 11.)

- **Identifying other forms of endocrine disruption, especially disruption of cortisol circadian rhythmicity.** If your normal 24-hour cycle of cortisol is disrupted, so is your daytime energy, sleep quality, and performance. Correction may involve a long-term effort but is rewarded by improved performance, better sleep quality, and higher morning and afternoon energy. (Endocrine disruption is discussed in detail in Chapter 12.)

- **Restoring healthy bowel flora with probiotics, indigestible prebiotic fibers, and fermented foods.** Not only are metabolic markers such as blood sugar, insulin, and triglycerides improved by healthy bowel flora, but bowel health itself is improved, including a reduced risk for intestinal cancers. Bowel regularity is also improved, freeing you from the discomfort of constipation. (The full approach to cultivating healthy bowel flora is discussed in Chapter 9.)

- **Achieving ideal weight.** Excess weight, especially that in visceral fat, is a source of exceptional health problems. Losing it is thereby accompanied by outsize health benefits, since this loss allows inflammation and hormonal distortions to recede. Reducing the physical burden of excess weight is also liberating and healthy for long-term joint health. (An extended discussion of how to achieve ideal weight and break a weight barrier can be found in Chapter 14.)

- **Breaking free from prescription medications.** By now, you have read about all the drug-freeing effects of grain elimination. I would argue that nothing does more to free you from dependence on medications than grain elimination, which then frees you from all the performance-impairing effects of prescription drugs. These include fatigue from antidepressants, mental fog caused by beta-blockers (for hypertension and migraine headaches), sleepiness and helplessness caused by chronic pain medications, and abdominal pain caused by anti-inflammatory drugs.

- **Addressing other common nutritional deficiencies.** Iron (including ferritin levels in athletes), zinc, magnesium, and vitamin B_{12} are all especially important. Deficiency of any of these nutrients can result in performance-impairing symptoms, such as impaired stamina with low iron and ferritin, muscle cramping during physical efforts due to magnesium deficiency, or struggles with memory and thinking with vitamin B_{12} deficiency. Correcting these deficiencies that commonly result from grain consumption reverses these phenomena. (Correction of grain-induced nutritional deficiencies is discussed in Chapter 8.)

- **Maintaining adequate sleep.** The enhanced sleep quality you experience with grain elimination does not mean that you need less sleep. Getting too little sleep is among the most common causes for impaired daytime performance, even with the high-octane potential of the grain-free. It really pays to not cut corners when it comes to sleep.

Yes, being confidently grain-free is the first step. And while so many wonderful changes in health occur with that step alone, you can appreciate that there are other factors that can impair or improve performance beyond grains. Attention to *each and every one* of these is required to achieve the highest level of performance your body and mind will allow.

GRAIN ELIMINATION EXCEEDS EXPECTATIONS

People often say, "I feel 20 years younger" after they adopt an ungrained life. When they post their "before" and "after" photos on Wheat Belly social media pages, they often do look 20 years younger, sometimes in as little as several weeks, with reductions in abdominal fat, facial swelling, redness, and rashes, and improved facial contours. Though we can't see it in photos, they relate wonderful stories of regaining youthful energy, a boost in mood, flexibility, mental alertness—all the features that make life richer, easier, more satisfying, and more successful.

Compound the health benefits of grain elimination with correction of the health impairments common to modern life, some caused by grains, others not, and the end result exceeds the sum of the parts: Your life can be better than you expected it to be.

EPILOGUE

WE'VE COVERED A lot of grassy ground on this journey.

If you were desperate and hungry, not having eaten in 10 days, you would readily and instinctively know that the shellfish you stumbled upon along a shoreline, the small game running across your path, or the wild berries hanging on a bush are all food.

What if you were desperate and hungry and found yourself standing in a field of wild grass? Would your mouth start to water in anticipation of isolating the seeds, bit by bit, separating them from the husk, drying, pulverizing, and then heating them as porridge or cereal, or baking them into bread? It is a substantial leap to make. In fact, most of us would have no idea how to survive on grasses as food and would probably starve to death in their midst.

This simple insight has been lost as humans have become better and better at manipulating products from the seeds of grasses and crafting them into something resembling food.

INCANTATIONS, SPELLS, AND NUTRITIONAL SCIENCE

Looking back from our enlightened nutritional perch of the 21st century, it is truly astounding that providers of dietary advice got the details so wrong: Limit fat, cut saturated fat, use low-fat dairy, replace saturated fats with polyunsaturated fats, eat fewer eggs, trim the fat off steak, don't reduce carbohydrates (it's unnecessary and dangerous), get more fiber, eat sugar in moderation, and, of course, the worst advice of all—eat lots of grains, preferably whole grains, as often as possible. It's a message that, if followed faithfully, requires increased exercise, vitamin fortification, prescription medication, and plus-size jeans to accommodate.

Such sweeping, systematic errors are not made in physics, nor biochemistry, nor astronomy—at least not since it became clear that the Earth revolved around the sun. When Copernicus published his theory challenging the prevailing view that the sun circled the Earth, his views sparked outrage, prompting accusations that his ideas violated scripture; everyone "knew," and had known since the time of Aristotle, that the Earth was the center of the universe. We now understand, of course, that Copernicus was right, and we've sent humans into space based on theories he advanced, no pesky sun to get in our way.

While other disciplines have yielded to the light of scientific investigation and practical application, nutritional science has somehow clung to archaic, outdated, magical notions, even in our enlightened Information Age. Accusations abound that the grain-free message is sacrilegious and contrary to everything dietitians "know" to be true, and predictions that it will fizzle out as a passing fad are common. But such defenses of the tired status quo are crumbling through insights offered by real science, as we have discussed at length in this book, and it's getting harder to ignore the countless successes experienced by those applying the grain-free message. It becomes increasingly difficult to dodge the knowledge that grains caused considerable health problems in the humans who first learned how to incorporate them into their diets. It becomes silly to deny that changes have been introduced into modern grains that have uncertain, sometimes fatal, implications for the humans who consume them. It gets awfully tough to dismiss cures of ulcerative colitis, rheumatoid arthritis, diabetes, and obesity as passing "fads."

Let dietitians and other defenders of the "healthy whole grain" incantation stir their cauldrons and worship their false idols, casting spells to regain health and blaming the suffering of the public on their impiety, while us grain-free folk enjoy the freedom and health of grainless enlightenment.

A DECLARATION OF GRAIN INDEPENDENCE

Can you begin to grasp the enormity of the implications of this new—no, *old*—lifestyle? If dozens, even hundreds, of human disease conditions recede or disappear with the elimination of grains, what does this say about the current model of dietary health, which encourages us to consume what amounts to little more than a tasty poison? We've discussed how weight gain, hormonal disruptions, diabetes, "high cholesterol," disrupted digestive health, unrelenting constipation, joint pain, autoimmune conditions, changes in bowel flora, and neurological health can all be blamed on a lifestyle of "healthy whole grains." In two generations we have, by relying on grains as a primary calorie source, watched such health conditions explode, made worse by the genetic manipulations of agribusiness. And with grain consumption accounting for more than 50 percent of all human calories, we are getting sicker and sicker, fatter and fatter, and we are being told that it is our own fault.

Seeing past the ignorance, indifference, and scientific charades of the conventional message is astoundingly powerful. There is truly no other dietary insight that packs such power, no single medication that can address the range of diseases addressed by grain elimination, nothing that can restore human life to its original state in the same way that a life without grains can.

The basic arguments made in this book about regaining health minus the darlings of nutritional advice, agribusiness, Big Food, and Big Pharma are, stated simply:

- You should eat no seeds of grasses, also known as "grains," or else you unavoidably compromise health in many ways.

- Years of consuming grain products inappropriate for human consumption disrupt physiology, metabolism, and health so profoundly that you will need to navigate a way back to health. It may involve addressing issues such as bowel flora and correcting nutritional deficiencies. It may require insight into endocrine disruptions. But a full path back can be charted for the majority of people and from the majority of conditions.

- While not directly attributable to grains, there are other health issues unique to modern life that need to be addressed to facilitate recovery of total health. Because elimination of grains yields such powerful health effects, many people discover renewed conviction to correct as many health deficiencies as possible. In this book, I've discussed several worthy of addressing that yield outsize benefits.

It's really very simple. It's so simple that it should be instinctive, achieved with just a week or so of starvation while struggling for survival against the elements. But few people wish to fight for survival by rubbing sticks together to build a fire while bound in dried skins, or by hand-carving a spear that they'll use to impale a wild creature, causing them to salivate in anticipation of consuming its organs and meat. Most of us are so thoroughly removed from such survival experiences that we have come to view O-shaped breakfast cereals created by pulverizing and gluing back together the product of the seeds of grasses as not only something to swallow for momentary sustenance, but also as something healthy.

We were wrong. We were, for 300 generations, terribly, tragically wrong. But we've been *most* wrong for the last 50 years, ever since grains were placed on the altar of dietary conviction. Just because something is tasty does not make it nutritious. Just because something is available does not mean it should serve to sustain the human population. Just because we've erred for several thousand years does not make it right.

So it's time we practiced a bit of magic ourselves and exorcised the chants, spells, and conjurations of conventional nutritional "science" from our lives.

GETTING AHEAD IN A GRAIN-FREE WORLD

No question: There are significant challenges ahead as more and more people embrace a life without grains.

After all, it has been the consumption of seeds of grasses, the seeds from a ubiquitous assortment of plants covering the earth, that has allowed the world's population to grow to its present size. This grand experiment began with a few million people in the early Neolithic period 10,000 years ago and has since ballooned to today's seven billion people populating every continent—a population that's anticipated to reach 15 billion by 2050. The world's billions are now cheaply and expeditiously fed, but they consume other resources. Because it is not politically correct to talk about world over-population, we instead talk about it in its various forms of environmental impact: global climate change, overfishing and acidification of the oceans, shrinkage of the coral reefs, thinning of the ozone layer, increasing salinity and erosion of topsoil—the big issues of our day that have the potential to change the planet that spawned us. All of these environmental issues are the consequences of so many humans exploiting life on this planet, and that population expansion was made possible by the seeds of grasses.

When there is starvation in Ethiopia or Bangladesh, we don't send in pork chops and pineapples; we send in the grains. When large business transactions are made in foodstuffs, they don't involve eggs, kale, or avocados; they involve millions of tons of grains. When livestock producers want to fatten up their animals faster and more cheaply, they replace forage with grains. The seeds of grasses now play an unprecedented role in sustaining and growing the human population.

Taking them away wholesale is, obviously, impossible, and certainly inadvisable. We cannot deny the world 50 percent of its calories. Worldwide starvation would result—yes, grains can be used to feed the desperate and hungry. Forgoing grains is something best undertaken individually, with full understanding of the reasons it is advisable to do so. I am *not* advocating legislative or economic action to dictate diet to the world, or even in the United States. This is a decision best reached through reason and scientific insight, not through more legislative action or a mandate. Removing grains is something achievable by individual choice and is most feasible in the developed world, where we have access to many other food choices. How this plays out on a worldwide stage is not something I, or anyone else, can predict.

But it will spark change—upheavals, in fact—concerning which foods we choose to consume, what crops farmers choose to grow, the economic consequences of these changes, how much health care we will or will not require, and the length of our lives. These are trends that will unfold over the next several decades and centuries, not by next January. But these revelations, reached through the emerging cross talk between scientific disciplines, will win out. They will win out because it is not just about losing a few pounds to fit into your skinny jeans, nor is it only about being freed from occasional heartburn or high blood sugars. These insights will win out because they ring instinctively true and because no other practice in health holds the potential for restoring the human condition so completely as elimination of grains.

This insight gives you an advantage. If you have greater energy, less sleeplessness, less joint pain and stiffness, less emotional and bowel turmoil, and fewer or no long-term health impairments, and you do not have to lug around 30, 50, 100, or 150 extra pounds, you can outrun, outperform, outsmart, and outdo humans trapped in this grain-consuming blunder.

Will we create a world of grain-eaters versus grain-deniers, a world in which we make judgments about people we meet based on whether or not they include grains in their daily diet? If I were given a choice between a grain-consuming or a grain-free business associate, all other things being equal I would choose the grain-free individual: He or she is more likely to perform consistently, is less likely to have life and work interrupted by health problems, and is likely to be more emotionally level, less likely to give in to impulse, and more rational. Hands down, I would opt to work with the grain-free.

IT'S NATURAL TO BE HEALTHY

I hope that by now you have begun, and perhaps even completed, your early grain-free experience. It may not have been easy. Perhaps it was tumultuous. Beyond the throes of withdrawal, maybe you had to endure the odd looks and sarcastic comments of family, friends, or coworkers. But once a grain-free life is achieved, the rest is wonderfully empowering and uplifting, an experience that gets better and better as you get further and further from something that should have been nothing more than fodder for your sheep.

Your experience will be different than that of the grain-consuming world. It will be breathtakingly better. Nature provided us with the basic necessities to enjoy excellent health; we're able to run, jump, climb, hunt, fish, compete, gather, love, and reproduce. Nature did not give us the instinctive tools to grow fat, become diabetic, erode joints, inflame organs, and suffer digestive turmoil—we accomplished all that ourselves. Had we adhered to the dietary script written for us over millions of years of adaptation to the varied environments on earth, none of the health struggles we experience today would have materialized. We might have died due to gangrene suffered from a wound received while tackling vicious prey, but we would not have succumbed to the subtle, chronic, and long-term disabling effects of the seeds of grasses. Humans as a species brought this mess—initially inadvertent, but now purposefully magnified by blundering misinterpretations of nutritional "science"—upon ourselves.

Lest we end on a dark note, let me remind you that buried in all of this is a powerful message of optimism. *You* are in control of your diet and health. You do not have to submit to influences that choose to put profit, convenience, and expedience before individual welfare.

You probably shower with soap, drink filtered water, live and work in a climate-controlled environment, and change your underwear every day. But beneath the veneer of modern habits, you are little different than an unwashed, hungry, desperate human, anxious about your next meal, concerned over the safety of your offspring, comforted by the nearness of the few dozen other members of your species you hold close and with whom you carve out survival in an inhospitable world. Once you understand what is true in diet and health, you are personally empowered to regain health in countless ways and are free to achieve at your highest levels.

You are grainless. And you are empowered.

APPENDIX A

Recipes for Total Health

THIS IS NOT a recipe section in the conventional sense. You will not find recipes for breakfast, lunch, or dinner here, nor for desserts. This is a small collection of recipes and methods to create "functional foods," which are foods meant to help you achieve specific goals.

The recipes here help provide better bowel health by providing sources of healthy bacterial species, such as *Lactobacillus*, in homemade yogurts, kefirs, and fermented vegetables. Other recipes show you how to make prebiotic fiber–rich foods to cultivate proliferation of healthy bowel flora. There is a basic recipe for making soup or stock, and there are recipes for making magnesium water to restore magnesium and electrolyte water to use whenever an electrolyte replacement solution is desired in place of sugary sports drinks. So don't expect to plan any meals from this recipe section. Just plan to learn a few new lessons about how to better manage health in tasty ways.

BREW YOUR OWN PROBIOTICS: FERMENTATION

Before there was refrigeration, there was fermentation—a way for humans to store food for more than a few days after picking or harvesting. This was how, for instance, our great grandparents managed to pick radishes, cucumbers, or asparagus in summer and then consume them throughout fall and winter. They allowed foods to ferment, which is the process of degradation by bacteria and fungi. If you eat kosher pickles, prosciutto, salami, and yogurt, you are already consuming fermented foods, whether you know it or not.

While fermented foods cannot replace a high-potency probiotic (especially if the probiotic contains a large variety of bacterial strains) during the first few weeks of grain elimination, they can be very helpful for *maintaining* healthy flora and bowel health over the long term.

There are some foods that you can easily make in your own home, thereby avoiding all the nasty and unnecessary ingredients used by food manufacturers and saving lots of money. Let's begin with yogurts and kefirs, both made from dairy products or coconut milk.

Yogurt and Kefir

If dairy is part of your diet, making your own yogurt and kefir allows you to use full-fat milk to start. Manufacturers have given in to the silly advice to reduce fat, which is desired by most ill-informed consumers, and as a result, it has become more and more difficult to find full-fat versions of dairy products on store shelves. Get around this by making your own.

People with some form of dairy intolerance have the option of starting with coconut milk products, or with almond or other nut milks. If you haven't tasted yogurt or kefir made with coconut milk, you are in for a great surprise. It has a unique, effervescent flavor that is perfectly compatible with the fruits, nuts, and seeds you add. Goat and sheep's milk are other alternatives for those with dairy intolerances. Some people who are intolerant to cow's milk find that they can tolerate yogurt and kefir due to the reduced lactose content in these foods and the changes to the structure of milk protein that occur during bacterial fermentation.

When you make your own yogurt or kefir, you control the ingredients used to add flavor and sweetness. You are unlikely to add, for instance, high-fructose corn syrup, sugar syrup, agave, food colorings, colored sprinkles, or animal crackers. You are more likely to add fresh or frozen organic blueberries, raspberries, blackberries, goji berries, walnuts, pecans, pistachios, chia seeds, pumpkin seeds, or sunflower seeds. You can ferment for longer to reduce the sugar content and increase microbial counts. And if you use full-fat dairy or coconut yogurt or kefir, you will be more satisfied and obtain all the health benefits of the fat.

In the past, making kefir or yogurt was a bit trickier, as it was necessary to prolong incubation at a temperature of around 110°F: too high for ambient room temperature, too low for an oven. Many people therefore purchased a yogurt maker or similar device to create kefirs and yogurts.

Things have gotten a bit simpler now that there are starter cultures for both kefir and yogurt that are able to conduct the process of lactic acid fermentation at room temperature. (See Appendix D.) One limitation: While manufacturers claim that cultures grow at room temperature, I have found that they work best if the temperature is kept around 85° to 90°F for the 48 hours or longer required to create the fermented end product. In a warm climate, this is no problem. In a cold climate (such as where I live, in Wisconsin), where room temperature might be more like 68°F, I've had success with storing the (oven-safe) vessel containing the fermenting kefir or yogurt in the oven and turning it up to, say, 300°F for 2 to 3 minutes every few hours while keeping the oven door closed. This is long enough to warm the oven and keep the temperature greater than ambient room temperature, but not long enough to heat the container, which will kill the starter culture and force me to start over. Of course, a yogurt maker, if you have one, works just fine.

Once started, you can continue to propagate your yogurt or kefir culture just by adding a tablespoon of your finished product to the next batch you make. This transfers the fermenting organisms to the new, uncultured batch and begins the process again, further saving on your costs.

Because lactic acid fermentation requires sugar, and coconut milk has next to none, it is necessary to add a bit of sugar to aid the process. But don't worry: As long as fermentation is allowed to proceed to completion, the sugar is converted to lactic acid, negating any effect it would have had on blood sugar levels.

HOMEMADE YOGURT AND KEFIR

1 can (14 ounces) coconut milk or 16 ounces full-fat milk

1 tablespoon sugar (if using coconut milk)

1 packet kefir or yogurt starter culture

If using cow, goat, or sheep's milk: Place the milk in a medium pan over low heat and warm it, stirring occasionally, until it is between 110° and 112°F. (Monitor the temperature with a candy thermometer.) Allow the milk to cool to room temperature before adding the culture.

In a medium to large bowl, combine the coconut or cooled cow, goat, or sheep's milk, sugar (if using coconut milk), and starter culture. Stir until they're combined, and then set aside, uncovered, at the temperature specified in the directions that came with your starter (with the caveats about "room temperature" discussed above). Allow the mixture to ferment for at least 24 hours. (Coconut milk may require 48 to 72 hours.) Ferment it for an additional 24 hours if you want to minimize the lactose or sugar content and enhance bacterial counts. Your kefir or yogurt is done when it is the approximate thickness of cream. (It will thicken further upon refrigeration.) Store in an airtight container in the refrigerator and consume within a week.

Fermented Vegetables

Fermenting vegetables is another wonderful way to create foods that are rich in healthy bacteria. Interestingly, some of the bacteria that emerge with fermentation are the same as those identified as among the healthiest strains for human bowel flora, such as *Lactobacillus plantarum*, *Lactobacillus brevis*, and *Bifidobacteria* species.

Fermentation refers to the proliferation of bacteria that serves to preserve food by producing lactate (responsible for the characteristic "bite" of fermented foods) while inhibiting growth of bacteria that are unsafe for consumption. This occurs in an anaerobic environment—an environment without oxygen. The key to successful fermentation is therefore keeping oxygen away from your fermenting vegetables. Fermentation should not be confused with *pickling* (soaking in vinegar and brine), which does not involve lactate production. Most commercial pickles and sauerkrauts are pickled, not fermented.

Consuming fermented vegetables at least a few times per week is a wonderful way to continue to inoculate your bowels with healthy bacterial strains, the same way humans have for thousands of years. Some basic ingredients are required.

- Vegetables. Onions, peppers, asparagus, cucumbers, radishes, garlic, carrots, cabbage, and green beans, preferably chopped into bite-size or slightly larger pieces, all work well. Vegetables should be raw, not cooked. Also, you can combine vegetables for unique flavors; carrots and onions work especially well together.

- Large jars or other containers, clean. (A sealable lid is not required, nor is sterilization necessary.)
- Sea salt or other salt.
- Herbs and spices. These will vary depending on the recipe and your personal taste. Favorites include peppercorns, dill, garlic cloves, coriander seeds, mustard seeds, and caraway seeds. Many people also use grape or other berry leaves.
- A clean plate, rock, or other heavy object that easily fits into the jar or container and is used to weigh down the fermenting vegetables.
- Water. Note that the water you use can't contain chlorine or chloramine, which inhibit the fermentation process. If your water is chlorinated, boiling it for 20 minutes will remove most of the chlorine; allow it to cool to room temperature before using. If your water contains chloramine (which is very common), you simply cannot use it, as it takes too long to boil off (more than 24 hours). (To determine which is used in your local water, contact your local water supplier or refer to the Environmental Protection Agency database found at http://cfpub.epa.gov/safewater/ccr/index.cfm.) If chloramine is present in your water, use spring or distilled water or water filtered via reverse osmosis or carbon filters. (For other filtration systems, refer to your product's specifications to determine whether chlorine and chloramine are removed by it.)

Fermentation is, like baking or making pottery, a world in and of itself. These instructions only serve as the most basic starting guide. For anyone interested in pursuing their fermentation efforts further, resources are listed in Appendix D.

BASIC FERMENTED VEGGIES

Vegetables, cut into bite-size pieces	Sea or other salt
Water (spring, distilled, filtered, or tap prepared per the instructions above)	Herbs and spices (if using)

Place the vegetables in a clean jar or container and cover with water, leaving at least 1 to 2 inches at the top after pressing the vegetables down.

Add salt, stir, and taste the mixture. Continue to add salt until the water is lightly to moderately salty to taste. (I believe the flavor is enhanced with a moderately salty brine.) Add your choice of herbs or spices. Stir to combine and to release any trapped air bubbles.

Cover with a plate or another clean object that fits within the jar and pushes the veggies below the water surface, then loosely cover with cloth, plastic wrap, or paper to keep flies and other pests out. The system should *not* be airtight, as the process of fermentation produces gases that will need to be released.

Set the container aside for at least 2 days before consuming. The time required varies with the vegetables and temperature, but it can go on for weeks to months. If longer time periods are going to be used, store it in a cool place. Optionally, after fermentation has occurred, add ½ cup of vinegar per quart of fermented mixture to enhance the flavor.

Should any white or other colored growth (mold) appear on top, skim it off. It does not harm the process.

SOUP AND STOCK

Grandma understood that saving bones, odd meat leftovers, fat, skin, and even stale vegetables to transform into delicious soup or stock was just part of eating well. The health benefits of this old practice of putting saved bones to use have only recently come to be appreciated, with particular benefits for bone and joint health.

This is just the bare-bones version of a recipe that can be varied in countless ways with different vegetables, some beans or lentils, added stewed tomatoes, etc. In this version, I include vinegar at the start to help leach the nutrients out of the bones. Don't worry: The acetic acid will boil off by the time your soup or stock is finished, and there should be no vinegary flavor remaining.

The recipe below is for soup. For stock, simply strain your mixture through cheesecloth and save the translucent liquid in the refrigerator, or freeze for long-term storage.

A large stockpot will be necessary, as well as several hours to mind the simmering mixture. While yield varies depending on how much bones, meat, and water you use, you will certainly have enough soup for several meals.

HEALTHY HOMEMADE SOUP

4 to 5 pounds bones (chicken, beef, pork, lamb, turkey, etc.)

2 medium onions, coarsely diced

8 carrots, sliced

4 to 6 ribs celery, sliced

1 sprig fresh thyme

1 bay leaf

½ teaspoon whole peppercorns

4 ounces tomato paste (optional)

Salt

¼ cup white or apple cider vinegar

If using raw bones: In a large roasting pan, roast the bones at 375°F for 30 to 60 minutes. (For soup, I like to add some meat to roast with the bones, preferably a fatty cut.) Let the bones cool and cube any meat. Transfer to a stockpot.

Add the onions, carrots, celery, thyme, bay leaf, peppercorns, tomato paste (if using), and salt to taste. Cover with water and add the vinegar.

Place the stockpot over high heat and bring the mixture to a boil, then reduce the heat and allow it to simmer, stirring occasionally, for at least 6 hours and as long as 48 hours or more. (Some prefer the richer flavors generated by pro-longed simmering. To keep veggies crisper, they can be added during the last 30 minutes of cooking time.)

Remove from the heat, allow the soup to cool slightly, and remove the bones. If you're storing it for later, allow the soup to cool, remove the bones, and do not skim off the gelatin or fat—it's good for you!

FAT BLASTERS

Fat Blasters are bite-size wallops of healthy fat that fill you up and keep you satisfied. You can eat them as a snack or even use them as a meal replacement. They can be especially useful when you are trying to lose weight. If you are trying to achieve ketosis, then these Fat Blasters can help you get there and stay there.

Note that because coconut oil's melting point is 76°F, these goodies are best stored in the refrigerator if you live in a warm climate or it's a warm time of year, or else you will have a gooey mess. But they can be safely left at room temperature if it's not higher than about 72°F.

These recipes yield approximately 18 squares if they're cut into 1½-inch pieces. I used a 9 x 5-inch baking pan, but any container that yields a similar surface area (45 square inches) can be used and will yield squares approximately ½-inch thick. Alternatively, you could pour the liquid mixture into approximately 12 paper or silicone cupcake liners, placed in muffin tins. The recipe can, of course, be multiplied to accommodate a larger pan or to increase thickness.

Because these Fat Blasters are nearly pure oil, sweeteners don't tend to dissolve easily, as they are not oil-soluble. Erythritol and stevia glycerite work well in this recipe, as they dissolve more readily. Other sweeteners also work, but you may be left with a gritty texture from undissolved sweetener crystals.

LEMON COCONUT FAT BLASTER

1 cup coconut oil, melted

¼ cup unsweetened shredded coconut

1 tablespoon lemon extract

Sweetener equivalent to ½ cup sugar (such as pure liquid or pure powdered stevia, stevia glycerite, erythritol, monk fruit, or xylitol)

Grease a 9 x 5-inch baking dish or similar-size container, or line a muffin pan with cupcake liners.

In a medium bowl, combine the coconut oil, coconut, lemon extract, and sweetener. Mix thoroughly.

Pour the mixture into the prepared pan and refrigerate for at least 1 hour. You can speed up the solidification process by placing it in the freezer for 30 minutes.

When it's solid, use a knife to cut it into 1½-inch squares. Store them covered in the refrigerator or anywhere below 72°F.

TOASTED COCONUT AND CHOCOLATE FAT BLASTER

1 cup coconut oil, melted

1 ounce 100% chocolate (unsweetened or Baker's), melted

½ teaspoon coconut extract

Sweetener equivalent to ½ cup sugar (such as pure liquid or pure powdered stevia, stevia glycerite, erythritol, monk fruit, or xylitol)

¼ cup unsweetened shredded coconut

Preheat the oven to 325°F.

Grease a 9 x 5-inch baking dish or similar-size container, or line a muffin pan with cupcake liners.

In a medium bowl, combine the coconut oil, chocolate, coconut extract, and sweetener. Mix thoroughly.

On a shallow baking sheet, spread the shredded coconut thinly. Bake for 4 to 5 minutes or until lightly browned. (Watch carefully: Coconut burns easily.) Transfer the coconut to the coconut oil mixture, and mix to thoroughly combine.

Pour the mixture into the prepared pan and refrigerate for at least 1 hour. You can speed up the solidification process by placing it in the freezer for 30 minutes.

When it's solid, use a knife to cut it into 1½-inch squares. Store them covered in the refrigerator or anywhere below 72°F.

RECIPES FOR BOWEL HEALTH, INCLUDING PREBIOTIC FIBERS

Here are some tasty ways to cultivate healthy bowel flora, increasing species that improve bowel habits, reduce colon cancer risk, and even achieve metabolic benefits such as reductions in blood sugar, triglycerides, and cholesterol values. Remember: Taking a probiotic or consuming fermented foods is not enough; they simply provide the microorganisms to populate your bowels. These prebiotic fibers nourish healthy bacteria, allowing them to dominate and outmuscle the undesirable species.

WHEAT WHACKER SMOOTHIE

This is no ordinary smoothie. The Wheat Whacker Smoothie contains ingredients that can help get you through the unpleasant withdrawal process that occurs when you remove opiates derived from wheat, rye, barley, and perhaps corn from your diet. It also starts you on the process of restoring prebiotic fibers.

A blender or food processor with a strong motor is recommended—it has to be strong enough to handle the tough green, unripe banana. Note that the banana must be *green and unripe,* providing fibers that are indigestible to humans but digestible by bowel flora. One green, unripe banana yields up to 27 grams (g) of indigestible fiber. (We aim for an intake of 10 to 20 g per day.)

For magnesium, I used a mixture of magnesium chloride and acetate with 133 milligrams (mg) of elemental magnesium per teaspoon. You can use another liquid or powder source of magnesium, but try to avoid magnesium oxide, as absorption is poor and diarrhea is a common side effect. The vitamin D dose can be adjusted to suit individual needs; I chose 5,000 international units (IU) because it's a common dosage for adult men and women, but feel free to adjust it. Although potassium is not added, the coconut milk and banana provide generous quantities (461 mg of potassium if carton coconut milk is used; 1,053 mg if canned coconut milk is used).

I include 5-hydroxytryptophan (5-HTP) to help deal with the cravings that some people experience during wheat withdrawal. I simply purchased 5-HTP capsules and emptied a single capsule (50 mg) into the mix. Because it raises brain serotonin, many people choose to take this supplement daily for its mood-elevating effects. (Anyone taking a prescription antidepressant or carbidopa for Parkinson's disease, however, should not use 5-HTP except under medical supervision, to avoid excessive serotonin levels.) Iodine addresses the reemerging problem of iodine deficiency as a cause for mild hypothyroidism that can stall weight loss. (If you have Hashimoto's thyroiditis, consult with your health-care provider before you supplement iodine.) Aloe vera is wonderfully soothing to the gastrointestinal system as the turmoil of prior wheat consumption subsides.

All the components of this smoothie can be modified—increased, decreased, or omitted—to suit your individual needs. If you are already taking vitamin D, for instance, there is no need to add it. Change the flavor by replacing the ground nutmeg and cinnamon with, say, a handful of blueberries, raspberries, or several strawberries. Also, if you'd like it sweeter, add your choice of benign sweetener (such as stevia, erythritol, or monk fruit) to taste.

Makes approximately 16 ounces (2 cups)

1½ cups unsweetened coconut, almond, or hemp milk (carton)

2 tablespoons coconut oil, melted

1 green, unripe banana, coarsely sliced

2 ounces aloe vera juice (whole leaf, filtered)

150 mg liquid magnesium (elemental magnesium)

5,000 IU vitamin D_3 liquid drops

250 to 500 micrograms iodine (potassium iodide) drops

50 mg 5-HTP

½ teaspoon ground nutmeg

1 teaspoon ground cinnamon

In a blender or food processor, combine all ingredients. Blend or process until the banana is reduced to a puree. Drink immediately.

COOKIE DOUGH BOWEL BLASTERS

Here's a way to get some additional prebiotic fibers from fructooligosaccharides (inulin) in a tasty cookie dough–like form. Though the yield will vary depending on the preparation you purchase, each serving will yield 2 to 3 g of prebiotic fibers. If you use Swerve as a sweetener, this will add an even greater quantity of prebiotic fibers.

To make chocolate-flavored cookie dough, add 1½ tablespoons of unsweetened cocoa powder.

Makes approximately 8 bars or 6 in cupcake liners

1 cup coconut oil

3 tablespoons almond butter

½ cup coconut flour

¼ cup cacao nibs

2 tablespoons inulin

Sweetener equivalent to ½ cup sugar (such as pure liquid or pure powdered stevia, stevia glycerite, erythritol, monk fruit, or xylitol)

1 teaspoon ground cinnamon

1 teaspoon vanilla extract

Grease a 9 x 5-inch baking dish or similar-size container, or line a muffin pan with 6 cupcake liners.

In a medium saucepan over low heat, melt the coconut oil. Stir in the almond butter, coconut flour, cacao nibs, inulin, sweetener, cinnamon, and vanilla. Continue to stir over low heat until thoroughly combined.

Pour the mixture into the prepared pan or cupcake liners. Cool in the refrigerator or freezer. Cut bars to the desired size and store in refrigerator.

SPICED RAW POTATO SMOOTHIE

Adding a raw potato to a smoothie is a way to add around 20 g of prebiotic fibers to your daily intake. Because it is raw, the quantity of digestible carbohydrates is negligible. In the beginning, 20 g of prebiotic fibers may be too much, so either set some of your smoothie aside for another time (covered and in the refrigerator, but for no more than 48 hours), or share with someone. You can also add a raw potato to other smoothie recipes and they will thicken up considerably. Be sure to pick a potato that has no green skin, and peel the potato before using; this avoids the low quantity of toxic solanine contained in the green-colored skin.

Because the potato is tough, you will need a high-powered blender or food processor for this. (I use a Vitamix, and it easily handles the job.) Depending on your sensitivity to sweetness, you may or may not need additional sweetener, such as stevia or erythritol.

Makes approximately 2 cups

1 medium raw potato, peeled and cubed

1 cup coconut milk (carton)

½ teaspoon ground cinnamon

½ teaspoon ground nutmeg

Sweetener equivalent to 1 tablespoon sugar (such as pure liquid or pure powdered stevia, stevia glycerite, erythritol, monk fruit, or xylitol)

In a blender or food processor, combine the potato, coconut milk, cinnamon, nutmeg, sweetener (if using), and ¼ cup water. Blend or process on high until liquefied. Add additional water, if necessary, to obtain desired thickness.

GREEN BANANA BLUEBERRY SMOOTHIE

This basic recipe can, of course, be changed in endless ways. Simply change the modest quantity of berries or add new ingredients, such as chia seeds or avocado.

Makes approximately 2 cups

1 green banana, coarsely sliced

½ cup blueberries (fresh or frozen)

1 cup coconut milk (carton)

2 tablespoons almond butter

Sweetener equivalent to 1 tablespoon sugar (optional, such as pure liquid or pure powdered stevia, stevia glycerite, erythritol, monk fruit, or xylitol)

In a blender or food processor, combine the banana, blueberries, coconut milk, almond butter, sweetener (if using), and ½ cup water. Blend or process until thoroughly combined. Add additional water, if necessary, to obtain desired consistency. Serve immediately.

SPINACH AND RAW SWEET POTATO SALAD WITH AVOCADO-LIME DRESSING

Here's another way to increase your daily prebiotic intake: in a salad that's filled with healthy ingredients and topped with a rich, creamy dressing.

Here, the sweet potato is cubed, but julienned can also work. Because the dressing contains avocado, it is best used immediately, or at least within 24 hours. The lime juice helps keep it from browning, but not for long.

Makes 4 servings as main dish or 6 as side; makes approximately 2 cups dressing

Salad

8 ounces spinach, raw and chopped or baby leaf	4 ounces white button mushrooms, sliced
1 medium raw sweet potato, peeled and chopped into ½-inch cubes	4 hard-cooked eggs, sliced
1 red onion, halved and thinly sliced	5 strips bacon, cooked, drained, and broken or chopped into pieces

In a large bowl, combine the spinach, sweet potato, onion, mushrooms, eggs, and bacon. Toss and top with the dressing (below).

Avocado-Lime Dressing

2 medium avocados, pitted, skin removed	1 clove garlic or 1 teaspoon dried garlic powder
½ cup extra-virgin olive oil	Juice of one small lime
¼ cup rice vinegar	½ teaspoon sea salt
3 tablespoons coarsely chopped fresh cilantro	

In a blender or food processor, combine the avocados, oil, vinegar, cilantro, garlic, lime juice, salt, and ¾ cup water. Blend or process until uniformly mixed. Use immediately or store in an airtight container in the refrigerator.

CHOPPED OLIVE, SUN-DRIED TOMATO, AND GARLIC HUMMUS

Garbanzo beans are another source of prebiotic fibers. Here, we liven them up as hummus combined with the flavors of garlic, ground red pepper, sun-dried tomatoes, pine nuts, and chives.

It is easy to exceed your carbohydrate tolerance by overconsuming garbanzo beans. But when eaten as a condiment (hummus) that's used as a dip for sliced peppers, jicama, celery, or flaxseed crackers, most people stay below the threshold for blood sugar trouble.

Makes approximately 2 cups

1 can (15.5 ounces) garbanzo beans, drained	2 tablespoons toasted sesame seed oil
2 cloves garlic	½ teaspoon ground red pepper
¼ cup extra-virgin olive oil	½ teaspoon sea salt
2 tablespoons freshly squeezed lemon juice	

Optional Toppings

1 tablespoon finely grated Romano or Parmesan cheese

2 tablespoons finely chopped sun-dried tomatoes

¼ cup kalamata olives

1 tablespoon pine nuts

1 tablespoon finely chopped chives

½ teaspoon paprika

Put the beans and garlic in a food chopper or food processor, and pulse until pureed. Scoop the mixture into a small bowl, then add the olive oil, lemon juice, sesame seed oil, ground red pepper, and salt. Mix thoroughly. Sprinkle with one or more of the toppings, if desired. Store in an airtight container in the refrigerator.

MAGNESIUM WATER

This simple recipe yields magnesium bicarbonate, a highly absorbable form of magnesium used to restore tissue magnesium, and the one with the least potential for diarrhea. To make it, you are going to react magnesium hydroxide (milk of magnesia) with carbonic acid (carbonation), yielding water and magnesium bicarbonate. The mixture will no longer be carbonated or have only a minor residual degree of carbonation. A 4-ounce serving provides 90 mg of elemental magnesium; 4 ounces twice per day thereby adds an additional 180 mg of elemental magnesium to your diet.

Note that the milk of magnesia *must* be unflavored, as flavorings block the reaction that yields magnesium bicarbonate (and you will be left with an unusable, unreacted mess). Be sure to label your bottle to prevent someone from unexpectedly guzzling it, which can result in diarrhea. Magnesium water does not need to be refrigerated if consumed within 2 weeks.

1 bottle (2 liters) seltzer (not club soda)

3 tablespoons unflavored milk of magnesia

Uncap the seltzer and pour off a few tablespoons. Shake the milk of magnesia, then measure out and slowly pour 3 tablespoons into the seltzer.

Cap securely, then shake until all of the sediment has dissolved. Allow the mixture to sit for 15 minutes and it will clarify. Drink 4 ounces twice per day.

ELECTROLYTE WATER

Rather than spending a couple of dollars on a sports drink that is little more than water with a few pennies' worth of electrolytes and plenty of sugar added, you can make your own for next to nothing. This can be used for a variety of purposes: to replenish electrolytes during heavy exercise, during a diarrheal illness, or just to drink throughout the day to obtain healthy doses of necessary electrolytes. For added flavor, squeeze a lemon or lime into the water or add a few drops of liquid stevia, pure powdered stevia, or erythritol.

The entire recipe (5 cups) contains approximately 90 mg of (elemental) magnesium, 600 mg of sodium, and 285 mg of potassium. You can multiply the ingredients to make a larger batch.

Makes 5 cups

1 quart water

4 ounces coconut water
    (unsweetened)

4 ounces Magnesium Water
    (page 341)

½ teaspoon baking soda (sodium
    bicarbonate)

In a large, clean container, combine the water, coconut water, Magnesium Water, and baking soda. Shake until dissolved. Drink as desired.

APPENDIX B

Grain Pain: Watch Out for Hidden Sources of Grains

THE MOST CONFIDENT way to minimize your exposure to the seeds of grasses is to focus on single-ingredient, natural foods. This includes vegetables such as spinach, kale, radicchio, and eggplant. It also includes fruits, poultry, beef, pork, fish, nuts, seeds, and dairy (such as cheese and unflavored yogurt). Single-ingredient natural foods have nothing to do with grains unless, of course, somebody added them.

When you venture outside of single-ingredient natural foods, such as when you eat in social situations, go to restaurants, or purchase prepared meals, there is always going to be the potential for inadvertent grain exposure, especially to wheat, barley, and cornstarch. Also be aware of the potential for cross-contamination from utensils, airborne particles, or liquids that were exposed to grains. This is most problematic for people with extreme gluten sensitivities or allergy to a grain component. If a food is labeled "gluten-free," then it should have been prepared in a facility where cross-contamination should not have occurred. Cross-contamination is especially tricky in restaurants; very few establishments have the ability to avoid it, though an increasing number are taking on the challenge as the market for these foods grows.

You will see from the lists on the following pages that grains come in an incredible variety of forms, and they're often hidden away in some additive, thickener, or coating. Couscous, matzo, orzo, graham, farro, panko, and bran are all made from wheat, for instance, while modified food starch is made from wheat or corn.

To qualify as gluten-free according to FDA criteria, products must be both free of gluten and produced in a gluten-free facility to prevent cross-contamination. The FDA's cutoff is no more than 20 parts per million (ppm). This means that the seriously sensitive need to be aware that even if an ingredient label does not list wheat or any buzzwords for wheat (such as "modified food starch"), it can *still* contain some measure of gluten.

When in doubt, contact the customer service department for the product to inquire whether it was made in a gluten-free facility. More and more manufacturers are starting to specify whether or not products are gluten-free on their Web sites.

Note that wheat-free is not the same thing as gluten-free. Wheat-free can mean, for instance, that barley malt or rye was used in place of wheat, but both are sources of gluten. The very gluten-sensitive, such as those with celiac, should not assume that wheat-free necessarily means gluten-free.

Identifying obvious sources of wheat, rye, and barley, such as breads, pastas, and pastries, is straightforward. Rye tends to be listed as "rye," while barley will usually be listed as "barley" or "barley malt."

Listed below are some not-so-obvious foods that can contain wheat. A question mark (?) following an item means it is either variable or uncertain (given manufacturers' reluctance to specify their sources).

Baguettes
Barley, barley malt
Beignets
Bran
Brioche
Bulgur
Burritos
Caramel coloring (?)
Caramel flavoring (?)
Couscous
Crepes
Croutons
Dextrimaltose
Durum wheat
Einkorn
Emmer
Emulsifiers
Farina
Farro
Focaccia

Fu (gluten in Asian foods)
Gnocchi
Graham flour
Gravies
Hydrolyzed vegetable protein
Hydrolyzed wheat starch
Kamut
Maltodextrin
Matzo
Modified food starch
Orzo
Panko (a bread crumb mixture used in Japanese cooking)
Ramen
Roux (wheat-based sauce or thickener)
Rusk
Rye
Seitan (nearly pure gluten used in place of meat)

Semolina

Soba (mostly buckwheat but
   usually also includes wheat)

Spelt

Stabilizers

Strudels

Tabboulehs

Tarts

Textured vegetable protein

Triticale

Triticum

Udon

Vital wheat gluten

Wheat bran

Wheat germ

Wraps

Identifying sources of corn is also not always so straightforward. While foods like corn on the cob, cornmeal, high-fructose corn syrup, and popcorn are obvious, there are also many hidden or not-so-obvious sources of corn.

Grits

Hominy

Hydrolyzed corn protein

Hydrolyzed corn starch

Maize

Mixed vegetable oil

Modified food starch

Polenta

Vegetable oil

Zea mays

One of the difficulties with corn products is that, in addition to the sources listed above, there are literally hundreds of common food ingredients derived from corn, such as dextrose, dextrin, maltodextrin, maltitol, polydextrose, ethanol, caramel coloring, and artificial flavorings. Most of these will not jump out at you as being made from corn. However, the process to generate them from corn reduces the protein content to negligible levels, and therefore they're generally not a grain-exposure problem for the majority of people (though these sugars pose other problems of their own).

Also note that many medications and nutritional supplements can contain wheat or corn. Be aware of the potential for corn-derived ingredients if there is suspicion of ongoing exposure.

The other grains, such as rice, teff, oats, and millet, tend to be more obvious. Just avoid a product if you see them listed on the ingredients list.

APPENDIX C

A Grain-Free Shopping List

IN THIS SECTION you will find a list of most of the ingredients you will need to follow a healthy and confident grain-free lifestyle, as well as some of the basic ingredients you'll need to begin fermenting foods and adding prebiotic fibers to your diet. Many of the ingredients listed are useful for re-creating grain-based foods that you or your family might miss because of tradition or habit, or you may find them useful to include at holidays and when entertaining. Pumpkin muffins or a blueberry cheesecake, for instance, can be easily re-created with grain-free ingredients and without added sugar. Many recipes consistent with this lifestyle can be found in the *Wheat Belly Cookbook* and the *Wheat Belly 30-Minute (or Less!) Cookbook*.

ALMOND MEAL, ALMOND FLOUR. Almond meal and almond flour are our preferred wheat flour replacements. Almond meal is ground from whole almonds, while almond flour is ground from blanched almonds. Anyone unfamiliar with almond meal or flour will be pleasantly surprised at the wonderful baked products you can create with them. I like to reserve the almond flour for when the lightest texture is desired, such as in a cake or pound cake, and use the coarser and less costly almond meal for everyday use.

ALMOND MILK, UNSWEETENED. Almond milk is the strained liquid from ground almonds. It is thinner than cow's milk. Look for unsweetened varieties to avoid the unnecessary added sugars. If you wish to make your own (which is delicious), start by soaking whole almonds in water for 24 hours. Drain and then puree the almonds, and then strain the puree through cheesecloth. Dilute with water, using twice the volume of water as almonds (for example, 2 cups of water to 1 cup of almonds) or to the desired thickness. Save the pulp for baking or thickening sauces.

BANANAS. We use green, unripe bananas in smoothies, yogurts, kefirs, ice cream, and iced coconut milk. Because an unripe banana's sugars are in an indigestible form, they provide nutrition for bowel flora.

BONES. Bones, saved from your meats or obtained from the butcher, are used for making soups and stocks.

CAULIFLOWER. Cauliflower is our go-to replacement for mashed potatoes, rice, stuffing, and dressing. A food chopper or food processor is helpful when you're creating these forms.

CHIA SEED. While it cannot be used as the primary flour in baking, it can be added (whole or ground) to generate a sturdier texture. You can also add it to thicken smoothies, yogurts, kefirs, and other dishes. Its peculiar capacity to expand when exposed to water makes it useful for making puddings, mousses, and jams.

CHOCOLATE. Use 100 percent chocolate—cocoa with cocoa butter but no sugar—to add a rich chocolate taste to a dish. People with dairy sensitivities can also use 100 percent chocolate to avoid exposure.

COCOA POWDER, UNSWEETENED. Unsweetened is the key here. Ghirardelli, Scharffen Berger, and Hershey's are all widely available brands.

COCONUT, SHREDDED AND UNSWEETENED; COCONUT FLAKES. Unsweetened coconut is a wonderful way to add texture, chewiness, and flavor to a variety of breads, muffins, and other baked foods. It's also a great topping for your grain-free cakes, cupcakes, and muffins. Coconut is also rich in potassium and fiber.

COCONUT FLOUR. Coconut flour, the flour that results from grinding dried coconut meat, is a staple in the grain-free kitchen. Coconut flour is best used as a secondary flour, added to nut flours and meals to create a finer texture. (It generates an excessively heavy, almost inedible end product if used alone.) Store it in an airtight container, as coconut flour is very water absorbent.

COCONUT MILK. Canned coconut milk is great for thickening and as a replacement for sour cream in recipes. Carton varieties are thinner and are useful anywhere you'd use milk, such as in coffee, as well as in baking. Native Forest, Natural Value, and Trader Joe's brands are all BPA-free. Anyone wishing to avoid the BPA can also thicken the carton version by adding shredded or flaked coconut that's been pulverized in a manual food chopper or food processor. Alternatively, you can make coconut milk of any consistency by grinding down the coconut meat with water and straining the coarse remains.

CULTURES. Dairy- or coconut-based starting cultures for yogurts and kefirs can be purchased, allowing you to make your own as part of a broader strategy of restoring and maintaining healthy bowel flora. (See Appendix D for sources.)

DRIED FRUIT. Dried apricots, cranberries, currants, blueberries, strawberries, dates, and figs are useful in small quantities in your grain-free baked products. Always buy them *unsweetened*, as those soaked in sugar or high-fructose corn syrup can present a substantial sugar load.

EGGS. If your budget permits, look for organic eggs obtained from free-range chickens. Truly healthy eggs have deep yellow, orange, or even red yolks, along with richer flavors.

EXTRACTS. Almond, coconut, vanilla, lemon, orange, and peppermint extracts (preferably natural) are useful for baking and for making Fat Blasters (see the recipes in Appendix A).

FLAXSEED. Flaxseed can be purchased either ground or whole, which you can then grind yourself. Flaxseed is rich in fiber and linolenic acid (plant-sourced omega-3), and is a versatile replacement flour when mixed with almond flour. The most baking-friendly variety is golden flaxseed, rather than brown. It is a great fiber to add for bowel health.

GHEE. Ghee is clarified butter: the oil from butter with the protein solids removed by heating. It is among the least problematic of dairy products, since most of the whey, casein, and lactose have been removed.

GUAR GUM. An optional thickener, it is useful for making wheat-free baked goods when improved cohesiveness and stiffness are desired. Guar is most useful for making ice cream or iced coconut desserts; it improves creaminess and mouthfeel.

INULIN. In its powdered form, this is an inexpensive and convenient way to add prebiotic fructooligosaccharides to smoothies, yogurt, and other foods.

NUT AND SEED BUTTERS. Almond butter, peanut butter, cashew butter, and sunflower seed butter can be purchased as preground butters or ground from whole nuts in your food processor or manual food chopper.

NUT MEALS/FLOURS. Ground almonds, pecans, walnuts, hazelnuts, cashews.

NUTS. Use chopped raw almonds, pecans, walnuts, pistachios, hazelnuts, Brazil nuts, and macadamias in baking. Buy dry-roasted nuts or nuts not roasted in unhealthy oils, such as hydrogenated cottonseed or hydrogenated soybean oils.

OILS. Keep extra-virgin olive, coconut, avocado, flaxseed, walnut, and extra-light olive oil on hand at all times.

POTATOES. Cooked potatoes send blood sugar through the roof, but *raw* potatoes are indigestible and do not. However, the indigestible fibers are nutritious for your bowel flora. Peel and chop into small cubes for a salad or reduce to a puree for sauces or smoothies.

SEEDS. Raw sunflower, raw pumpkin, sesame, and chia are all good choices. Seeds can be ground into flours and used in baking, used whole in grain-free granola, or included for texture and crunch in grain-free cookies and bars.

SHIRATAKI NOODLES. Noodles and pasta replacements made from the flour of the konjac root are safe, posing virtually no blood sugar challenge. Shirataki is packaged in liquid in single-serving bags, usually found in the grocery store refrigerator section, not on the shelves with the pasta. The water needs to be drained and the noodles rinsed (don't mind the slightly fishy odor) and then boiled briefly to warm.

SWEETENERS. Pure liquid stevia, stevia glycerite, pure powdered stevia, powdered stevia with inulin (not maltodextrin), powdered erythritol, Swerve (inulin and erythritol), Truvía (erythritol and rebiana, an isolate of stevia), Wheat Free Market sweetener (erythritol and monk fruit), and xylitol are the best choices.

XANTHAN GUM. A fiber thickener, it's useful for making wheat-free doughs sturdier and more cohesive. It's also useful for making ice cream or iced coconut desserts.

APPENDIX D

Resources

ADVANCED LIPOPROTEIN TESTING

These are the laboratories that provide advanced lipoprotein testing that represents an improvement over standard cholesterol, or lipid, testing. These tests are run at the locations listed below, but the blood specimen is obtained in your local laboratory. Your health-care provider will have to either arrange for such a test through the local laboratory or contact one of the laboratories below to identify a local laboratory familiar with the process. It is really very easy, but it will require a few minutes of effort on your doctor's part.

Interpretation of the results requires additional training and nutritional sophistication. One option is to contact the testing laboratory and ask for the sales representative for your area; he or she will often know the local health-care practitioners who are most skilled at use of their test and can share their names with you.

Atherotech
www.atherotech.com

Vertical Auto Profile (VAP) Cholesterol Test

Berkeley HeartLab
www.bhlinc.com

Gel electropheresis (GGE)

Health Diagnostic Laboratory Inc.
www.hdlabinc.com

Liposcience
www.liposcience.com/nmr-lipoprofile-test

NMR LipoProfile

SpectraCell

www.spectracell.com

There are also testing laboratories that provide lipoprotein and other testing, such as 25-hydroxy vitamin D and thyroid tests, without a doctor's order.

Direct Labs

www.directlabs.com

Health Check USA

www.healthcheckusa.com

Lab Testing Direct

www.labtestingdirect.com

FERMENTATION

Books

Katz, Sandor. *The Art of Fermentation: An In-Depth Exploration of Essential Concepts and Processes from around the World.* White River Junction, VT: Chelsea Green Publishing, 2012.
    Katz's beautifully written and illustrated book is the bible for all things fermented, including fascinating discussions about the lore, cultural idiosyncrasies, health, and science behind the process. He leaves no stone unturned.

Lewin, Alex. *Real Food Fermentation.* Minneapolis: Quarry Books, 2012.
    A practical, just-getting-started book useful for fermentation beginners.

Supplies and Yogurt and Kefir Starter Cultures

Cultures for Health
www.culturesforhealth.com
Phone: 800-962-1959

Yógourmet
www.yogourmet.com
Phone: 800-863-5606

GASTROINTESTINAL TESTING

If you are confirming a diagnosis of celiac disease; identifying an unusual autoimmune response to gliadin, secalin, or hordein (important in neurological syndromes); or exploring intolerances to other foods that might underlie persistent inflammation or autoimmunity despite grain elimination, these labs can assist you.

Enterolab
www.enterolab.com
Stool testing for reactions against grains and other foods.

Metametrix Clinical Laboratory
http://metametrix.com
The Metametrix panel tests for 90 IgG antibodies to foods. There is also an abbreviated test kit for at-home finger-stick testing that tests for intolerances to 30 different foods.

GRAIN-FREE COOKBOOKS

Davis, William, MD. *Wheat Belly Cookbook: 150 Recipes to Lose the Wheat, Lose the Weight, and Find Your Path Back to Health*. Emmaus, PA: Rodale, 2013.

Davis, William, MD. *Wheat Belly 30-Minute (or Less!) Cookbook: 200 Quick and Simple Recipes to Lose the Wheat, Lose the Weight, and Find Your Path Back to Health*. Emmaus, PA: Rodale, 2013.

Emmerich, Maria. *The Art of Healthy Eating—Savory: Grain Free Low Carb Reinvented*. Amazon Digital Services, 2012.

Staley, Bill, and Hayley Mason. *Gather: The Art of Paleo Entertaining*. Las Vegas: Victory Belt Publishing, 2013.

Walker, Danielle. *Against All Grain: Delectable Paleo Recipes to Eat Well & Feel Great*. Las Vegas: Victory Belt Publishing, 2013.

HOME BLOOD TESTING KITS

ZRT Test Kits
www.zrtlab.com
Phone: 866-600-1636
ZRT Labs provides at-home test kits for a wide variety of tests, including 25-hydroxy vitamin D to assess vitamin D status and a thyroid panel (free T3, free T4, TSH, and thyroid peroxidase antibodies). Not available in New York.

INDIGESTIBLE PREBIOTIC FIBERS

Products on the market that provide inulin, fructooligosaccharides, or other prebiotic fiber include:

Quest bars

www.questproteinbar.com

> Quest bars are low-carbohydrate bars that contain 16 to 17 grams of fructooligosaccharides per bar. They also contain whey, so beware if you have dairy intolerance issues or are struggling with weight loss.

Swerve

www.swervesweetener.com

> Swerve is a sweetener mix of erythritol and fructooligosaccharides, a form of indigestible prebiotic fiber. One teaspoon provides 5 grams of prebiotic fiber.

LIQUID TRIGLYCERIDE FISH OIL

Preferred sources of liquid triglyceride fish oil include the brands below. There are other brands, but I believe that these are the best in terms of purity and lack of contaminants and oxidative breakdown products, as well as taste and smell.

People often express reluctance at using liquid fish oil, as they are fearful of fishy smell or taste. These products are actually nearly scentless except for the lemon or orange oil added by manufacturers. Be sure to cap and refrigerate, as they become rancid if kept at room temperature.

Ascenta NutraSea

www.ascentahealth.com

Nordic Naturals

www.nordicnaturals.com

Pharmax

Pharmax products are usually sold through health-care practitioners, but they can also be obtained directly through retailers such as Amazon.

ENDNOTES

CHAPTER 1

1   C. Roberts and K. Manchester, "Dental Disease," in *The Archaeology of Disease* (New York: Cornell University Press, 2005), 63–83; M. N. Cohen and G. M. M. Crane-Kramer, editors' summation, in *Ancient Health: Skeletal Indicators of Agricultural and Economic Intensification* (Gainesville: University Press of Florida, 2007), 320–43; L. Cordain, "Cereal Grains: Humanity's Double-Edged Sword," in *Evolutionary Aspects of Nutrition and Health*, ed. A. P. Simopoulos (Basel: Karger, 1999);84: 19–73.

2   Cohen, *Ancient Health*, 320–43.

3   "Global and Regional Food Consumption Patterns and Trends," World Health Organization, accessed April 10, 2014, http://www.who.int/dietphysicalactivity /publications/trs916/en/gsfao_global.pdf.

4   R. Batista et al., "Microarray Analyses Reveal That Plant Mutagenesis May Induce More Transcriptomic Changes Than Transgene Insertion," *Proceedings of the National Academy of Sciences of the United States of America* 105, no. 9 (2008): 3640–45.

5   S. Pearce et al., "Molecular Characterization of Rht-1 Dwarfing Genes in Hexaploid Wheat," *Plant Physiology* 157 (December 2011): 1820–31.

6   P. Sabelli and P. M. Shewry, "Characterization and Organization of Gene Families at the Gli-1 Loci of Bread and Durum Wheat by Restriction Fragment Analysis," *Theoretical and Applied Genetics* 83 (1991): 209–16.

7   H. C. Van den Broeck et al., "Presence of Celiac Disease Epitopes in Modern and Old Hexaploid Wheat Varieties: Wheat Breeding May Have Contributed to Increased Prevalence of Celiac Disease," *Theoretical and Applied Genetics* 121 (2010): 1527–39.

8   A. Rubio-Tapia et al., "Increased Prevalence and Mortality in Undiagnosed Celiac Disease," *Gastroenterology* 137, no. 1 (July 2009): 88–93.

9   C. Zioudrou, R. A. Streaty, and W. A. Klee, "Opioid Peptides Derived from Food Proteins. The Exorphins," *Journal of Biological Chemistry* 254, no. 7 (April 10, 1979): 2446–49.

10 J. M. Tjon, J. van Bergen, and F. Koning, "Celiac Disease: How Complicated Can It Get?" *Immunogenetics* 62, no. 10 (October 2010): 641–51.

11 X. Gao et al., "High Frequency of HMW-GS Sequence Variation through Somatic Hybridization between *Agropyron elongatum* and Common Wheat," *Planta* 23, no. 2 (January 2010): 245–50.

12 W. J. Peumans, H. M. Stinissen, and A. R. Carlier, "Isolation and Partial Characterization of Wheat-Germ-Agglutinin-Like Lectins from Rye (*Secale cereale*) and Barley (*Hordeum vulgare*) Embryos," *Biochemical Journal* 203, no. 1 (April 1, 1982): 239–43.

13 V. Lorenzsonn and W. A. Olsen, "In Vivo Responses of Rat Intestinal Epithelium to Intraluminal Dietary Lectins," *Gastroenterology* 82 (1982): 838–48.

14 P. B. Holm, K. N. Kristiansen, and H. B. Pedersen, "Transgenic Approaches in Commonly Consumed Cereals to Improve Iron and Zinc Content and Bioavailability," *Journal of Nutrition* 132, no. 3 (March 2002): 514S–6S.

15 R. Gibson, "Zinc Nutrition in Developing Countries," *Nutrition Research Reviews* 7 (1994): 151–73; L. H. Allen, "The Nutrition CRSP: What Is Marginal Malnutrition and Does It Affect Human Function?" *Nutrition Reviews* 51 (1993): 255–67.

16 C. Larré et al., "Assessment of Allergenicity of Diploid and Hexaploid Wheat Genotypes: Identification of Allergens in the Albumin/Globulin Fraction," *Journal of Proteomics* 74, no. 8 (August 12, 2011): 1279–89.

17 E. A. Pastorello et al., "Wheat IgE-Mediated Food Allergy in European Patients: Alpha-Amylase Inhibitors, Lipid Transfer Proteins and Low-Molecular-Weight Glutenins. Allergenic Molecules Recognized by Double-Blind, Placebo-Controlled Food Challenge," *Internal Archives of Allergy and Immunology* 144, no. 1 (2007): 10–22.

18 P. Carrera-Bastos et al., "The Western Diet and Lifestyle and Diseases of Civilization," *Research Reports in Clinical Cardiology* 2 (2011): 15–35.

19 J. Woodburn, "An Introduction to Hadza Ecology," in *Man the Hunter*, ed. R. B. Lee and I. Devore (New Bruswick (USA): Aldine Transaction, 2009), 49.

20 H. Pontzer et al., "Hunter-Gatherer Energetics and Human Obesity," *PLoS One* 7, no. 7 (2012): e40503.

21 L. R. Dugas et al., "Energy Expenditure in Adults Living in Developing Compared with Industrialized Countries: A Meta-Analysis of Doubly Labeled Water Studies," *American Journal of Clinical Nutrition* 93 (2011): 427–41.

22 G. V. Mann et al., "Cardiovascular Disease in the Masai," *Journal of Atherosclerosis Research* 8, no. 4 (1964): 289–312; G. V. Mann et al., "Atherosclerosis in the Masai," *American Journal of Epidemiology* 95, no. 1 (January 1972): 26–37.

23 K. Milton, "Hunter-Gatherer Diets: Wild Foods Signal Relief from Diseases of Affluence," in *Human Diet: Its Origin and Evolution*, ed. P. S. Ungar and M. F. Teaford (Westport, Connecticut: Bergin & Garvey, 2002), 111–22.

24 W. C. Knowler et al., "Diabetes Incidence and Prevalence in Pima Indians: A 19-Fold Greater Incidence than in Rochester, Minnesota," *American Journal of Epidemiology* 108, no. 6 (December 1978): 497–505; W. C. Knowler et al., "Diabetes Incidence in Pima Indians: Contributions of Obesity and Parental Diabetes," *American Journal of Epidemiology* 113, no. 2 (February 1981): 144–56.

25 M. Story et al., "The Epidemic of Obesity in American Indian Communities and the Need for Childhood Obesity-Prevention Programs," *American Journal of Clinical Nutrition* 69, no. 4 (1999): 747S–54S.

26 G. M. Egeland, Z. Cao, and T. K. Young, "Hypertriglyceridemic-Waist Phenotype and Glucose Intolerance among Canadian Inuit: The International Polar Year Inuit Health Survey for Adults 2007–2008," *Canadian Medical Association Journal* 183, no. 9 (June 14, 2011): E553–58, doi:10.1503/cmaj.101801; H. V. Kuhnlein et al., "Arctic Indigenous Peoples Experience the Nutrition Transition with Changing Dietary Patterns and Obesity," *Journal of Nutrition* 134, no. 6 (June 2004): 1447–53.

27 P. Zimmet et al., "The Effect of Westernization on Native Populations. Studies on a Micronesian Community with a High Diabetes Prevalence," *Australian and New Zealand Journal of Medicine* 8, no. 2 (April 1978): 141–46.

28 "Progress Can Kill: How Imposed Development Destroys the Health of Tribal People," Survival International, 2007, http://assets.survivalinternational.org/static /lib/downloads/source/progresscankill/full_report.pdf.

29 J. Day, A. Bailey, and D. Robinson, "Biological Variations Associated with Change in Lifestyle among the Pastoral and Nomadic Tribes of East Africa," *Annals of Human Biology* 6, no. 1 (January–February 1979): 29–39; D. L. Christensen et al., "Obesity and Regional Fat Distribution in Kenyan Populations: Impact of Ethnicity and Urbanization," *Annals of Human Biology* 35, no. 2 (March–April 2008): 232–49.

30 F. J. Fernandes-Costa, J. Marshall, and C. Ritchie, "Transition from a Hunter-Gatherer to a Settled Lifestyle in the !Kung San: Effect on Iron, Folate, and Vitamin B$_{12}$ Nutrition," *American Journal of Clinical Nutrition* 40, no. 5 (December 1984): 1295–303.

31 S. G. Gimeno et al., "Cardiovascular Risk Factors among Brazilian Karib Indigenous Peoples: Upper Xingu, Central Brazil, 2000-3," *Journal of Epidemiology and Community Health* 63, no. 4 (April 2009): 299–304.

32 S. G. Agostinho Gimeno et al., "Metabolic and Anthropometric Profile of Aruák Indians: Mehináku, Waurá and Yawalapití in the Upper Xingu, Central Brazil, 2000-2002," *Cadernos de Saúde Pública* 23, no. 8 (August 2007): 1946–54.

33 D. R. Matthews and P. C. Matthews, "Banting Memorial Lecture 2010. Type 2 Diabetes as an 'Infectious' Disease: Is This the Black Death of the 21st Century?" *Diabetic Medicine* 28, no. 1 (January 2011): 2–9.

34 W. A. Price, *Nutrition and Physical Degeneration* (Lemon Grove, California: The Price-Pottenger Nutrition Foundation, 1939; reprinted 2008).

35 K. O'Dea, "Marked Improvement in Carbohydrate and Lipid Metabolism in Diabetic Australian Aborigines after Temporary Reversion to Traditional Lifestyle," *Diabetes* 33, no. 6 (June 1984): 596–603.

36 K. O'Dea, "Preventable Chronic Diseases among Indigenous Australians: The Need for a Comprehensive National Approach" (paper presented at the 2005 Australian Judges Conference in Darwin, January 2005), http://melbourneinstitute.com /downloads/conferences/archive/s7b/kerin-odea-p.pdf.

37 "Progress Can Kill: How Imposed Development Destroys the Health of Tribal People," Survival International, 2007, http://assets.survivalinternational.org/static /lib/downloads/source/progresscankill/full_report.pdf.

38 W. Wadd, *Comments on Corpulency, Lineaments of Leanness, Mems on Diet and Dietetics* (Ebers and Co.: London, 1829), 65.

CHAPTER 2

1 Y. Minami et al., "Isolation and Amino Acid Sequence of a Protein-Synthesis Inhibitor from the Seeds of Rye (*Secale cereale*)," *Bioscience, Biotechnology, and Biochemistry* 62, no. 6 (June 1998): 1152–56.

2 V. Lorenzsonn and W. A. Olsen, "In Vivo Responses of Rat Intestinal Epithelium to Intraluminal Dietary Lectins," *Gastroenterology* 82, no. 5, pt. 1 (May 1982): 838–48.

3 K. Fälth-Magnusson and K. E. Magnusson, "Elevated Levels of Serum Antibodies to the Lectin Wheat Germ Agglutinin in Celiac Children Lend Support to the Gluten-Lectin Theory of Celiac Disease," *Pediatric Allergy and Immunology* 6, no. 2 (1995): 98–102.

4 A. Pusztai et al., "Antinutritive Effects of Wheat-Germ Agglutinin and Other N-Acetylglucosamine-Specific Lectin," *British Journal of Nutrition* 70, no. 1 (July 1993): 313–21; D. L. Freed, "Lectins," *British Medical Journal* 290, no. 6468 (February 23, 1985): 584–86.

5 R. Cianci et al., "New Insights on the Role of T Cells in the Pathogenesis of Celiac Disease," *Journal of Biological Regulators and Homeostatic Agents* 26, no. 2 (April–June 2012): 171–79.

6 J. L. Messina, J. Hamlin, and J. Larner, "Insulin-Mimetic Actions of Wheat Germ Agglutinin and Concanavalin A on Specific mRNA Levels," *Archives of Biochemistry and Biophysics* 254, no. 1 (April 1987): 110–15.

7 T. Jönsson et al., "Agrarian Diet and Diseases of Affluence—Do Evolutionary Novel Dietary Lectins Cause Leptin Resistance?" *BMC Endocrine Disorders* 5 (December 10, 2005): 10.

8 J. Chocola et al., "Structural and Functional Analysis of the Human Vasoactive Intestinal Peptide Receptor Glycosylation. Alteration of Receptor Function by Wheat Germ Agglutinin," *Journal of Biological Chemistry* 268, no. 4 (February 5, 1993): 2312–18; A. El Battari et al. "The Vasoactive Intestinal Peptide Receptor on

Intact Human Colonic Adenocarcinoma Cells (HT29-D4). Evidence for Its Glycoprotein Nature," *Biochemical Journal* 242, no. 1 (February 15, 1987): 185–91.

9   M. R. Nicol et al., "Vasoactive Intestinal Peptide (VIP) Stimulates Cortisol Secretion from the H295 Human Adrenocortical Tumour Cell Line Via VPAC1 Receptors," *Journal of Molecular Endocrinology* 32, no. 3 (June 2004): 869–77.

10 L. Souza-Moreira et al., "Neuropeptides as Aleiotropic Modulators of the Immune Response," *Neuroendocrinology* 94, no. 2 (2011): 89–100.

11 C. Abad and J. A. Waschek, "Immunomodulatory Roles of VIP and PACAP in Models of Multiple Sclerosis," *Current Pharmaceutical Design* 17, no. 10 (2011): 1025–35.

12 D. Wu, D. Lee, Y. K. Sung, "Prospect of Vasoactive Intestinal Peptide Therapy for COPD/PAH and Asthma: A Review," *Respiratory Research* 12 (April 11, 2011): 45.

13 K. J. Gross and C. Pothoulakis, "Role of Neuropeptides in Inflammatory Bowel Disease," *Inflammatory Bowel Diseases* 13, no. 7 (July 2007): 918–32.

14 F. Garcia-Garcia et al., "Sleep-Inducing Factors," *CNS and Neurological Disorders—Drug Targets* 8, no. 4 (August 2009): 235–44.

15 S. Herness and F. L. Zhao, "The Neuropeptides CCK and NPY and the Changing View of Cell-to-Cell Communication in the Taste Bud," *Physiology and Behavior* 97, no. 5 (July 14, 2009): 581–91.

16 R. Saraceno et al., "The Role of Neuropeptides in Psoriasis," *British Journal of Dermatology* 155, no. 5 (November 2006): 876–82.

17 C. J. Adler et al., "Sequencing Ancient Calcified Dental Plaque Shows Changes in Oral Microbiota with Dietary Shifts of the Neolithic and Industrial Revolutions," *Nature Genetics* 45, no. 4 (April 2013): 450–55.

18 P. Lingström, J. van Houte, and S. Kashket, "Food Starches and Dental Caries," *Critical Reviews in Oral Biology and Medicine* 11, no. 3 (2000): 366–80.

19 "Dental Decay: The Evolution of Oral Diversity," Wellcome Trust/Sanger Institute, February 17, 2013, http://www.sanger.ac.uk/about/press/2013/130217.html.

20 L. Cordain, "Cereal Grains: Humanity's Double-Edged Sword," *World Review of Nutrition and Dietetics* 84 (1999): 19–73.

21 R. Y. Tito et al., "Insights from Characterizing Extinct Human Gut Microbiomes," *PLoS ONE* 7, no. 12 (2012): e51146, doi:10.1371/journal.pone.0051146; C. De Filippo et al., "Impact of Diet in Shaping Gut Microbiota Revealed by a Comparative Study in Children from Europe and Rural Africa," *Proceedings of the National Academy of Sciences* 107 (2010): 14691.

22 A. Swidsinski et al., "Active Crohn's Disease and Ulcerative Colitis Can Be Specifically Diagnosed and Monitored Based on the Biostructure of the Fecal Flora," *Inflammatory Bowel Diseases* 14, no. 2 (February 2008): 147–61.

23 G. H. Perry et al., "Diet and the Evolution of Human Amylase Gene Copy Number Variation," *Nature Genetics* 39, no. 10 (October 2007): 1256–60.

24 A. Helgason et al., "Refining the Impact of TCF7L2 Gene Variants on Type 2 Diabetes and Adaptive Evolution," *Nature Genetics* 39, no. 2 (February 2007): 218–25.

25 K. S. Juntunen et al., "Structural Differences between Rye and Wheat Breads but Not Total Fiber Content May Explain the Lower Postprandial Insulin Response to Rye Bread," *American Journal of Clinical Nutrition* 78, no. 5 (November 2003): 957–64.

26 S. M. Stenman et al., "Degradation of Coeliac Disease–Inducing Rye Secalin by Germinating Cereal Enzymes: Diminishing Toxic Effects in Intestinal Epithelial Cells," *Clinical and Experimental Immunology* 161, no. 2 (August 2010): 242–49; E. Vainio and E. Varionen, "Antibody Response against Wheat, Rye, Barley, Oats, and Corn: Comparison between Gluten-Sensitive Patients and Monoclonal Antigliadin Antibodies," *Internal Archives of Allergy and Immunity* 106, no. 2 (February 1995): 134–38.

27 W. J. Peumans, H. M. Stinissen, and A. R. Carlier, "Isolation and Partial Characterization of Wheat-Germ-Agglutinin-Like Lectins from Rye (*Secale cereale*) and Barley (*Hordeum vulgare*) Embryos," *Biochemical Journal* 203, no. 1 (April 1, 1982): 239–43.

28 T. Y. Curtis et al., "Free Amino Acids and Sugars in Rye Grain: Implications for Acrylamide Formation," *Journal of Agricultural and Food Chemistry* 58 (2010): 1959–69; J. Postles et al., "Effects of Variety and Nutrient Availability on the Acrylamide-Forming Potential of Rye Grain," *Journal of Cereal Science* 57, no. 3 (May 2013): 463–70.

29 L. Caporael, "Ergotism: The Satan Loosed in Salem?" *Science* 192 (1976): 21–26.

30 I. Comino et al., "Significant Differences in Coeliac Immunotoxicity of Barley Varieties," *Molecular Nutrition and Food Research* 56, no. 11 (November 2012): 1697–707.

31 J. Snegaroff et al., "Barley 3-Hordein: Glycosylation at an Atypical Site, Disulfide Bridge Analysis, and Reactivity with IgE from Patients Allergic to Wheat," *Biochimica et Biophysica Acta* 1834, no. 1 (January 2013): 395–403.

32 E. A. Pechenkina et al., "Skeletal Biology of the Central Peruvian Coast: Consequences of Changing Population Density and Progressive Dependence on Maize Agriculture," in *Ancient Health: Skeletal Indicators of Agricultural and Economic Intensification*, ed. M. N. Cohen and G. M. M. Crane-Kramer (Gainesville: University Press of Florida, 2007), 92–112; M. P. Alfonso, V. G. Standen, and V. Castro, "The Adoption of Agriculture among Northern Chile Populations in the Azapa Valley, 9000-1000 BP," in *Ancient Health: Skeletal Indicators of Agricultural and Economic Intensification*, ed. M. N. Cohen and G. M. M. Crane-Kramer (Gainesville: University Press of Florida, 2007), 245.

33 S. E. Byrnes, J. C. Miller, and G. S. Denyer, "Amylopectin Starch Promotes the Development of Insulin Resistance in Rats," *Journal of Nutrition* 125, no. 6 (June 1995): 1430–37.

34 E. Vainio and E. Varionen, "Antibody Response against Wheat, Rye, Barley, Oats, and Corn: Comparison between Gluten-Sensitive Patients and Monoclonal Antigliadin Antibodies," *International Archives of Allergy and Immunology* 106, no. 2 (February 1995): 134–38; E. N. Mills et al., "Structural, Biological, and Evolutionary Relationships of Plant Food Allergens Sensitizing via the Gastrointestinal Tract," *Critical Reviews in Food Science and Nutrition* 44, no. 5 (2004): 379–407; E. A. Pastorello et al., "Maize Food Allergy: Lipid-Transfer Proteins, Endochitinases, and Alpha-Zein Precursor Are Relevant Maize Allergens in Double-Blind Placebo-Controlled Maize-Challenge-Positive Patients," *Analytical and Bioanalytical Chemistry* 395, no. 1 (September 2009): 93–102.

35 M. P. Valencia Zavala et al., "Maize (*Zea mays*): Allergen or Toleragen? Participation of the Cereal in Allergic Disease and Positivity Incidence in Cutaneous Tests," *Revista Alergia Mexico* 53, no. 6 (November–December 2006): 207–11.

36 Vainio, "Antibody Response against Wheat, Rye, Barley, Oats, and Corn," 134–38.

37 F. Cabrera-Chavez et al., "Maize Prolamins Resistant to Peptic-Tryptic Digestion Maintain Immune-Recognition by IgA from Some Celiac Disease Patients," *Plant Foods for Human Nutrition* 67, no. 1 (March 2012): 24–30.

38 J. Spiroux de Vendômois et al., "A Comparison of the Effects of Three GM Corn Varieties on Mammalian Health," *International Journal of Biological Sciences* 5 (2009): 706–26.

39 G. E. Seralini et al., "Long Term Toxicity of a Roundup Herbicide and a Roundup-Tolerant Genetically Modified Maize," *Food and Chemical Toxicology* 50, no. 11 (November 2012): 4221–31.

40 B. P. Mezzomo et al., "Hematotoxicity of *Bacillus thuringiensis* as Spore-Crystal Strains Cry1Aa, Cry1Ab, Cry1Ac or Cry2Aa in Swiss Albino Mice," *Journal of Hematology and Thromboembolic Diseases* 1 (2013): 1.

41 J. Spiroux de Vendômois et al., "A Comparison of the Effects of Three GM Corn Varieties on Mammalian Health," 706–26.

42 W. Xu et al., "Analysis of Caecal Microbiota in Rats Fed with Genetically Modified Rice by Real-Time Quantitative PCR," *Journal of Food Science* 76, no. 1 (January–February 2011): M88–93.

43 S. Thongprakaisang et al., "Glyphosate Induces Human Breast Cancer Cells Growth via Estrogen Receptors," *Food and Chemical Toxicology* 59C (June 10, 2013): 129–36; V. L. de Liz Oliveira Cavalli et al., "Roundup Disrupts Male Reproductive Functions by Triggering Calcium-Mediated Cell Death in Rat Testis and Sertoli Cells," *Free Radical Biology and Medicine* 65 (December 2013): 335–46; C. Gasnier et al., "Glyphosate-Based Herbicides Are Toxic and Endocrine Disruptors in Human Cell Lines," *Toxicology* 262, no. 3 (August 21, 2009): 184–91.

44 S. S. Yadav et al., "Toxic and Genotoxic Effects of Roundup on Tadpoles of the Indian Skittering Frog (*Euflictis cyanophlyctis*) in the Presence and Absence of Predator Stress," *Aquatic Toxicology* 132–133 (May 15, 2013): 1–8.

45 J. R. Lukacs, "Climate, Subsistence, and Health in Prehistoric India," in *Ancient Health: Skeletal Indicators of Agricultural and Economic Intensification*, ed. M. N. Cohen and G. M. M. Crane-Kramer (Gainesville: University Press of Florida, 2007), 245.

46 J. S. Sandhu and D. R. Fraser, "Effect of Dietary Cereals on Intestinal Permeability in Experimental Enteropathy in Rats," *Gut* 24, no. 9 (September 1983): 825–30.

47 "Arsenic in Rice and Rice Products," US Food and Drug Administration, http://www.fda.gov/Food/FoodborneIllnessContaminants/Metals/ucm319870.htm.

48 F. Faita et al., "Arsenic-Induced Genotoxicity and Genetic Susceptibility to Arsenic-Related Pathologies," *International Journal of Environmental Research and Public Health* 10, no. 4 (April 12, 2013): 1527–46.

49 Y. Chen et al., "Arsenic Exposure at Low-to-Moderate Levels and Skin Lesions, Arsenic Metabolism, Neurological Functions, and Biomarkers for Respiratory and Cardiovascular Diseases: Review of Recent Findings from the Health Effects of Arsenic Longitudinal Study (HEALS) in Bangladesh," *Toxicology and Applied Pharmacology* 239, no. 2 (September 1, 2009): 184–92.

50 Vainio, "Antibody Response against Wheat, Rye, Barley, Oats, and Corn," 134–38; I. Comino et al., "Diversity in Oat Potential Immunogenicity: Basis for the Selection of Oat Varieties with No Toxicity in Coeliac Disease," *Gut* 60, no. 7 (July 2011): 915–22.

51 M. L. Mishkind et al., "Localization of Wheat Germ Agglutinin-Like Lectins in Various Species of the Gramineae," *Science* 220, no. 4603 (June 17, 1983): 1290–92.

52 J. D. Axtell et al., "Digestibility of Sorghum Proteins," *Proceedings of the National Academy of Sciences* 78, no. 3 (1981): 1333–35.

CHAPTER 3

1 "Feed Grains: Yearbook Tables," USDA Economic Research Service, http://www.ers.usda.gov/data-products/feed-grains-database/feed-grains-yearbook-tables.aspx#26766.

2 D. Pimentel and M. Pimentel, "Sustainability of Meat-Based and Plant-Based Diets and the Environment," *American Journal of Clinical Nutrition* 78, no. 3 (2003): 660S–3S.

3 D. Morgan, *Merchants of Grain* (Lincoln, NE: Authors Guild, 2000): 181.

4   http://www.supremecourt.gov/Search.aspx?FileName=/docketfiles/13-303.htm.
5   "Agribusiness," Center for Responsive Politics, http://www.opensecrets.org/lobby /indus.php?id=A&year=2012.

CHAPTER 4

1   "Gastrointestinal," AstraZeneca Annual Report and Form 20-F Information 2011, http://www.astrazeneca-annualreports.com/2011/business_review/therapy_area_ review/gastrointestinal.
2   C. Bourne et al., "Emergent Adverse Effects of Proton Pump Inhibitors," *La Presse Médicale* 42, no. 2 (February 2013): e53–62.
3   I. M. Tieyjeh et al., "The Association between Histamine 2 Receptor Antagonist Use and *Clostridium difficile* Infection: A Systematic Review and Meta-Analysis," *PLoS ONE* 8, no. 3 (2013): e56498.
4   S. Biswas et al., "Potential Immunological Consequences of Pharmacological Suppression of Gastric Acid Production in Patients with Multiple Sclerosis," *BMC Medicine* 10 (June 7, 2012): 57.
5   M. I. Vazquez-Roque et al., "A Controlled Trial of Gluten-Free Diet in Patients with Irritable Bowel Syndrome-Diarrhea: Effects on Bowel Frequency and Intestinal Function," *Gastroenterology* 145 (2013): 320–28.
6   C. Ebert et al., "Inhibitory Effect of the Lectin Wheat Germ Agglutinin (WGA) on the Proliferation of AR42J cells," *Acta Histochemica* 111, no. 4 (2009): 335–42; R. Santer et al., "The Role of Carbohydrate Moieties of Cholecystokinin Receptors in Cholecystokinin Octapeptide Binding: Alteration of Binding Data by Specific Lectins," *Biochimica et Biophysica Acta* 1051, no. 1 (January 23, 1990): 78–83.
7   A. Sonnenberg and A. D. Müller, "Constipation and Cathartics as Risk Factors of Colorectal Cancer: A Meta-Analysis," *Pharmacology* 47, sup. 1 (1993): 224–33.
8   C. Catassi et al., "Non-Celiac Gluten Sensitivity: The New Frontier of Gluten Related Disorders," *Nutrients* 5, no. 10 (September 26, 2013): 3839–53.
9   U. Volta et al., "Serological Tests in Gluten Sensitivity (Non Celiac Gluten Intolerance)," *Journal of Clinical Gastroenterology* 46 (2012): 680–85.
10 S. R. Lynch, B. S. Skikne, and J. D. Cook, "Food Iron Absorption in Idiopathic Hemochromatosis," *Blood* 74, no. 6 (November 1, 1989): 2187–93.
11 P. B. Holm, K. N. Kristiansen, and H. B. Pedersen, "Transgenic Approaches in Commonly Consumed Cereals to Improve Iron and Zinc Content and Bioavailability," *Journal of Nutrition* 132, no. 3 (March 2002): 514S–6S.
12 H. Monzón et al., "Mild Enteropathy as a Cause of Iron-Deficiency Anaemia of Previously Unknown Origin," *Digestive and Liver Disease* 43, no. 6 (June 2011): 448– 53; L. Davidsson, "Approaches to Improve Iron Bioavailability from Complementary Foods," *Journal of Nutrition* 133, no. 5, sup. 1 (May 2003): 1560S–2S.
13 N. Elhakim et al., "Fortifying Baladi Bread in Egypt: Reaching More Than 50 Million People through the Subsidy Program," *Food and Nutrition Bulletin* 33, sup. 4 (December 2012): S260–71.
14 N. J. Wierdsma et al., "Vitamin and Mineral Deficiencies are Highly Prevalent in Newly Diagnosed Celiac Disease Patients," *Nutrients* 5, no. 10 (September 30, 2013): 3975–92; L. R. Sáez et al., "Refractory Iron-Deficiency Anemia and Gluten Intolerance—Response to Gluten-Free Diet," *Revista Española de Enfermedades Digestivas* 103, no. 7 (July 2011): 349–54.
15 N. Roohani et al., "Zinc and Its Importance for Human Health: An Integrative Review," *Journal of Research in Medical Sciences* 18, no. 2 (February 2013): 144–57.
16 H. H. Sandstead, "Human Zinc Deficiency: Discovery to Initial Translation," *Advances in Nutrition* 4, no. 1 (January 1, 2013): 76–81.

17 P. B. Holm, "Transgenic Approaches in Commonly Consumed Cereals," 514S–6S.

18 International Zinc Nutrition Consultative Group (IZiNCG) et al., "International Zinc Nutrition Consultative Group (IZiNCG) Technical Document #1. Assessment of the Risk of Zinc Deficiency in Populations and Options for Its Control," *Food and Nutrition Bulletin* 25 (2004): S99–203.

19 A. S. Prasad, "Discovery of Human Zinc Deficiency: Its Impact on Human Health and Disease," *Advances in Nutrition* 4, no. 2 (March 1, 2013): 176–90.

20 R. B. Ervin and J. Kennedy-Stephenson, "Mineral Intakes of Elderly Adult Supplement and Non-Supplement Users in the Third National Health and Nutrition Examination Survey," *Journal of Nutrition* 132 (2002): 3422–27; N. J. Wierdsma, "Vitamin and Mineral Deficiencies," 3975–92.

21 R. S. Gibson, "History Review of Progress in the Assessment of Dietary Zinc Intake as an Indicator of Population Zinc Status," *Advances in Nutrition* 3 (2012): 772–82.

22 Institute of Medicine, *Dietary Reference Intakes for Vitamin A, Vitamin K, Arsenic, Boron, Chromium, Copper, Iodine, Iron, Manganese, Molybdenum, Nickel, Silicon, Vanadium, and Zinc* (Washington, DC: National Academies Press, 2001).

23 N. J. Wierdsma, "Vitamin and Mineral Deficiencies," 3975–92.

24 O. Jokinen et al., "Lectin Binding to the Porcine and Human Ileal Receptor of Intrinsic Factor-Cobalamin," *Glycoconjugate Journal* 6, no. 4 (1989): 525–38.

25 W. Hunger-Battefeld et al., "Prevalence of Polyglandular Autoimmune Syndrome in Patients with Diabetes Mellitus Type 1," *Medizinische Klinik* 104, no. 3 (March 15, 2009): 183–91.

26 L. H. Allen et al., "Considering the Case for Vitamin B_{12} Fortification of Flour," *Food and Nutrition Bulletin* 31, sup. 1 (March 2010): S36–46.

27 J. A. Arnason et al., "Do Adults with High Gliadin Antibody Concentrations Have Subclinical Gluten Intolerance?" *Gut* 33, no. 2 (February 1992): 194–97.

28 S. F. Choumenkovitch et al., "Folic Acid Intake from Fortification in United States Exceeds Predictions," *Journal of Nutrition* 132 (2002): 2792–98; J. B. Mason et al., "A Temporal Association between Folic Acid Fortification and an Increase in Colorectal Cancer Rates May Be Illuminating Important Biological Principles: A Hypothesis," *Cancer Epidemiology, Biomarkers, and Prevention* 16 (2007): 1325.

29 R. Vieth, "Vitamin D Supplementation, 25-Hydroxyvitamin D Concentrations, and Safety," *American Journal of Clinical Nutrition* 69, no. 5 (May 1999): 842–56.

30 M. A. Cabral et al., "Prevalence of Vitamin D Deficiency During the Summer and Its Relationship with Sun Exposure and Skin Phototype in Elderly Men Living in the Tropics," *Journal of Clinical Interventions in Aging* 8 (2013): 1347–51.

31 A. J. Lucendo and A. García-Manzanares, "Bone Mineral Density in Adult Coeliac Disease: An Updated Review," *Revista Espanola de Enfermedades Digestivas* 105, no. 3 (May 2013): 154–62.

32 C. De Filippo et al., "Impact of Diet in Shaping Gut Microbiota Revealed by a Comparative Study in Children from Europe and Rural Africa," *Proceedings of the National Academy of Sciences of the United States of America* 107, no. 33 (2010): 14691–96.

33 K. Brown et al., "Diet-Induced Dysbiosis of the Intestinal Microbiota and the Effects on Immunity and Disease," *Nutrients* 4, no. 8 (August 2012): 1095–119.

34 A. W. Walker et al., "Dominant and Diet-Responsive Groups of Bacteria within the Human Colonic Microbiota," *The ISME Journal: Multidisciplinary Journal of Microbial Ecology* 5 (2011): 220–30; G. D. Wu et al., "Linking Long-Term Dietary Patterns with Gut Microbial Enterotypes," *Science* 334 (2011): 105–8.

35 A. H. Sachdev and M. Pimentel, "Gastrointestinal Bacterial Overgrowth: Pathogenesis and Clinical Significance," *Therapeutic Advances in Chronic Disease* 4, no. 5 (September 2013): 223–31.

36 A. Tursi, G. Brandimarte, and G. Giorgetti, "High Prevalence of Small Intestinal Bacterial Overgrowth in Celiac Patients with Persistence of Gastrointestinal Symptoms after Gluten Withdrawal," *American Journal of Gastroenterology* 98, no. 4 (April 2003): 839–43; R. Khoshini et al., "A Systematic Review of Diagnostic Tests for Small Intestinal Bacterial Overgrowth," *Digestive Diseases and Sciences* 53, no. 6 (June 2008): 1443–54.

37 M. D. Howell et al., "Iatrogenic Gastric Acid Suppression and the Risk of Nosocomial Clostridium difficile Infection," *Archives of Internal Medicine* 170, no. 9 (May 10, 2010): 784–90.

38 M. C. Arrieta, L. Bistritz, and J. B. Meddings, "Alterations in Intestinal Permeability," *Gut* 55 (2006): 1512–20.

39 D. Bernardo et al., "Is Gliadin Really Safe for Non-Coeliac Individuals? Production of Interleukin 15 in Biopsy Culture from Non-Coeliac Individuals Challenged with Gliadin Peptides," *Gut* 56, no. 6 (June 2007): 889–90; M. Londei et al., "Gliadin as a Stimulator of Innate Responses in Celiac Disease," *Molecular Immunology* 42, no. 8 (May 2005): 913–18.

40 W. Wang et al., "Human Zonulin, a Potential Modulator of Intestinal Tight Junctions," *Journal of Cell Science* (2000): 1134435–40.

41 O. D. Anderson et al., "A New Class of Wheat Gliadin Genes and Proteins," *PLoS ONE* 7, no. 12 (2012): e52139; J. S. Sandhu and D. R. Fraser, "Effect of Dietary Cereals on Intestinal Permeability in Experimental Enteropathy in Rats," *Gut* 24, no. 9 (September 1983): 825–30.

CHAPTER 5

1 I. R. Korponay-Szabó et al., "Deamidated Gliadin Peptides Form Epitopes That Transglutaminase Antibodies Recognize," *Journal of Pediatric Gastroenterology and Nutrition* 46, no. 3 (March 2008): 253–61.

2 O. Lo Iacono et al., "Anti-Tissue Transglutaminase Antibodies in Patients with Abnormal Liver Tests: Is It Always Coeliac Disease?" *American Journal of Gastroenterology* 100, no. 11 (November 2005): 2472–77.

3 A. J. Williams et al., "The High Prevalence of Autoantibodies to Tissue Transglutaminase in First-Degree Relatives of Patients with Type 1 Diabetes Is Not Associated with Islet Autoimmunity," *Diabetes Care* 24, no. 3 (March 2001): 504–9.

4 D. B. Mueller et al., "Influence of Early Nutritional Components on the Development of Murine Autoimmune Diabetes," *Annals of Nutrition and Metabolism* 54, no. 3 (2009): 208–17.

5 S. S. Mehr et al., "Rice: A Common and Severe Cause of Food Protein-Induced Enterocolitis Syndrome," *Archives of Disease in Childhood* 94, no. 3 (March 2009): 220–23.

6 D. O. Funda et al., "Gluten-Free Diet Prevents Diabetes in NOD Mice," *Diabetes/ Metabolism Research and Reviews* 15, no. 5 (September–October 1999): 323–27.

7 D. B. Mueller, "Influence of Early Nutritional Components," 208–17.

8 D. Hansen et al., "High Prevalence of Coeliac Disease in Danish Children with Type I Diabetes Mellitus," *Acta Paediatrica* 90, no. 11 (November 2001): 1238–43.

9 G. Barera et al., "Occurrence of Celiac Disease after Onset of Type 1 Diabetes: A 6-Year Prospective Longitudinal Study," *Pediatrics* 109, no. 5 (May 2002): 833–38.

10 W. E. Barbeau et al., "Elevated CD8 T Cell Responses in Type 1 Diabetes Patients to a 13 Amino Acid Coeliac-Active Peptide from α-Gliadin," *Clinical and Experimental Immunology* (published electronically September 10, 2013): doi:10.1111/cei.12203.

11 K. Vehik et al., "Increasing Incidence of Type 1 Diabetes in 0- to 17-Year-Old Colorado Youth," *Diabetes Care* 30, no. 3 (March 2007): 503–9.

12 J. Jiskra et al., "IgA and IgG Antigliadin, IgA Anti-Tissue Transglutaminase and Antiendomysial Antibodies in Patients with Autoimmune Thyroid Diseases and Their Relationship to Thyroidal Replacement Therapy," *Physiological Research* 52, no. 1 (2003): 79–88.

13 C. Betterle et al., "Celiac Disease in North Italian Patients with Autoimmune Addison's Disease," *European Journal of Endocrinology* 154, no. 2 (February 2006): 275–79.

14 R. Rosmond and P. Björntorp, "The Interactions between Hypothalamic-Pituitary-Adrenal Axis Activity, Testosterone, Insulin-Like Growth Factor I and Abdominal Obesity with Metabolism and Blood Pressure in Men," *International Journal of Obesity and Related Metabolic Disorders* 22, no. 12 (December 1998): 1184–96.

15 M. N. Silverman and E. M. Sternberg, "Glucocorticoid Regulation of Inflammation and Its Behavioral and Metabolic Correlates: From HPA Axis to Glucocorticoid Receptor Dysfunction," *Annals of the New York Academy of Sciences* 1261 (July 2012): 55–63.

16 C. Zioudrou, R. A. Streaty, and W. A. Klee, "Opioid Peptides Derived from Food Proteins. The Exorphins," *Journal of Biological Chemistry* 254, no. 7 (April 10, 1979): 2446–49.

17 M. T. Bardella et al., "Body Composition and Dietary Intakes in Adult Celiac Disease Patients Consuming a Strict Gluten-Free Diet," *American Journal of Clinical Nutrition* 72, no. 4 (October 2000): 937–39.

18 A. Vojdani, T. O'Bryan, and J. A. Green, "Immune Response to Dietary Proteins, Gliadin, and Cerebellar Peptides in Children with Autism," *Nutritional Neuroscience* 7, no. 3 (June 2004): 151–61; E. Lahat et al., "Prevalence of Celiac Antibodies in Children with Neurologic Disorders," *Pediatric Neurology* 22, no. 5 (May 2000): 393–96.

19 N. M. Lau et al., "Markers of Celiac Disease and Gluten Sensitivity in Children with Autism," *PLoS ONE* 8, no. 6 (June 18, 2013): e66155.

20 F. C. Dohan, D. R. Levitt, and L. D. Kushnir, "Abnormal Behavior after Intracerebral Injection of Polypeptides from Wheat Gliadin: Possible Relevance to Schizophrenia," *Pavlovian Journal of Biological Science* 13, no. 2 (1978): 73–82; O. Okusaga et al., "Elevated Gliadin Antibody Levels in Individuals with Schizophrenia," *World Journal of Biological Psychiatry* 14, no. 7 (September 2013): 509–15; F. Dickerson et al., "Markers of Gluten Sensitivity and Celiac Disease in Recent-Onset Psychosis and Multi-Episode Schizophrenia," *Biological Psychiatry* 68, no. 1 (July 1, 2010): 100–4.

21 A. E. Kalaydijan et al., "The Gluten Connection: The Association between Schizophrenia and Celiac Disease," *Acta Psychiatrica Scandinavica* 113, no. 2 (February 2006): 82–90; J. Jackson et al., "A Gluten-Free Diet in People with Schizophrenia and Anti-Tissue Transglutaminase or Anti-Gliadin Antibodies," *Schizophrenia Research* 140, no. 1–3 (September 2012): 262–63.

22 F. Dickerson et al., "Markers of Gluten Sensitivity and Celiac Disease in Bipolar Disorder," *Bipolar Disorders* 13, no. 1 (February 2011): 52–58; F. Dickerson et al., "Markers of Gluten Sensitivity in Acute Mania: A Longitudinal Study," *Psychiatry Research* 196, no. 1 (March 30, 2012): 68–71.

23 U. Volta et al., "Serological Tests in Gluten Sensitivity (Nonceliac Gluten Intolerance)," *Journal of Clinical Gastroenterology* 46, no. 8 (September 2012): 680–85.

24 S. Choi et al., "Meal Ingestion, Amino Acids, and Brain Neurotransmitters: Effects of Dietary Protein Source on Serotonin and Catecholamine Synthesis Rates," *Physiology and Behavior* 98, no. 1–2 (August 4, 2009): 156–62.

25 T. R. Sharma et al., "Psychiatric Comorbidities in Patients with Celiac Disease: Is There Any Concrete Biological Association?" *Asian Journal of Psychiatry* 4, no. 2 (June 2011): 150–51.

26 A. Alaedini et al., "Immune Cross-Reactivity in Celiac Disease: Anti-Gliadin Antibodies Bind to Neuronal Synapsin I," *Journal of Immunology* 178, no. 10 (May 15, 2007): 6590–95.

27 G. Gobbi et al., "Coeliac Disease, Epilepsy, and Cerebral Calcifications. The Italian Working Group on Coeliac Disease and Epilepsy," *Lancet* 340, no. 8817 (August 22, 1992): 439–43.

28 W. T. Hu et al., "Cognitive Impairment and Celiac Disease," *Archives of Neurology* 63, no. 10 (October 2006): 1440–46.

29 P. K. Crane et al., "Glucose Levels and Risk of Dementia," *New England Journal of Medicine* 369, no. 6 (August 8, 2013): 540–48.

30 S. Choi, "Meal Ingestion, Amino Acids, and Brain Neurotransmitters," 156–62.

31 K. Pol et al., "Whole Grain and Body Weight Changes in Apparently Healthy Adults: A Systematic Review and Meta-Analysis of Randomized Controlled Studies," *American Journal of Clinical Nutrition* 98, no. 4 (October 2013): 872–84.

32 M. Dall et al., "Gliadin Fragments and a Specific Gliadin 33-mer Peptide Close KATP Channels and Induce Insulin Secretion in INS-1E Cells and Rat Islets of Langerhans," *PLoS ONE* 8, no. 6 (2013): e66474, doi:10.1371/journal.pone.0066474.

33 M. R. Cohen et al., "Naloxone Reduces Food Intake in Humans," *Psychosomatic Medicine* 47, no. 2 (March/April 1985): 1332–38; A. Drewnowski et al., "Naloxone, an Opiate Blocker, Reduces the Consumption of Sweet High-Fat Foods in Obese and Lean Female Binge Eaters," *American Journal of Clinical Nutrition* 61 (1995): 1206–12.

34 Z. Shi et al., "Vegetable-Rich Food Pattern Is Related to Obesity in China," *International Journal of Obesity* 32, no. 6 (June 2008): 975–84.

35 N. M. Morton and J. R. Seckl, "11beta-Hydroxysteroid Dehydrogenase Type 1 and Obesity," *Frontiers of Hormone Research* 36 (2008): 146–64.

36 T. Jönsson et al., "Agrarian Diet and Diseases of Affluence—Do Evolutionary Novel Dietary Lectins Cause Leptin Resistance?" *BMC Endocrine Disorders* 5 (December 10, 2005): 10.

37 "2011 National Diabetes Fact Sheet," Centers for Disease Control, http://www.cdc.gov/diabetes/pubs/factsheet11.htm.

38 "IDF Diabetes Atlas, 6th Edition" International Diabetes Federation, http://www.idf.org/diabetesatlas.

39 B. M. Popkin and K. J. Duffey, "Does Hunger and Satiety Drive Eating Anymore? Increasing Eating Occasions and Decreasing Time between Eating Occasions in the United States," *American Journal of Clinical Nutrition* 91, no. 5 (May 2010): 1342–47.

40 "Dietary Guidelines for Americans, 2010," US Department of Agriculture, http://www.health.gov/dietaryguidelines/dga2010/DietaryGuidelines2010.pdf.

41 K. Foster-Powell, S. Holt, and J. Brand-Miller, "International Table of Glycemic Index and Glycemic Load Values: 2002," *American Journal of Clinical Nutrition* 76 (2002): 5–56.

42 B. Beck et al., "Effects of Long-Term Ingestion of Aspartame on Hypothalamic Neuropeptide Y, Plasma Leptin and Body Weight Gain and Composition," *Physiology and Behavior* 75, no. 1–2 (February 1, 2002): 41–47.

43 P. Marchetti et al., "The Pancreatic Beta Cells in Human Type 2 Diabetes," *Advances in Experimental Medicine and Biology* 771 (2012): 288–309.

44 Ibid.

45 Z. Michailidou et al., "Omental 11beta-Hydroxysteroid Dehydrogenase 1 Correlates with Fat Cell Size Independently of Obesity," *Obesity* 15, no. 5 (May 2007): 1155–63.

46 G. Williams, "Aromatase Up-Regulation, Insulin, and Raised Intracellular Oestrogens in Men, Induce Adiposity, Metabolic Syndrome, and Prostate Disease, via Aberrant ER-α and GPER Signalling," *Molecular and Cellular Endocrinology* 351, no. 2 (April 4, 2012): 269–78.

47 F. Roelfsema et al., "Prolactin Secretion in Healthy Adults Is Determined by Gender, Age, and Body Mass Index," *PLoS One* 7, no. 2 (2012): e31305; G. Fanciulli et al., "Serum Prolactin Levels after Administration of the Alimentary Opioid Peptide Gluten Exorphin B4 in Male Rats," *Nutritional Neuroscience* 7, no. 1 (February 2004): 53–55.

48 R. E. Johnson and M. H. Murah, "Gynecomastia: Pathophysiology, Evaluation, and Management," *Mayo Clinic Proceedings* 84, no. 11 (November 2009): 1010–15.

49 N. Molteni, M. T. Bardella, and P. A. Bianchi, "Obstetric and Gynecological Problems in Women with Untreated Celiac Sprue," *Journal of Clinical Gastroenterology* 12, no. 1 (February 1990): 37–39; K. S. Sher, et al., "Infertility, Obstetric and Gynaecological Problems in Coeliac Sprue," *Digestive Diseases* 12, no. 3 (May–June 1994): 186–90; J. R. Green et al., "Reversible Insensitivity to Androgens in Men with Untreated Gluten Enteropathy," *Lancet* 1, no. 8006 (February 5, 1977): 280–82.

50 R. J. Santen et al., "History of Aromatase: Saga of an Important Biological Mediator and Therapeutic Target," *Endocrine Reviews* 30, no. 4 (June 2009): 343–75.

51 A. Lautenbach, A. Budde, and C. D. Wrann, "Obesity and the Associated Mediators Leptin, Estrogen and IGF-I Enhance the Cell Proliferation and Early Tumorigenesis of Breast Cancer Cells," *Nutrition and Cancer* 61, no. 4 (2009): 484–91; Endogenous Hormones and Breast Cancer Collaborative Group et al., "Endogenous Sex Hormones and Breast Cancer in Postmenopausal Women: Reanalysis of Nine Prospective Studies," *Journal of the National Cancer Institute* 94 (2002): 606–16.

52 P. Kok et al., "Prolactin Release Is Enhanced in Proportion to Excess Visceral Fat in Obese Women," *Journal of Clinical Endocrinology and Metabolism* 89, no. 9 (September 2004): 4445–49.

53 A. Lautenbach, "Obesity and the Associated Mediators," 484–91.

54 A. Veronelli et al., "Sexual Dysfunction Is Frequent in Premenopausal Women with Diabetes, Obesity, and Hypothyroidism, and Correlates with Markers of Increased Cardiovascular Risk. A Preliminary Report," *Journal of Sexual Medicine* 6, no. 6 (June 2009): 1561–68.

55 D. Bustos et al., "Autoantibodies in Argentine Women with Recurrent Pregnancy Loss," *American Journal of Reproductive Immunology* 55, no. 3 (March 2006): 201–7.

56 R. Pasquali, L. Patton, and A. Gambineri, "Obesity and Infertility," *Current Opinion in Endocrine, Diabetes, and Obesity* 14, no. 6 (December 2007): 482–87; C. J. Brewer and A. H. Balen, "The Adverse Effects of Obesity on Conception and Implantation," *Reproduction* 140, no. 3 (September 2010): 347–64.

57 J. W. Rich-Edwards et al., "Adolescent Body Mass Index and Infertility Caused by Ovulatory Disorder," *American Journal of Obstetrics and Gynecology* 171 (1994): 171–77.

58 A. Gambineri et al., "Obesity and the Polycystic Ovary Syndrome," *International Journal of Obesity and Related Metabolic Disorders* 26 (2002): 883–96.

59 M. Quinkler et al., "Androgen Generation in Adipose Tissue in Women with Simple Obesity—a Site-Specific Role for 17beta-Hydroxysteroid Dehydrogenase Type 5," *Journal of Endocrinology* 183, no. 2 (November 2004): 331–42.

60 P. O. Kwiterovich, "Clinical Relevance of the Biochemical, Metabolic, and Genetic Factors That Influence Low-Density Lipoprotein Heterogeneity," *American Journal of Cardiology* 90, sup. (2002): 30i-47i.

61 T. J. Lyons, "Glycation and Oxidation: A Role in the Pathogenesis of Atherosclerosis," *American Journal of Cardiology* 71, no. 6 (February 25, 1993): 26B–31B.

62 S. Lindeberg, "Risks with the Paleolithic Diet," in *Food and Western Disease* (Oxford: Wiley-Blackwell, 2010), 99.

63 A. Frustaci et al., "Celiac Disease Associated with Autoimmune Myocarditis," *Circulation* 105, no. 22 (June 4, 2002): 2611–18.

64 M. Curione et al., "Idiopathic Dilated Cardiomyopathy Associated with Coeliac Disease: The Effect of a Gluten-Free Diet on Cardiac Performance," *Digestive and Liver Disease* 34, no. 12 (December 2002): 866–69.

65 D. Saadeh et al., "Diet and Allergic Diseases among Population Aged 0 to 18 Years: Myth or Reality?" *Nutrients* 5, no. 9 (August 29, 2013): 3399–423.

66 T. E. Hansen, B. Evjenth, and J. Holt, "Increasing Prevalence of Asthma, Allergic Rhinoconjunctivitis and Eczema among Schoolchildren: Three Surveys During the Period 1985–2008," *Acta Paediatrica* 102, no. 1 (January 2013): 47–52.

67 S. Quirce and A. Diaz-Perales, "Diagnosis and Management of Grain-Induced Asthma," *Allergy, Asthma, and Immunology Research* 5, no. 6 (November 2013): 348–56.

68 D. J. Hogan et al., "Questionnaire Survey of Pruritus and Rash in Grain Elevator Workers," *Contact Dermatitis* 14, no. 3 (March 1986): 170–75.

69 A. M. Minford, A. MacDonald, and J. M. Littlewood, "Food Intolerance and Food Allergy in Children: A Review of 68 Cases," *Archives of Disease in Childhood* 57, no. 10 (October 1982): 742–47.

70 L. Cordain, "Implications for the Role of Diet in Acne," *Seminars in Cutaneous Medicine and Surgery* 24, no. 2 (June 2005): 84–91.

71 L. Cordain et al., "Acne Vulgaris: A Disease of Western Civilization," *Archives of Dermatology* 138 (2002): 1584–90.

72 Ibid.

73 H. Liljeberg Elmståhl and I. Björk, "Milk as a Supplement to Mixed Meals May Elevate Postprandial Insulinaemia," *European Journal of Clinical Nutrition* 55, no. 11 (November 2001): 994–99.

74 G. Gaitanis et al., "Skin Diseases Associated with Malassezia Yeasts: Facts and Controversies," *Clinical Dermatology* 31, no. 4 (July–August 2013): 455–63.

75 J. Skayland et al., "In Vitro Screening for Putative Psoriasis-Specific Antigens among Wheat Proteins and Peptides," *British Journal of Dermatology* 166, no. 1 (January 2012): 67–73.

76 G. Michaëlsson et al., "Patients with Psoriasis Often Have Increased Serum Levels of IgA Antibodies to Gliadin," *British Journal of Dermatology* 129, no. 6 (December 1993): 667–73.

77 R. Saraceno, "The Role of Neuropeptides in Psoriasis," 876–82.

78 G. Michaëlsson et al., "Psoriasis Patients with Antibodies to Gliadin Can Be Improved by a Gluten-Free Diet," *British Journal of Dermatology* 142, no. 1 (January 2000): 44–51.

79 R. Beasley, "The International Study of Asthma and Allergies in Childhood (ISAAC) Steering Committee. Worldwide Variation in Prevalence of Symptoms of Asthma, Allergic Rhinoconjunctivitis, and Atopic Eczema: ISAAC," *Lancet* 351 (1998): 1225–32.

80 T. E. Hansen, B. Evjenth, and J. Holt, "Increasing Prevalence of Asthma, Allergic Rhinoconjunctivitis and Eczema among Schoolchildren: Three Surveys During the Period 1985–2008," 47–52.

81 C. Ciacci et al., "Allergy Prevalence in Adult Celiac Disease," *Journal of Allergy and Clinical Immunology* 113, no. 6 (June 2004): 1199–203.

82 E. A. Pastorello et al., "Wheat IgE-Mediated Food Allergy in European Patients: Alpha-Amylase Inhibitors, Lipid Transfer Proteins and Low-Molecular-Weight Glutenins," *International Archives of Allergy and Immunology* 144, no. 1 (2007): 10–22.

83 D. Wray, "Gluten-Sensitive Recurrent Aphthous Stomatitis," *Digestive Diseases and Sciences* 26, no. 8 (August 1981): 737–40.

CHAPTER 6

1 S. D. Phinney et al., "Capacity for Moderate Exercise in Obese Subjects after Adaptation to a Hypocaloric, Ketogenic Diet," *Journal of Clinical Investigation* 66, no. 5 (November 1980): 1152–61.

2   M. W. Brands and M. M. Manhiani, "Sodium-Retaining Effect of Insulin in Diabetes," *American Journal of Physiology—Regulatory, Integrative, and Comparative Physiology* 303, no. 11 (December 2012): R1101–9.

3   K. L. Caldwell et al., "Iodine Status of the US Population, National Health and Nutrition Examination Survey 2003-2004," *Thyroid* 18, no. 11 (November 2008): 1207–14.

4   I. F. Mao, M. L. Chen, and Y. C. Ko, "Electrolyte Loss in Sweat and Iodine Deficiency in a Hot Environment," *Archives of Environmental Health* 56, no. 3 (May–June 2001): 271–77.

5   N. A. Qureshi and A. M. Al-Bedah, "Mood Disorders and Complementary and Alternative Medicine: A Literature Review," *Journal of Neuropsychiatric Disease and Treatment* 9 (2013): 639–58.

6   C. Cangiano et al., "Eating Behavior and Adherence to Dietary Prescriptions in Obese Adult Subjects Treated with 5-Hydroxytryptophan," *American Journal of Clinical Nutrition* 56, no. 5 (November 1992): 863–67; T. Jukic et al., "The Use of a Food Supplementation with D-Phenylalanine, L-Glutamine and L-5-Hydroxytriptophan in the Alleviation of Alcohol Withdrawal Symptoms," *Collegium Antropologicum* 35, no. 4 (December 2011): 1225–30.

7   V. Darbinyan et al., "Clinical Trial of *Rhodiola rosea* L. Extract SHR-5 in the Treatment of Mild to Moderate Depression," *Nordic Journal of Psychiatry* 61, no. 5 (2007): 343–48; Q. G. Chen et al., "The Effects of *Rhodiola rosea* Extract on 5-HT Level, Cell Proliferation and Quantity of Neurons at Cerebral Hippocampus of Depressive Rats," *Phytomedicine* 16, no. 9 (September 2009): 830–38.

8   J. A. Murray et al., "Effect of a Gluten-Free Diet on Gastrointestinal Symptoms in Celiac Disease," *American Journal of Clinical Nutrition* 79, no. 4 (April 2004): 669–73; J. Cheng et al., "Body Mass Index in Celiac Disease: Prevalence, Clinical Characteristics, and Effect of a Gluten-Free Diet," *Journal of Clinical Gastroenterology* 44, no. 4 (April 2010): 267–71; N. Venkatasubramani, G. Telega, and S. L. Werlin, "Obesity in Pediatric Celiac Disease," *Journal of Pediatric Gastroenterology and Nutrition* 51, no. 3 (September 2010): 295–97; M. T. Bardella et al., "Body Composition and Dietary Intakes in Adult Celiac Disease Patients Consuming a Strict Gluten-Free Diet," *American Journal of Clinical Nutrition* 72, no. 4 (October 2000): 937–39; E. Smecuol et al., "Longitudinal Study on the Effect of Treatment on Body Composition and Anthropometry of Celiac Disease Patients," *American Journal of Gastroenterology* 92, no. 4 (April 1997): 639–43.

9   B. R. Douglas et al., "Coffee Stimulation of Cholecystokinin Release and Gallbladder Contraction in Humans," *American Journal of Clinical Nutrition* 52, no. 3 (September 1990): 553–56.

10   A. M. Riordan et al., "Treatment of Active Crohn's Disease by Exclusion Diet: East Anglian Multicentre Controlled Trial," *Lancet* 342 (1993): 1131–34.

11   H. S. Said et al., "Dysbiosis of Salivary Microbiota in Inflammatory Bowel Disease and Its Association with Oral Immunological Biomarkers," *DNA Research* (published electronically September 7, 2013); F. Fava and S. Danese, "Intestinal Microbiota in Inflammatory Bowel Disease: Friend of Foe?" *World Journal of Gastroenterology* 17, no. 5 (February 7, 2011): 557–66.

12   G. R. Greenberg, "Antibiotics Should Be Used as First-Line Therapy for Crohn's Disease," *Inflammatory Bowel Diseases* 10 (2004): 318–20.

13   D. Jonkers et al., "Probiotics in the Management of Inflammatory Bowel Disease: A Systematic Review of Intervention Studies in Adult Patients," *Drugs* 72, no. 6 (April 16, 2012): 803–23.

14   E. Miele et al., "Effect of a Probiotic Preparation (VSL#3) on Induction and Maintenance of Remission in Children with Ulcerative Colitis," *American Journal of Gastroenterology* 104, no. 2 (February 2009): 437–43.

15 W. Kruis, "Review Article: Antibiotics and Probiotics in Inflammatory Bowel Disease," *Alimentary Pharmacology and Therapeutics* 20, sup. 4 (2004): 75–78.

16 J. O. Lindsay et al., "Clinical, Microbiological, and Immunological Effects of Fructo-Oligosaccharide in Patients with Crohn's Disease," *Gut* 55 (2006): 348–55.

17 F. Fava, "Intestinal Microbiota," 557–66.

18 A. Belluzzi et al., "Effect of an Enteric-Coated Fish-Oil Preparation on Relapses in Crohn's Disease," *New England Journal of Medicine* 334, no. 24 (June 13, 1996): 1557–60.

19 V. A. Jones, "Comparison of Total Parenteral Nutrition and Elemental Diet in Induction of Remission of Crohn's Disease. Long-Term Maintenance of Remission by Personalized Food Exclusion Diets," *Digestive Diseases and Sciences* 32, sup. 12 (December 1987): 100S–7S.

20 S. Mishkin, "Dairy Sensitivity, Lactose Malabsorption, and Elimination Diets in Inflammatory Bowel Disease," *American Journal of Clinical Nutrition* 65, no. 2 (February 1997): 564–67.

21 J. S. Barrett et al., "Comparison of the Prevalence of Fructose and Lactose Malabsorption across Chronic Intestinal Disorders," *Alimentary Pharmacology and Therapeutics* 30, no. 2 (July 1, 2009): 165–74.

22 G. DePalma et al., "Intestinal Dysbiosis and Reduced Immunoglobulin-Coated Bacteria Associated with Coeliac Disease in Children," *BMC Microbiology* 10 (February 24, 2010): 63.

23 A. Tursi, G. Brandimarte, and G. Giorgetti, "High Prevalence of Small Intestinal Bacterial Overgrowth in Celiac Patients with Persistence of Gastrointestinal Symptoms after Gluten Withdrawal," *American Journal of Gastroenterology* 98 (2003): 839–43.

24 T. Malterre, "Digestive and Nutritional Considerations in Celiac Disease: Could Supplementation Help?" *Alternative Medicine Review* 14, no. 3 (September 2009): 247–57.

25 M. C. Lomer, G. C. Parkes, and J. D. Sanderson, "Review Article: Lactose Intolerance in Clinical Practice—Myths and Realities," *Alimentary Pharmacology and Therapeutics* 27 (2008): 93–103.

26 I. Hafström et al., "A Vegan Diet Free of Gluten Improves the Signs and Symptoms of Rheumatoid Arthritis: The Effects on Arthritis Correlate with a Reduction in Antibodies to Food Antigens," *Rheumatology* (2001): 1175–79.

27 A. M. Clark et al., "Weight Loss in Obese Infertile Women Results in Improvement in Reproductive Outcome for all Forms of Fertility Treatment," *Human Reproduction* 13 (1998): 1502–5.

28 D. S. Kiddy et al., "Improvement in Endocrine and Ovarian Function During Dietary Treatment of Obese Women with Polycystic Ovary Syndrome," *Clinical Endocrinology* 36 (1992): 105–11.

29 J. R. Green et al., "Reversible Insensitivity to Androgens in Men with Untreated Gluten Enteropathy," *Lancet* 1, no. 8006 (February 5, 1977): 280–82.

30 E. Camacho et al., "Age-Associated Changes in Hypothalamic–Pituitary–Testicular Function in Middle-Aged and Older Men Are Modified by Weight Change and Lifestyle Factors: Longitudinal Results from the European Male Ageing Study," *European Journal of Endocrinology* 168 (2013): 445–55.

31 M. J. Farthing et al., "Male Gonadal Function in Coeliac Disease: 1. Sexual Dysfunction, Infertility, and Semen Quality," *Gut* 23, no. 7 (July 1982): 608–14; M. J. Farthing, L. H. Rees, and A. M. Dawson, "Male Gonadal Function in Coeliac Disease: III. Pituitary Regulation," *Clinical Endocrinology* 19, no. 6 (December 1983): 661–71.

CHAPTER 7

1   G. Jarzynska and J. Falandysz, "Selenium and 17 Other Largely Essential and Toxic Metals in Muscle and Organ Meats of Red Deer (*Cervus elaphus*)—Consequences to

Human Health," *Environment International* 37, no. 5 (July 2011): 882–88; N. Waegeneers et al., "Accumulation of Trace Elements in Cattle from Rural and Industrial Areas in Belgium," *Food Additives and Contaminants Part A* 26, no. 3 (March 2009): 326–32.

2   M. H. Ward, "Too Much of a Good Thing? Nitrate from Nitrogen Fertilizers and Cancer: President's Cancer Panel—October 21, 2008," *Reviews on Environmental Health* 24, no. 4 (2009): 357–63; D. C. Paik et al., "The Epidemiological Enigma of Gastric Cancer Rates in the US: Was Grandmother's Sausage the Cause?" *International Journal of Epidemiology* 30, no. 1 (February 2001): 181–82.

3   R. C. Massey et al., "Volatile, Non-Volatile and Total N-Nitroso Compounds in Bacon," *Food Additives and Contaminants* 8, no. 5 (1991): 585–98; J. Haorah et al., "Determination of Total N-Nitroso Compounds and Their Precursors in Frankfurters, Fresh Meat, Dried Salted Fish, Sauces, Tobacco, and Tobacco Smoke Particulates," *Journal of Agricultural and Food Chemistry* 49, no. 12 (December 2001): 6068–78.

4   H. Malekinejad, P. Scherpenisse, and A. A. Bergwerff, "Naturally Occurring Estrogens in Processed Milk and in Raw Milk (from Gestated Cows)," *Journal of Agricultural and Food Chemistry* 54, no. 26 (December 27, 2006): 9785–91.

5   "Sodium Intake in Populations: Assessment of Evidence, 2013," Institute of Medicine, http://www.iom.edu/Reports/2013/Sodium-Intake-in-Populations-Assessment-of-Evidence/Report-Brief051413.aspx.

6   I. A. Lang et al., "Association of Urinary Bisphenol A Concentration with Medical Disorders and Laboratory Abnormalities in Adults," *Journal of the American Medical Association* 300, no. 11 (September 17, 2008): 1303–10.

7   D. Mozaffarian, A. Aro, and W. C. Willett, "Health Effects of Trans-Fatty Acids: Experimental and Observational Evidence," *European Journal of Clinical Nutrition* 63, sup. 2 (May 2009): S5–21.

8   J. Uribarri et al., "Advanced Glycation End Products in Foods and a Practical Guide to Their Reduction in the Diet," *Journal of the American Dietetic Association* 110, no. 6 (June 2010): 911–16.e12.

9   B. Simonato et al., "Immunochemical and Mass Spectrometry Detection of Residual Proteins in Gluten Fined Red Wine," *Journal of Agricultural and Food Chemistry* 59, no. 7 (April 13, 2011): 3101–10.

CHAPTER 8

1   S. R. Lynch, "Why Nutritional Iron Deficiency Persists as a Worldwide Problem," *Journal of Nutrition* 141, no. 4 (April 1, 2011): 763S–8S.

2   L. Davidsson, "Approaches to Improve Iron Bioavailability from Complementary Foods," *Journal of Nutrition* 133, no. 5, sup. 1 (May 2003): 1560S–2S.

3   P. Santiago, "Ferrous versus Ferric Oral Iron Formulations for the Treatment of Iron Deficiency: A Clinical Overview," *Scientific World Journal* 2012 (2012): 846824.

4   D. Y. Liu et al., "Investigation of the Amount of Dissolved Iron in Food Cooked in Chinese Iron Pots and Estimation of Daily Iron Intake," *Biomedical and Environmental Sciences* 3, no. 3 (September 1990): 276–80; H. C. Brittin and C. E. Nossaman, "Iron Content of Food Cooked in Iron Utensils," *Journal of the American Dietetic Association* 86, no. 7 (July 1986): 897–901.

5   R. S. Gibson, "History Review of Progress in the Assessment of Dietary Zinc Intake as an Indicator of Population Zinc Status," *Advances in Nutrition* 3 (2012): 772–82.

6   W. Maret, "Zinc and Human Disease," *Metal Ions in Life Sciences* 13 (2013): 389–414.

7   F. H. Nielsen, "Magnesium, Inflammation, and Obesity in Chronic Disease," *Nutrition Reviews* 68, no. 6 (June 2010): 333–40; D. Thomas, "A Study on the Mineral Depletion of the Foods Available to Us as a Nation Over the Period 1940 to 1991," *Nutrition and Health* 17, no. 2 (2003): 85–115.

8   T. Bohn et al., "Phytic Acid Added to White-Wheat Bread Inhibits Fractional Apparent Magnesium Absorption in Humans," *American Journal of Clinical Nutrition* 79, no. 3 (March 2004): 418–23.

9   L. Cohen, "Recent Data on Magnesium and Osteoporosis," *Magnesium Research* 1 (1988): 85–87.

10 A. Rosanoff, C. M. Weaver, and R. K. Rude, "Suboptimal Magnesium Status in the United States: Are the Health Consequences Underestimated?" *Nutrition Reviews* 70, no. 3 (March 2012): 153–64; N. Hovdenak and K. Haram, "Influence of Mineral and Vitamin Supplements on Pregnancy Outcome," *European Journal of Obstetrics Gynecology and Reproductive Biology* 164, no. 2 (October 2012): 127–32.

11 G. Stendig-Lindberg, R. Tepper, and I. Leichter, "Trabecular Bone Density in a Two Year Controlled Trial of Peroral Magnesium in Osteoporosis," *Magnesium Research* 6, no. 2 (1993): 155–63.

12 S. J. Genuis and T. P. Bouchard, "Combination of Micronutrients for Bone (COMB) Study: Bone Density after Micronutrient Intervention," *Journal of Environmental and Public Health* 2012 (2012): 354151.

13 L. Kass, J. Weekes, and L. Carpenter, "Effect of Magnesium Supplementation on Blood Pressure: A Meta-Analysis," *European Journal of Clinical Nutrition* 66, no. 4 (April 2012): 411–18.

14 J. MacLaughlin and M. F. Holick, "Aging Decreases the Capacity of Human Skin to Produce Vitamin D_3," *Journal of Clinical Investigation* 76, no. 4 (October 1985): 1536–38; A. Valcour et al., "Effects of Age and Serum 25-OH-Vitamin D on Serum Parathyroid Hormone Levels," *Journal of Clinical Endocrinology and Metabolism* 97, no. 11 (November 2012): 3989–95.

15 C. C. Sung et al., "Role of Vitamin D in Insulin Resistance," *Journal of Biomedicine and Biotechnology* 2012 (2012): 634195; B. Schöttker et al., "Strong Associations of 25-Hydroxyvitamin D Concentrations with All-Cause, Cardiovascular, Cancer, and Respiratory Disease Mortality in a Large Cohort Study," *American Journal of Clinical Nutrition* 97, no. 4 (April 2013): 782–93; M. F. Holick, "Sunlight and Vitamin D for Bone Health and Prevention of Autoimmune Diseases, Cancers, and Cardiovascular Disease," *American Journal of Clinical Nutrition* 80, sup. 6 (December 2004): 1678S–88S.

16 S. Afzal, S. E. Bojesen, and B. G. Nordestgaard, "Low 25-Hydroxyvitamin D and Risk of Type 2 Diabetes: A Prospective Cohort Study and Meta-Analysis," *Clinical Chemistry* (published electronically December 11, 2012).

17 P. S. George, E. R. Pearson, and M. D. Witham, "Effect of Vitamin D Supplementation on Lycaemic Control and Insulin Resistance: A Systematic Review and Meta-Analysis," *Diabetic Medicine* 29, no. 8 (August 2012): e142–50; J. L. Rosenblum et al., "Calcium and Vitamin D Supplementation Is Associated with Decreased Abdominal Visceral Adipose Tissue in Overweight and Obese Adults," *American Journal of Clinical Nutrition* 95, no. 1 (January 2012): 101–18.

18 A. Valcour et al., "Effects of Age and Serum 25-OH-Vitamin D on Serum Parathyroid Hormone Levels," *Journal of Clinical Endocrinology and Metabolism* 97, no. 11 (November 2012): 3989–95.

19 M. B. Smith et al., "Vitamin D Excess Is Significantly Associated with Risk of Atrial Fibrillation," *Circulation* 124 (2011): A14699.

20 T. Rafferty, C. A. O'Morain, and M. O'Sullivan, "Vitamin D: New Roles and Therapeutic Potential in Inflammatory Bowel Disease," *Current Drug Metabolism* 13, no. 9 (November 2012): 1294–302; A. Tavakkoli et al., "Vitamin D Status and Concomitant Autoimmunity in Celiac Disease," *Journal of Clinical Gastroenterology* 47, no. 6 (July 2013): 515–19.

21 S. K. Raatz et al., "Issues of Fish Consumption for Cardiovascular Disease Risk Reduction," *Nutrients* 5, no. 4 (March 28, 2013): 1081–97; J. Mariani et al.,

"N-3 Polyunsaturated Fatty Acids to Prevent Atrial Fibrillation: Updated Systematic Review and Meta-Analysis of Randomized Controlled Trials," *Journal of the American Heart Association* 2, no. 1 (February 19, 2013): e005033; E. A. Miles and P. C. Calder, "Influence of Marine n-3 Polyunsaturated Fatty Acids on Immune Function and a Systematic Review of Their Effects on Clinical Outcomes in Rheumatoid Arthritis," *British Journal of Nutrition* 107, sup. 2 (June 2012): S171–84; A. Laviano et al., "Omega-3 Fatty Acids in Cancer," *Current Opinion in Clinical Nutrition and Metabolic Care* 16, no. 2 (March 2013): 156–61.

22 M. De Lorgeril et al., "Recent Findings on the Health Effects of Omega-3 Fatty Acids and Statins, and Their Interactions: Do Statins Inhibit Omega-3?" *BMC Medicine* 11 (2013): 5.

23 P. P. Smyth and L. H. Duntas, "Iodine Uptake and Loss—Can Frequent Strenuous Exercise Induce Iodine Deficiency?" *Hormone and Metabolic Research* 37, no. 9 (September 2005): 555–58.

24 T. Remer, A. Neubert, and F. Manz, "Increased Risk of Iodine Deficiency with Vegetarian Nutrition," *British Journal of Nutrition* 81, no. 1 (January 1999): 45–49.

25 W. R. Ghent et al., "Iodine Replacement in Fibrocystic Disease of the Breast," *Canadian Journal of Surgery* 36, no. 5 (October 1993): 453–60.

26 B. C. Blount et al., "Urinary Perchlorate and Thyroid Hormone Levels in Adolescent and Adult Men and Women Living in the United States," *Environmental Health Perspectives* 114, no. 12 (December 2006): 1865–71; C. Schmutzler et al., "Endocrine Disruptors and the Thyroid Gland—A Combined in Vitro and in Vivo Analysis of Potential New Biomarkers," *Environmental Health Perspectives* 115, sup. 1 (December 2007): 77–83.

27 P. K. Dasgupta, Y. Liu, and J. V. Dyke, "Iodine Nutrition: Iodine Content of Iodized Salt in the United States," *Environmental Science and Technology* 42, no. 4 (February 15, 2008): 1315–23.

28 B. S. Oberlin et al., "Vitamin B_{12} Deficiency in Relation to Functional Disabilities," *Nutrients* 5, no. 11 (November 12, 2013): 4462–75.

29 R. Carmel, "Biomarkers of Cobalamin (Vitamin B-12) Status in the Epidemiologic Setting: A Critical Overview of Context, Applications, and Performance Characteristics of Cobalamin, Methylmalonic Acid, and Holotranscobalamin II," *American Journal of Clinical Nutrition* 94, no. 1 (July 2011): 348S–58S.

30 E. L. Doets et al., "Systematic Review on Daily Vitamin B_{12} Losses and Bioavailability for Deriving Recommendations on Vitamin B_{12} Intake with the Factorial Approach," *Annals of Nutrition and Metabolism* 62, no. 4 (2013): 311–22.

31 S. J. Eussen et al., "Oral Cyanocobalamin Supplementation in Older People with Vitamin B12 Deficiency: A Dose-Finding Trial," *Archives of Internal Medicine* 164, no. 10 (May 23, 2005): 1167–72.

32 A. Sharabi et al., "Replacement Therapy for Vitamin B12 Deficiency: Comparison between the Sublingual and Oral Route," *British Journal of Clinical Pharmacology* 56, no. 6 (December 2003): 635–38.

33 K. Okuda, "Intestinal Absorption and Concurrent Chemical Changes of Methylcobalamin," *Journal of Laboratory and Clinical Medicine* 81 (1973): 557–67.

34 "National Nutrient Database for Standard Reference, Release 26," US Department of Agriculture Agricultural Research Service, http://ndb.nal.usda.gov/ndb/foods.

35 R. Green, "Indicators for Assessing Folate and Vitamin B-12 Status and for Monitoring the Efficacy of Intervention Strategies," *American Journal of Clinical Nutrition* 94, no. 2 (August 2011): 666S–72S.

36 Institute of Medicine, Food and Nutrition Board, *Dietary Reference Intakes: Thiamin, Riboflavin, Niacin, Vitamin B_6, Folate, Vitamin B_{12}, Pantothenic Acid, Biotin, and Choline* (National Academy Press: Washington, DC, 1998).

37 "National Nutrient Database for Standard Reference, Release 26," US Department of Agriculture Agricultural Research Service, http://ndb.nal.usda.gov/ndb/foods.

38 M. Ebbing et al., "Cancer Incidence and Mortality after Treatment with Folic Acid and Vitamin B₁₂," *JAMA* 302, no. 19 (2009): 2119–26; J. B. Mason et al., "A Temporal Association between Folic Acid Fortification and an Increase in Colorectal Cancer Rates May Be Illuminating Important Biological Principles: A Hypothesis," *Cancer Epidemiology, Biomarkers, and Prevention* 16 (2007): 1325.

39 A. E. Czeizel et al., "Prevention of Neural-Tube Defects with Periconceptional Folic Acid, Methylfolate, or Multivitamins?" *Annals of Nutrition and Metabolism* 58, no. 4 (October 2011): 263–71.

40 M. Fava and D. Mischoulon, "Folate in Depression: Efficacy, Safety, Differences in Formulations, and Clinical Issues," *Journal of Clinical Psychiatry* 70, sup. 5 (2009): 12–17.

41 A. C. Nilsson et al., "Including Indigestible Carbohydrates in the Evening Meal of Healthy Subjects Improves Glucose Tolerance, Lowers Inflammatory Markers, and Increases Satiety after a Subsequent Standardized Breakfast," *Journal of Nutrition* 138 (2008): 732–39.

CHAPTER 9

1 R. Khoshini et al., "A Systematic Review of Diagnostic Tests for Small Intestinal Bacterial Overgrowth," *Digestive Diseases and Sciences* 53 (2008): 1443–54.

2 A. H. Sachdev and M. Pimentel, "Gastrointestinal Bacterial Overgrowth: Pathogenesis and Clinical Significance," *Therapeutic Advances in Chronic Disease* 4, no. 5 (September 2013): 223–31.

3 A. Parodi et al., "Small Intestinal Bacterial Overgrowth in Rosacea: Clinical Effectiveness of Its Eradication," *Clinical Gastroenterology and Hepatology* 6 (2008): 759–64; L. Weinstock and A. Walters, "Restless Legs Syndrome Is Associated with Irritable Bowel Syndrome and Small Intestinal Bacterial Overgrowth," *Sleep Medicine* 12 (2011): 610–13.

4 H. M. Dodd and M. J. Gasson, "Bacteriocins of Lactic Acid Bacteria" in *Genetics and Biotechnology of Lactic Acid Bacteria*, M. J. Gasson and W. M. de Vos WM, eds. (Blackie Academic and Professional: London, 1994): 211–52.

5 L. R. Fitzpatrick, "Probiotics for the Treatment of *Clostridium difficile* Associated Disease," *World Journal of Gastrointestinal Pathophysiology* 4, no. 3 (August 15, 2013): 47–52.

6 V. Venugopalan, K. A. Shriner, and A. Wong-Beringer, "Regulatory Oversight and Safety of Probiotic Use," *Emerging Infectious Diseases* 16, no. 11 (November 2010): 1661–65.

7 G. D'Argenio and G. Mazzacca, "Short-Chain Fatty Acid in the Human Colon. Relation to Inflammatory Bowel Diseases and Colon Cancer," *Advances in Experimental Medicine and Biology* 472 (1999): 149–58.

8 J. M. Wong and D. J. Jenkins, "Carbohydrate Digestibility and Metabolic Effects," *Journal of Nutrition* 137, sup. 11 (November 2007): 2539S–46S.

9 G. Laden and R. Wrangham, "The Rise of the Hominids as an Adaptive Shift in Fallback Foods: Plant Underground Storage Organs (USOs) and Australopith Origins," *Journal of Human Evolution* 49, no. 4 (October 2005): 482–98.

10 J. G. Muir and K. O'Dea, "Measurement of Resistant Starch: Factors Affecting the Amount of Starch Escaping Digestion in Vitro," *American Journal of Clinical Nutrition* 56, no. 1 (July 1992): 123–27; D. J. Jenkins et al., "Digestibility of Carbohydrate Foods in an Ileostomate: Relationship to Dietary Fiber, in Vitro Digestibility, and Glycemic Response," *American Journal of Gastroenterology* 82 (1987): 709–17; M. M. Murphy, J. S. Douglass, and A. Birkett, "Resistant Starch Intakes in the United States," *Journal of the American Dietetic Association* 108, no. 1 (2008): 67–78.

11 J. Slavin, "Fiber and Prebiotics: Mechanisms and Health Benefits," *Nutrients* 5, no. 4 (April 22, 2013): 1417–35.

12 K. J. Heller, "Probiotic Bacteria in Fermented Foods: Product Characteristics and Starter Organisms," *American Journal of Clinical Nutrition* 73, sup. 2 (February 2001): 374S–79S.

13 S. W. Rizkalla et al., "Chronic Consumption of Fresh but Not Heated Yogurt Improves Breath-Hydrogen Status and Short-Chain Fatty Acid Profiles: A Controlled Study in Healthy Men with or without Lactose Maldigestion," *American Journal of Clinical Nutrition* 72, no. 6 (December 2000): 1474–79; U. Schillinger, "Isolation and Identification of Lactobacilli from Novel-Type Probiotic and Mild Yoghurts and Their Stability During Refrigerated Storage," *International Journal of Food Microbiology* 47, no. 1–2 (March 1, 1999): 79–87.

14 A. N. Ananthakrishnan, "Environmental Risk Factors for Inflammatory Bowel Disease," *Journal of Gastroenterology and Hepatology* 9, no. 6 (June 2013): 367–74.

15 A. Tjonneland et al., "Linoleic Acid, a Dietary n-6 Polyunsaturated Fatty Acid, and the Aetiology of Ulcerative Colitis: A Nested Case-Control Study within a European Prospective Cohort Study," *Gut* 58 (2009): 1606–11; S. John et al., "Dietary n-3 Polyunsaturated Fatty Acids and the Aetiology of Ulcerative Colitis: A UK Prospective Cohort Study," *European Journal of Gastroenterology and Hepatology* 22 (2010): 602–6.

16 T. Nambu, T. Bamba, and S. Hosoda, "Promotion of Healing by Orally Administered Glutamine in Elemental Diet after Small Intestinal Injury by X-Ray Radiation," *Asia Pacific Journal of Clinical Nutrition* 1, no. 3 (September 1992): 175–82; A. L. Buchman, "Glutamine: Commercially Essential or Conditionally Essential? A Critical Appraisal of the Human Data," *American Journal of Clinical Nutrition* 74, no. 1 (July 2001): 25–32.

17 A. N. Ananthakrishnan, "Environmental Risk Factors for Inflammatory Bowel Disease," *Journal of Gastroenterology and Hepatology* 9, no. 6 (June 2013): 367–74.

18 Ibid.

19 L. Langmead et al., "Randomized, Double-Blind, Placebo-Controlled Trial of Oral Aloe Vera Gel for Active Ulcerative Colitis," *Alimentary Pharmacology and Therapeutics* 19 (2004): 739–47.

20 H. Hanai et al., "Curcumin Maintenance Therapy for Ulcerative Colitis: Randomized, Multicenter, Double-Blind, Placebo-Controlled Trial," *Clinical Gastroenterology and Hepatology* 4, no. 12 (2006): 1502–6.

21 L. Langmead and D. S. Rampton, "Review Article: Complementary and Alternative Therapies for Inflammatory Bowel Disease," *Alimentary Pharmacology and Therapeutics* 23, no. 3 (February 1, 2006): 341–49.

22 M. R. Yago et al., "Gastric Reacidification with Betaine HCl in Healthy Volunteers with Rabeprazole-Induced Hypochlorhydria," *Molecular Pharmaceutics* 10, no. 11 (November 4, 2013): 4032–37.

23 A. Rasyid and A. Lelo, "The Effect of Curcumin and Placebo on Human Gall-Bladder Function: An Ultrasound Study," *Alimentary Pharmacology and Therapeutics* 13, no. 2 (1999): 245–49.

CHAPTER 10

1 E. C. Westman et al., "The Effect of a Low-Carbohydrate Ketogenic Diet versus a Low-Glycemic Index Diet on Glycemic Control in Type 2 Diabetes Mellitus," *Nutrition and Metabolism* 5 (December 19, 2008): 36; T. A. Hussain et al., "Effect of Low-Calorie versus Low-Carbohydrate Ketogenic Diet in Type 2 Diabetes," *Nutrition* 28, no. 10 (October 2012): 1016–21.

2   S. Kayaniyil et al., "Prospective Associations of Vitamin D with β-Cell Function and Glycemia: The PROspective Metabolism and ISlet cell Evaluation (PROMISE) Cohort Study," *Diabetes* 60, no. 11 (November 2011): 2947–53.

3   S. L Volpe, "Magnesium in Disease Prevention and Overall Health," *Advances in Nutrition* 4, no. 3 (May 1, 2013): 378S–83S.

4   S. Jehle et al., "Partial Neutralization of the Acidogenic Western Diet with Potassium Citrate Increases Bone Mass in Postmenopausal Women with Osteopenia," *Journal of the American Society of Nephrology* 17 (2006): 3213–22.

5   C. L. Bodinham et al., "Dietary Fibre Improves First-Phase Insulin Secretion in Overweight Individuals," *PLoS ONE* 7, no. 7 (2012): e40834.

6   P. Ranasinghe et al., "Medicinal Properties of 'True' Cinnamon (*Cinnamomum zeylanicum*): A Systematic Review," *BMC Complementary and Alternative Medicine* 13, no. 1 (October 22, 2013): 275.

7   P. J. Barter et al., "Apo B versus Cholesterol in Estimating Cardiovascular Risk and in Guiding Therapy: Report of the Thirty-Person/Ten-Country Panel," *Journal of Internal Medicine* 259 (2006): 247–58.

8   R. Fears, "The Contribution of the Cholesterol Biosynthetic Pathway to Intermediary Metabolism and Cell Function," *Biochemical Journal* 199, no. 1 (October 1, 1981): 1–7.

9   E. S. Ford and S. Capewell, "Trends in Total and Low-Density Lipoprotein Cholesterol among US Adults: Contributions of Changes in Dietary Fat Intake and Use of Cholesterol-Lowering Medications," *PLoS ONE* 8, no. 5 (May 22, 2013): e65228.

10 A. D. Sniderman et al., "A Meta-Analysis of Low-Density Lipoprotein Cholesterol, Non-High-Density Lipoprotein Cholesterol, and Apolipoprotein B as Markers of Cardiovascular Risk," *Circulation: Cardiovascular Quality and Outcomes* 4, no. 3 (May 2011): 337–45; A. F. Stalenhoef and J. de Graaf, "Association of Fasting and Nonfasting Serum Triglycerides with Cardiovascular Disease and the Role of Remnant-Like Lipoproteins and Small Dense LDL," *Current Opinion in Lipidology* 19 (2008): 355–61; B. Lamarche et al., "Apolipoprotein A-I and B Levels and the Risk of Ischemic Heart Disease During a Five-Year Follow-Up of Men in the Québec Cardiovascular Study," *Circulation* 94, no. 3 (August 1, 1996): 273–78; P. O. Kwiterovich, "Clinical Relevance of the Biochemical, Metabolic, and Genetic Factors That Influence Low-Density Lipoprotein Heterogeneity," *American Journal of Cardiology* 90, sup. (2002): 30i–47i.

11 G. Sobal et al., "Why Is Glycated LDL More Sensitive to Oxidation Than Native LDL? A Comparative Study," *Prostaglandins, Leukotrienes and Essential Fatty Acids* 63, no. 4 (October 2000): 177–86; N. Younis et al., "Glycation as an Atherogenic Modification of LDL," *Current Opinion in Lipidology* 19, no. 4 (August 2008): 378-84.

12 I. Marques-Lopes et al., "Postprandial de novo Lipogenesis and Metabolic Changes Induced by a High-Carbohydrate, Low-Fat Meal in Lean and Overweight Men," *American Journal of Clinical Nutrition* 73, no. 2 (February 2001): 253–61.

13 R. M. Krauss, "Dietary and Genetic Effects on Low-Density Lipoprotein Heterogeneity," *Annual Review of Nutrition* 21 (2001): 283–95.

14 R. Jorde and G. Grimnes, "Vitamin D and Metabolic Health with Special Reference to the Effect of Vitamin D on Serum Lipids," *Progress in Lipid Research* 50, no. 4 (October 2011): 303–12.

15 B. De Roos, Y. Mavrommatis, and I. A. Brouwer, "Long-Chain n-3 Polyunsaturated Fatty Acids: New Insights into Mechanisms Relating to Inflammation and Coronary Heart Disease," *British Journal of Pharmacology* 158, no. 2 (September 2009): 413–28.

16 L. Duntas and D. Micic, "Adiposopathy and Thyroid Disease: Tracing the Pathway to Cardiovascular Risk," *Expert Review of Cardiovascular Therapy* 10, no. 6 (June 2012): 797–803.

17 M. Kumar et al., "Cholesterol-Lowering Probiotics as Potential Biotherapeutics for Metabolic Diseases," *Experimental Diabetes Research* 2012 (2012): 902917.

18 F. K. Santos et al., "Systematic Review and Meta-Analysis of Clinical Trials of the Effects of Low Carbohydrate Diets on Cardiovascular Risk Factors," *Obesity Reviews* 13, no. 11 (November 2012): 1048–66.

19 D. K. Rajpal and J. R. Brown, "Modulating the Human Gut Microbiome as an Emerging Therapeutic Paradigm," *Science Progress* 96, pt. 3 (2013): 224–36.

20 D. W. Zhang et al., "Curcumin and Diabetes: A Systematic Review," *Current Opinion in Lipidology* 19, no. 4 (August 2008): 378–84.

21 S. C. Gupta et al., "Discovery of Curcumin, a Component of Golden Spice, and Its Miraculous Biological Activities," *Clinical and Experimental Pharmacology and Physiology* 39, no. 3 (March 2012): 283–99.

22 H. P. Ammon, "Boswellic Acids in Chronic Inflammatory Diseases," *Planta Medica* 72, no. 12 (October 2006): 1100–16.

23 V. Sterk, B. Büchele, and T. Simmet, "Effect of Food Intake on the Bioavailability of Boswellic Acids from a Herbal Preparation in Healthy Volunteers," *Planta Medica* 70, no. 12 (December 2004): 1155–60.

24 J. C. Bai et al., "Long-Term Effect of Gluten Restriction on Bone Mineral Density of Patients with Coeliac Disease," *Alimentary Pharmacology and Therapeutics* 11, no. 1 (February 1997): 157–64.

25 R. Burge et al., "Incidence and Economic Burden of Osteoporosis-Related Fractures in the United States, 2005-2025," *Journal of Bone and Mineral Research* 22, no. 3 (March 2007): 465–75.

26 E. Dennison, M. A. Mohamed, and C. Cooper, "Epidemiology of Osteoporosis," *Rheumatic Diseases Clinics of North America* 32 (2006): 617–29.

27 I. Kurtz et al., "Effect of Diet on Plasma Acid-Base Composition in Normal Humans," *Kidney International* 24 (1983): 670–80.

28 S. J. Genuis and T. P. Bouchard, "Combination of Micronutrients for Bone (COMB) Study: Bone Density after Micronutrient Intervention," *Journal of Environment and Public Health* 2012 (2012): 354151.

29 M. F. Holick, "Vitamin D: The Underappreciated D-Lightful Hormone That Is Important for Skeletal and Cellular Health," *Current Opinion in Endocrinology and Diabetes* 9 (2002): 87–98.

30 D. J. Jenkins et al., "Effect of High Vegetable Protein Diets on Urinary Calcium Loss in Middle-Aged Men and Women," *European Journal of Clinical Nutrition* 57, no. 2 (February 2003): 376–82.

31 R. D. Jackson et al., "Calcium Plus Vitamin D Supplementation and the Risk of Fractures," *New England Journal of Medicine* 354, no. 7 (February 16, 2006): 669–83.

32 H. A. Bischoff-Ferrari et al., "A Pooled Analysis of Vitamin D Dose Requirements for Fracture Prevention," *New England Journal of Medicine* 367, no. 1 (July 5, 2012): 40–49.

33 A. A. Ginde et al., "Defining Vitamin D Status by Secondary Hyperparathyroidism in the US Population," *Journal of Endocrinological Investigation* 35, no. 1 (January 2012): 42–48; K. M. Hill et al., "An Onflection Point of Serum 25-Hydroxyvitamin D for Maximal Suppression of Parathyroid Hormone Is Not Evident from Multi-Site Pooled Data in Children and Adolescents," *Journal of Nutrition* 140, no. 11 (November 2010): 1983–88.

34 R. Vieth, "Vitamin D Supplementation, 25-Hydroxyvitamin D Concentrations, and Safety," *American Journal of Clinical Nutrition* 69, no. 5 (May 1999): 842–56.

35 D. J. Jenkins et al., "Effect of High Vegetable Protein Diets on Urinary Calcium Loss in Middle-Aged Men and Women," *European Journal of Clinical Nutrition* 57, no. 2 (February 2003): 376–82.

36 Q. Xiao et al., "Dietary and Supplemental Calcium Intake and Cardiovascular Disease Mortality: The National Institutes of Health-AARP Diet and Health Study," *JAMA Internal Medicine* 173, no. 8 (April 22, 2013): 639–46; K. Michaëlsson et al., "Long Term Calcium Intake and Rates of All Cause and Cardiovascular Mortality: Community Based Prospective Longitudinal Cohort Study," *BMJ* 346 (February 12, 2013): f228.

37 S. A. Jamal and S. M. Moe, "Calcium Builds Strong Bones, and More Is Better—Correct? Well, Maybe Not," *Clinical Journal of the American Society of Nephrology* 7, no. 11 (November 2012): 1877–83.

38 K. L. Tucker et al., "Potassium, Magnesium, and Fruit and Vegetable Intakes Are Associated with Greater Bone Mineral Density in Elderly Men and Women," *American Journal of Clinical Nutrition* 69, no. 4 (April 1999): 727–36.

39 D. Feskanich et al., "Vitamin K Intake and Hip Fractures in Women: A Prospective Study," *American Journal of Clinical Nutrition* 69 (1999): 74–79.

40 A. M. Cheung et al., "Vitamin K Supplementation in Postmenopausal Women with Osteopenia (ECKO Trial): A Randomized Controlled Trial," *PLoS Medicine* 5, no. 10 (October 14, 2008): e196.

41 L. A. Braam et al., "Vitamin K1 Supplementation Retards Bone Loss in Postmenopausal Women between 50 and 60 Years of Age," *Calcified Tissue International* 73, no. 1 (July 2003): 21–26.

42 L. J. Schurgers et al., "Role of Vitamin K and Vitamin K-Dependent Proteins in Vascular Calcification," *Zeitschrift fur Kardiologie* 90, sup. 3 (2001): 57–63.

43 J. Iwamoto, T. Takeda, and S. Ichimura, "Effect of Menatetrenone on Bone Mineral Density and Incidence of Vertebral Fractures in Postmenopausal Women with Osteoporsis: A Comparison with the Effect of Etidronate," *Journal of Orthopaedic Science* 6 (2001): 487–92.

44 T. Ushiroyama, A. Ikeda, and M. Ueki, "Effect of Continuous Combined Therapy with Vitamin K(2) and Vitamin D(3) on Bone Mineral Density and Coagulofibrinolysis Function in Postmenopausal Women," *Maturitas* 41 (2002): 211–21.

45 N. Koitaya et al., "Effect of Low Dose Vitamin K2 (MK-4) Supplementation on Bio-Indices in Postmenopausal Japanese Women," *Journal of Nutritional Science and Vitaminology* 55, no. 1 (February 2009): 15–21.

46 S. Kanellakis et al., "Changes in Parameters of Bone Metabolism in Postmenopausal Women Following a 12-Month Intervention Period using Dairy Products Enriched with Calcium, Vitamin D, and Phylloquinone (Vitamin K(1)) or Menaquinone-7 (Citamin K(2)): The Postmenopausal Health Study II," *Calcified Tissue International* 90, no. 4 (April 2012): 251–62, doi:10.1007/s00223-012-9571-z; M. H. Knapen et al., "Three-Year Low-Dose Menaquinone-7 Supplementation Helps Decrease Bone Loss in Healthy Postmenopausal Women," *Osteoporosis International* 24, no. 9 (September 2013): 2499–507.

47 M. J. Shearer, A. Bach, and M. Kohlmeier, "Chemistry, Nutritional Sources, Tissue Distribution, and Metabolism of Vitamin K with Special Reference to Bone Health," *Journal of Nutrition* 126, sup. 4 (April 1996): 1181S-6S; J. Conly and K. Stein, "Reduction of Vitamin K2 Concentrations in Human Liver Associated with the Use of Broad Spectrum Antimicrobials," *Clinical and Investigative Medicine* 17, no. 6 (December 1994): 531–39.

48 L. Cohen, "Recent Data on Magnesium and Osteoporosis," *Magnesium Research* 1 (1988): 85–87.

49 *A Report of the Panel on Micronutrients. Dietary Reference Intakes for Vitamin A, Vitamin K, Arsenic, Boron, Chromium, Copper, Iodine, Iron, Manganese, Molybdenum, Nickel, Silicon, Vanadium, and Zinc*, National Academy of Sciences (Washington DC: National Academy Press, 2001).

50 G. Stendig-Lindberg, R. Tepper, and I. Leichter, "Trabecular Bone Density in a Two Year Controlled Trial of Peroral Magnesium in Osteoporosis," *Magnesium Research* 6, no. 2 (1993): 155–63.

51 S. J. Genuis and T. P. Bouchard, "Combination of Micronutrients for Bone (COMB) Study: Bone Density after Micronutrient Intervention," *Journal of Environment and Public Health* 2012 (2012): 354151.

52 S. A. New et al., "Dietary Influences on Bone Mass and Bone Metabolism: Further Evidence of a Positive Link between Fruit and Vegetable Consumption and Bone Health?" *American Journal of Clinical Nutrition* 71, no. 1 (January 2000): 142–51.

53 S. Jehle et al., "Partial Neutralization of the Acidogenic Western Diet with Potassium Citrate Increases Bone Mass in Postmenopausal Women with Osteopenia," *Journal of the American Society of Nephrology* 17 (2006): 3213–22.

54 K. A. Bolam et al, "The Effect of Physical Exercise on Bone Density in Middle-Aged and Older Men: A Systematic Review," *Osteoporosis International* 24, no. 11 (November 2013): 2749–62.

55 M. Martyn-St. James and S. Carroll, "Effects of Different Impact Exercise Modalities on Bone Mineral Density in Premenopausal Women: A Meta-Analysis," *Journal of Bone and Mineral Metabolism* 28, no. 3 (May 2010): 251–67.

56 K. Engelke et al., "Exercise Maintains Bone Density at Spine and Hip EFOPS: A 3-Year Longitudinal Study in Early Postmenopausal Women," *Osteoporosis International* 17, no. 1 (January 2006): 133–42.

57 G. L. Anderson et al., "Effects of Conjugated Equine Estrogen in Postmenopausal Women with Hysterectomy: The Women's Health Initiative Randomized Controlled Trial," *JAMA* 291, no. 14 (April 14, 2004): 1701–12; J. Marjoribanks et al., "Long Term Hormone Therapy for Perimenopausal and Postmenopausal Women," *Cochrane Database of Systematic Reviews* 7 (July 11, 2012): CD004143.

58 K. Stephenson, P. F. Neuenschwander, and A. K. Kurdowska, "The Effects of Compounded Bioidentical Transdermal Hormone Therapy on Hemostatic, Inflammatory, Immune Factors; Cardiovascular Biomarkers; Quality-of-Life Measures; and Health Outcomes in Perimenopausal and Postmenopausal Women," *International Journal of Pharmaceutical Compounding* 17, no. 1 (January–February 2013): 74–85.

59 V. Seifert-Klauss et al., "Progesterone and Bone: A Closer Link Than Previously Realized," *Climacteric* 15, sup. 1 (April 2012): 26–31.

60 Y. J. Wang et al., "Effects of Low-Dose Testosterone Undecanoate Treatment on Bone Mineral Density and Bone Turnover Markers in Elderly Male Osteoporosis with Low Serum Testosterone," *International Journal of Endocrinology* 2013 (2013): 570413.

61 D. Von Mühlen et al., "Effect of Dehydroepiandrosterone Supplementation on Bone Mineral Density, Bone Markers, and Body Composition in Older Adults: The DAWN Trial," *Osteoporosis International* 19, no. 5 (May 2008): 699–707; D. T. Villareal, J. O. Holloszy, and W. M. Kohrt, "Effects of DHEA Replacement on Bone Mineral Density and Body Composition in Elderly Women and Men," *Clinical Endocrinology* 53, no. 5 (November 2000): 561–68; K. S. Nair et al., "DHEA in Elderly Women and DHEA or Testosterone in Elderly Men," *New England Journal of Medicine* 355, no. 16 (October 19, 2006): 1647–59.

CHAPTER 11

1 "Body Burden: The Pollution in Newborns," Environmental Working Group, July 14, 2005, http://www.ewg.org/research/body-burden-pollution-newborns/test-results.

2 B. C. Blount et al., "Perchlorate Exposure of the US Population, 2001-2002," *Journal of Exposure Science and Environmental Epidemiology* 17, no. 4 (July 2007): 400–7.

3 H. Sasano, M. Rojas, and S. G. Silverberg, "Analysis of Lectin Binding in Benign and Malignant Thyroid Nodules," *Archives of Pathology & Laboratory Medicine* 113, no. 2 (February 1989): 186–89.

4 M. N. Akcay and G. Akcay, "The Presence of the Antigliadin Antibodies in Autoimmune Thyroid Diseases," *Hepatogastroenterology* 50, sup. 2 (December 2003): cclxxix–cclxxx; J. Jiskra et al., "IgA and IgG Antigliadin, IgA Anti-Tissue Transglutaminase and Antiendomysial Antibodies in Patients with Autoimmune Thyroid Diseases and Their Relationship to Thyroidal Replacement Therapy," *Physiology Research* 52, no. 1 (2003): 79–88.

5 R. Shimizu et al., "Structure-Activity Relationships of 44 Halogenated Compounds for Iodotyrosine Deiodinase-Inhibitory Activity," *Toxicology* 314, no. 1 (December 2013): 22–29.

6 J. R. Garber et al., "Clinical Practice Guidelines for Hypothyroidism in Adults: Cosponsored by the American Association of Clinical Endocrinologists and the American Thyroid Association," *Endocrine Practice* 18, no. 6 (November–December 2012): 988–1028.

7 B. O. Asvold et al., "Thyrotropin Levels and Risk of Fatal Coronary Heart Disease: The HUNT Study," *Archives of Internal Medicine* 168, no. 8 (April 28, 2008): 855–60.

8 A. C. Gore, "Neuroendocrine Targets of Endocrine Disruptors," *Hormones* 9, no. 1 (2010): 16–27.

9 L. H. Duntas and G. Brenta, "The Effect of Thyroid Disorders on Lipid Levels and Metabolism," *Medical Clinics of North America* 96, no. 2 (March 2012): 269–81.

10 S. Andersen et al., "Narrow Individual Variation in Serum T4 and T3 in Normal Subjects: A Clue to the Understanding of Subclinical Thyroid Disease," *Journal of Clinical Endocrinology and Metabolism* 87 (2002): 1068–72.

11 B. O. Asvold et al., "Thyrotropin Levels and Risk of Fatal Coronary Heart Disease: The HUNT Study," *Archives of Internal Medicine* 168, no. 8 (April 2008): 855–60.

12 A. Carlé et al., "Thyroid Peroxidase and Thyroglobulin Auto-Antibodies in Patients with Newly Diagnosed Overt Hypothyroidism," *Autoimmunity* 39, no. 6 (September 2006): 497–503.

13 Ibid.

14 F. Economidou et al., "Thyroid Function During Critical Illness," *Hormones* 10, no. 2 (April–June 2011): 117–24.

15 C. D. Clark, B. Bassett, and M. R. Burge, "Effects of Kelp Supplementation on Thyroid Function in Euthyroid Subjects," *Endocrine Practice* 9, no. 5 (September–October 2003): 363–69.

16 M. Sund-Levander, C. Forsberg, and L. K. Wahren, "Normal Oral, Rectal, Tympanic, and Axillary Body Temperature in Adult Men and Women: A Systematic Literature Review," *Scandinavian Journal of Caring Science* 16 (2002): 122–28; K. P. McGann et al., "The Influence of Gender and Race on Mean Body Temperature in a Population of Healthy Older Adults," *Archives of Family Medicine* 2, no. 12 (December 1993): 1265–67.

17 G. S. Kelly, "Body Temperature Variability (Part 1): A Review of the History of Body Temperature and Its Variability Due to Site Selection, Biological Rhythms, Fitness, and Aging," *Alternative Medicine Review* 11, no. 4 (2006): 278–93.

18 C. G. Cattaneo et al., "The Accuracy and Precision of Body Temperature Monitoring Methods during Regional and General Anesthesia," *Anesthesia and Analgesia* 90 (2000): 938–45; G. S. Kelly, "Body Temperature Variability (Part 1): A Review of the History of Body Temperature and Its Variability Due to Site Selection, Biological Rhythms, Fitness, and Aging," 278–93.

19 P. Saravanan et al., "Psychological Well-Being in Patients on 'Adequate' Doses of l-Thyroxine: Results of a Large, Controlled Community-Based Questionnaire

Study," *Clinical Endocrinology* 57, no. 5 (2002): 577–85; R. Bunevicius et al., "Effects of Thyroxine as Compared with Thyroxine plus Triiodothyronine in Patients with Hypothyroidism," *New England Journal of Medicine* 340, no. 6 (February 11, 1999): 424–29; B. C. Appelhof et al., "Combined Therapy with Levothyroxine and Liothyronine in Two Ratios, Compared with Levothyroxine Monotherapy in Primary Hypothyroidism: A Double-Blind, Randomized, Controlled Clinical Trial," *Journal of Clinical Endocrinology and Metabolism* 90, no. 5 (2005): 2666–74; T. D. Hoang, C. H. Olsen, and V. Q. Mai, "Desiccated Thyroid Extract Compared with Levothyroxine in the Treatment of Hypothyroidism: A Randomized, Double-Blind, Crossover Study," *Journal of Clinical Endocrinology and Metabolism* 98, no. 5 (May 2013): 1982–90.

20 A. Gaby, "'Sub-Laboratory' Hypothyroidism and the Empirical Use of Armour Thyroid," *Alternative Medicine Review* 9, no. 2 (June 2004): 157–79.

21 F. Economidou et al., "Thyroid Function during Critical Illness," *Hormones* 10, no. 2 (April–June 2011): 117–24.

22 U. Querfeld, "Vitamin D and Inflammation," *Pediatric Nephrology* 28, no. 4 (April 2013): 605–10.

23 G. Tamer et al., "Relative Vitamin D Insufficiency in Hashimoto's Thyroiditis," *Thyroid* 21, no. 8 (August 2011): 891–96.

24 O. M. Camurdan et al., "Vitamin D Status in Children with Hashimoto Thyroiditis," *Journal of Pediatric Endocrinology and Metabolism* 25, no. 5–6 (2012): 467–70.

CHAPTER 12

1   A. C. Gore, "Neuroendocrine Targets of Endocrine Disruptors," *Hormones* 9, no. 1 (2010): 16–27; S. De Coster and N. van Larebeke, "Endocrine-Disrupting Chemicals: Associated Disorders and Mechanisms of Action," *Journal of Environmental and Public Health* 2012 (2012): 713696.

2   G. B. Post, P. D. Cohn, and K. R. Cooper, "Perfluorooctanoic Acid (PFOA), an Emerging Drinking Water Contaminant: A Critical Review of Recent Literature," *Environmental Research* 116 (July 2012): 93–117.

3   M. Deschodt-Lanckman et al., "Wheat Germ Agglutinin Inhibits Basal- and Stimulated-Adenylate Cyclase Activity as well as the Binding of [3H] Caerulein to Rat Pancreatic Plasma Membranes," *Journal of Cyclic Nucleotide Research* 3, no. 3 (June 1977): 177–87; R. Masnikosa et al., "Characterisation of Insulin-Like Growth Factor Receptors and Insulin Receptors in the Human Placenta Using Lectin Affinity Methods," *Growth Hormones and IGF Research* 16 (2006): 174–84; P. Cuatrecasas and G. P. Tell, "Insulin-Like Activity of Concanavalin A and Wheat Germ Agglutinin—Direct Interactions with Insulin Receptors," *Proceedings of the National Academy of Sciences* 70, no. 2 (February 1973): 485–89.

4   M. N. Akçay and G. Akçay, "The Presence of the Antigliadin Antibodies in Autoimmune Thyroid Diseases," *Hepatogastroenterology* 50, sup. 2 (December 2003): cclxxix–cclxxx.

5   C. Jaeger et al., "Comparative Analysis of Organ-Specific Autoantibodies and Celiac Disease—Associated Antibodies in Type 1 Diabetic Patients, Their First-Degree Relatives, and Healthy Control Subjects," *Diabetes Care* 24, no. 1 (January 2001): 27–32.

6   M. Prázny et al., "Screening for Associated Autoimmunity in Type 1 Diabetes Mellitus with Respect to Diabetes Control," *Physiological Research* 54, no. 1 (2005): 41–48.

7   J. W. Fahey, Y. Zhang, and P. Talalay, "Broccoli Sprouts: An Exceptionally Rich

Source of Inducers of Enzymes That Protect against Chemical Carcinogens," *Proceedings of the National Academy of Sciences* 94, no. 19 (September 16, 1997): 10367–72; D. F. Romagnolo et al., "Phytoalexins in Cancer Prevention," *Frontiers in Bioscience* 17 (June 1, 2012): 2035–58.

8   W. J. Inder, G. Dimeski, and A. Russell, "Measurement of Salivary Cortisol in 2012—Laboratory Techniques and Clinical Indications," *Clinical Endocrinology* 77, no. 5 (November 2012): 645–51.

9   K. Stephenson, P. F. Neuenschwander, and A. K. Kurdowska, "The Effects of Compounded Bioidentical Transdermal Hormone Therapy on Hemostatic, Inflammatory, Immune Factors; Cardiovascular Biomarkers; Quality-of-Life Measures; and Health Outcomes in Perimenopausal and Postmenopausal Women," *International Journal of Pharmaceutical Compounding* 17, no. 1 (January–February 2013): 74–85.

10 M. E. Bauer et al., "Psychoneuroendocrine Interventions Aimed at Attenuating Immunosenescence: A Review," *Biogerontology* 14, no. 1 (February 2013): 9–20.

CHAPTER 13

1   Y. Shapira, N. Agmon-Levin, and Y. Schoenfeld, "Defining and Analyzing Geoepidemiology and Human Autoimmunity," *Journal of Autoimmunity* 34, no. 3 (May 2010): J168–77.

2   I. M. Lacroix and E. C. Li-Chan, "Investigation of the Putative Associations between Dairy Consumption and Incidence of Type 1 and Type 2 Diabetes," *Critical Reviews in Food Science and Nutrition* 54, no. 4 (2014): 411–32.

3   A. Alaedini et al., "Immune Cross-Reactivity in Celiac Disease: Anti-Gliadin Antibodies Bind to Neuronal Synapsin I," *Journal of Immunology* 178, no. 10 (May 15, 2007): 6590–95; M. Hadjivassiliou et al., "Autoantibodies in Gluten Ataxia Recognize a Novel Neuronal Transglutaminase," *Annals of Neurology* 64, no. 3 (September 2008): 332–43; K. Karská et al., "Calreticulin—the Potential Autoantigen in Celiac Disease," *Biochemical and Biophysical Research Communications* 209, no. 2 (April 17, 1995): 597–605.

4   A. Fasano, "Zonulin, Regulation of Tight Junctions, and Autoimmune Diseases," *Annals of the New York Academy of Sciences* 1258, no. 1 (2012): 25–33.

5   A. Antico et al., "Can Supplementation with Vitamin D Reduce the Risk or Modify the Course of Autoimmune Diseases? A Systematic Review of the Literature," *Autoimmunity Reviews* 12, no. 2 (December 2012): 127–36.

6   B. Franchi et al., "Vitamin D at the Onset of Type 1 Diabetes in Italian Children," *European Journal of Pediatrics* 173, no. 4 (April 2014): 477–82.

7   E. Hyppönen et al., "Intake of Vitamin D and Risk of Type 1 Diabetes: A Birth-Cohort Study," *Lancet* 358, no. 9292 (November 3, 2001): 1500–3.

8   C. Y. Yang et al., "The Implication of Vitamin D and Autoimmunity: A Comprehensive Review," *Clinical Reviews in Allergy and Immunology* 45, no. 2 (October 2013): 217–26; N. Agmon-Levin et al., "Vitamin D in Systemic and Organ-Specific Autoimmune Diseases," *Clinical Reviews in Allergy and Immunology* 45, no. 2 (October 2013): 256–66.

9   P. C. Calder, "Omega-3 Fatty Acids and Inflammatory Processes," *Nutrients* 2, no. 3 (March 2010): 355–74.

10 P. R. Fortin et al., "Validation of a Meta-Analysis: The Effects of Fish Oil in Rheumatoid Arthritis," *Journal of Clinical Epidemiology* 48 (1995): 1379–90.

11 B. Chassaing and A. T. Gewirtz, "Gut Microbiota, Low-Grade Inflammation, and Metabolic Syndrome," *Toxicologic Pathology* 42, no. 1 (January 2014): 49–53.

12 G. De Palma et al., "Intestinal Dysbiosis and Reduced Immunoglobulin-Coated Bacteria Associated with Coeliac Disease in Children," *BMC Microbiology* 10 (2010): 63.

13 S. Brugman et al., "Antibiotic Treatment Partially Protects against Type 1 Diabetes in the Bio-Breeding Diabetes-Prone Rat. Is the Gut Flora Involved in the Development of Type 1 Diabetes?" *Diabetologia* 49, no. 9 (September 2006): 2105–8.

14 A. W. Walker et al., "High-Throughput Clone Library Analysis of the Mucosa-Associated Microbiota Reveals Dysbiosis and Differences between Inflamed and Non-Inflamed Regions of the Intestine in Inflammatory Bowel Disease," *BMC Microbiology* 11 (2011): 7.

15 T. H. Frazier et al., "Gut Microbiota, Intestinal Permeability, Obesity-Induced Inflammation, and Liver Injury," *Journal for Parenteral and Enteral Nutrition* 35, sup. 5 (September 2011): 14S–20S.

16 L. Järup, "Hazards of Heavy Metal Contamination," *British Medical Bulletin* 68 (2003): 167–82.

17 A. Vojdani, "Detection of IgE, IgG, IgA and IgM Antibodies against Raw and Processed Food Antigens," *Nutrition and Metabolism* 6 (May 12, 2009): 22.

CHAPTER 14

1 S. Liu et al., "Relation between Changes in Intakes of Dietary Fiber and Grain Products and Changes in Weight and Development of Obesity among Middle-Aged Women," *American Journal of Clinical Nutrition* 78, no. 5 (November 2003): 920–27.

2 Q. Yang, "Gain Weight by 'Going Diet?' Artificial Sweeteners and the Neurobiology of Sugar Cravings: Neuroscience 2010," *Yale Journal of Biology and Medicine* 83, no. 2 (June 2010): 101–18.

3 N. B. Bueno et al., "Very-Low-Carbohydrate Ketogenic Diet v. Low-Fat Diet for Long-Term Weight Loss: A Meta-Analysis of Randomised Controlled Trials," *British Journal of Nutrition* 110, no. 7 (October 2013): 1178–87.

4 N. Santesso et al., "Effects of Higher- versus Lower-Protein Diets on Health Outcomes: A Systematic Review and Meta-Analysis," *European Journal of Clinical Nutrition* 66, no. 7 (July 2012): 780–88.

5 P. W. Siri-Tarino et al., "Saturated Fat, Carbohydrate, and Cardiovascular Disease," *American Journal of Clinical Nutrition* 91, no. 3 (March 2010): 502–9.

6 L. Fontana et al., "Low Bone Mass in Subjects on a Long-Term Raw Vegetarian Diet," *Archives of Internal Medicine* 165, no. 6 (March 28, 2005): 684–89; C. Koebnick et al., "Consequences of a Long-Term Raw Food Diet on Body Weight and Menstruation: Results of a Questionnaire Survey," *Annals of Nutrition and Metabolism* 43, no. 2 (1999): 69–79.

7 A. C. Gore, "Neuroendocrine Targets of Endocrine Disruptors," *Hormones* 9, no. 1 (January–March 2010): 16–27.

8 Y Liu et al., "Association between Perceived Insufficient Sleep, Frequent Mental Distress, Obesity and Chronic Diseases among US Adults, 2009 Behavioral Risk Factor Surveillance System," *BMC Public Health* 13 (January 29, 2013): 84.

9 M. P. St-Onge, "The Role of Sleep Duration in the Regulation of Energy Balance: Effects on Energy Intakes and Expenditure," *Journal of Clinical Sleep Medicine* 9, no. 1 (January 15, 2013): 73–80.

10 A. V. Nedeltcheva et al., "Sleep Curtailment Is Accompanied by Increased Intake of Calories from Snacks," *American Journal of Clinical Nutrition* 89, no. 1 (January 2009): 126–33.

11 R. Killick, S. Banks, and P. Y. Liu, "Implications of Sleep Restriction and Recovery on Metabolic Outcomes," *Journal of Clinical Endocrinology and Metabolism* 97, no. 11 (November 2012): 3876–90.

12 L. F. Drager et al., "Obstructive Sleep Apnea: A Cardiometabolic Risk in Obesity and the Metabolic Syndrome," *Journal of the American College of Cardiology* 62, no. 7 (August 13, 2013): 569–76.

13 E. Grossman, M. Laudon, and N. Zisapel, "Effect of Melatonin on Nocturnal Blood Pressure: Meta-Analysis of Randomized Controlled Trials," *Journal of Vascular Health and Risk Management* 7 (2011): 577–84.

14 R. J. Wyatt et al., "Effects of 5-Hydroxytryptophan on the Sleep of Normal Human Subjects," *Electroencephalography and Clinical Neurophysiology* 30 (1971): 505–9.

15 J. F. Trepanowski et al., "Impact of Caloric and Dietary Restriction Regimens on Markers of Health and Longevity in Humans and Animals: A Summary of Available Findings," *Nutrition Journal* 10 (October 7, 2011): 107.

16 K. M. Beavers et al., "Effect of an 18-Month Physical Activity and Weight Loss Intervention on Body Composition in Overweight and Obese Older Adults," *Obesity* (August 20, 2013): doi:10.1002/oby.20607.

17 E. B. Parr, V. G. Coffey, and J. A. Hawley, "'Sarcobesity': A Metabolic Conundrum," *Maturitas* 74, no. 2 (February 2013): 109–13.

18 S. Romero-Arenas, M. Martinez-Pascual, and P. E. Alcaraz, "Impact of Resistance Circuit Training on Neuromuscular, Cardiorespiratory and Body Composition Adaptations in the Elderly," *Aging Disease* 4, no. 5 (October 1, 2013): 256–63.

19 D. Vaidya et al., "Association of Baseline Sex Hormone Levels with Baseline and Longitudinal Changes in Waist-to-Hip Ratio: Multi-Ethnic Study of Atherosclerosis," *International Journal of Obesity* 36, no. 12 (December 2012): 1578–84.

20 D. G. Stein, "The Case for Progesterone," *Annals of the New York Academy of Sciences* 1052 (June 2005): 152–69.

21 K. Stephenson, P. F. Neuenschwander, and A. K. Kurdowska, "The Effects of Compounded Bioidentical Transdermal Hormone Therapy on Hemostatic, Inflammatory, Immune Factors; Cardiovascular Biomarkers; Quality-of-Life Measures; and Health Outcomes in Perimenopausal and Postmenopausal Women," *International Journal of Pharmaceutical Compounding* 17, no. 1 (January–February 2013): 74–85.

22 G. Huang et al., "Testosterone Dose-Response Relationships in Hysterectomized Women with or without Oophorectomy: Effects on Sexual Function, Body Composition, Muscle Performance, and Physical Function in a Randomized Trial," *Menopause* (published electronically November 25, 2013).

23 D. M. Schulte et al., "Caloric Restriction Increases Serum Testosterone Concentrations in Obese Male Subjects by Two Distinct Mechanisms," *Hormone and Metabolic Research* 46, no. 4 (April 2014): 283–86.

24 G. Corona et al., "Dehydroepiandrosterone Supplementation in Elderly Men: A Meta-Analysis Study of Placebo-Controlled Trials," *Journal of Clinical Endocrinology and Metabolism* 98, no. 9 (September 2013): 3615–26.

25 R. Muckelbauer et al., "Association between Water Consumption and Body Weight Outcomes: A Systematic Review," *American Journal of Clinical Nutrition* 98, no. 2 (August 2013): 282–99.

26 E. M. Dewulf et al., "Insight into the Prebiotic Concept: Lessons from an Exploratory, Double Blind Intervention Study with Inulin-Type Fructans in Obese Women," *Gut* 62, no. 8 (August 2013): 1112–21.

27 J. A. Greenberg et al., "Coffee, Tea, and Diabetes: The Role of Weight Loss and Caffeine," *International Journal of Obesity* 29, no. 9 (September 2005): 1121–29.

28 J. J. Shelmet et al., "Ethanol Causes Acute Inhibition of Carbohydrates, Fat, and Protein Oxidation and Insulin Resistance," *Journal of Clinical Investigation* 81, no. 4 (April 1988): 1137–45.

CHAPTER 15

1 J. Bergstrom et al., "Diet, Muscle Glycogen, and Physical Performance," *Acta Physiologica* 71 (1967): 140–50.

2   S. D. Phinney et al., "Capacity for Moderate Exercise in Obese Subjects after Adaptation to a Hypocaloric Ketogenic Diet," *Journal of Clinical Investigation* 66 (1980): 1152–61.

3   S. D. Phinney et al., "The Human Metabolic Response to Chronic Ketosis without Caloric Restriction: Physical and Biochemical Adaptation," *Metabolism* 32 (1983): 757–68.

INDEX

Underscored page numbers indicate boxed text.
Boldface references indicate illustrations and photographs.